NURSING DIAGNOSIS

PROCESS AND APPLICATION

NURSING DIAGNOSIS

PROCESS AND APPLICATION

SECOND EDITION

Marjory Gordon, R.N., Ph.D., F.A.A.N.

Professor of Nursing
Boston College

McGRAW-HILL BOOK COMPANY

New York   St. Louis   San Francisco   Auckland   Bogotá
Hamburg   Johannesburg   London   Madrid   Mexico   Milan   Montreal
New Delhi   Panama   Paris   São Paulo   Singapore   Sydney   Tokyo   Toronto

This book was set in Helvetica by J. M. Post Graphics, Corp.
The editor was Sally J. Barhydt;
the production supervisor was Leroy A. Young;
the cover was designed by Scott Chelius.
Project supervision was done by The Total Book.
R. R. Donnelley & Sons Company was printer and binder.

Notice

As new medical and nursing research and clinical experience broaden our knowledge, changes in treatment and drug therapy are required. The editors and the publisher of this work have made every effort to ensure that the drug dosage schedules herein are accurate and in accord with the standards accepted at the time of publication. Readers are advised, however, to check the product information sheet included in the package of each drug they plan to administer to be certain that changes have not been made in the recommended dose or in the contraindications for administration. This recommendation is of particular importance in regard to new or infrequently used drugs.

NURSING DIAGNOSIS
Process and Application

1 2 3 4 5 6 7 8 9 0 D O C D O C 8 9 3 2 1 0 9 8 7

ISBN 0-07-023828-6

Library of Congress Cataloging-in-Publication Data

Gordon, Marjory.
  Nursing diagnosis, process and application.

  Bibliography: p.
  Includes index.
  1. Diagnosis. 2. Nursing. I. Title. [DNLM:
1. Nursing Assessment. 2. Nursing Process.
WY 100 G664n]
RT48.G67 1987   610.73   86-20944
ISBN 0-07-023828-6

ABOUT THE AUTHOR

Dr. MARJORY GORDON is a Professor and Coordinator of Adult Nursing at Boston College, Chestnut Hill, Massachusetts. Her teaching responsibilities include classroom and clinical teaching of students preparing as clinical specialists in adult nursing. She has recently completed a three-year, federally funded project on teaching diagnostic reasoning and plans to continue research in this area. Publications have primarily been in the area of nursing diagnosis, and Dr. Gordon is currently President of the North American Nursing Diagnosis Association. In 1984 she was honored by this Association for distinguished contributions to nursing diagnosis. She is a Fellow of the American Academy of Nursing and received a Sigma Theta Tau Founders Award for high professional standards in 1978. Through workshops, lectures, and seminars she has helped nurses in this and other countries to examine the usefulness of nursing diagnosis in their practice.

Dr. Gordon was born in Cleveland, Ohio, of Scottish-Irish parents and moved to New York City when she began her nursing education. She has a diploma from The Mount Sinai Hospital School of Nursing and baccalaureate and master's degrees from Hunter College of the City University of New York. Her doctoral work was done at Boston College in educational psychology with a dissertation in the area of diagnostic reasoning.

To My Parents
and
to Nurses Past, Present,
and Future

Like hues and harmonies of evening—
Like clouds in starlight widely spread—
Like memory of music fled—
Like aught that for its grace may be
Dear, and yet dearer for its mystery.

Thy light alone—like mist o'er mountain driven,
or music by the night—wind sent
through strings of some still instrument,
or moonlight on a midnight stream,
Gives grace and truth to life's unquiet dream.

P. B. Shelley
Hymn to Intellectual Beauty

CONTENTS

PREFACE

This second edition of *Nursing Diagnosis: Process and Application* attests to the widespread interest of nurses in this topic. The success of the first edition has been attributed to its in-depth treatment of nursing diagnosis and the assistance it provided beginning professional nursing students in acquiring a solid foundation upon which to build clinical experience in diagnosis. A career in professional nursing requires competency in diagnostic reasoning and in the use of diagnostic categories. Knowledge of terms is necessary, yet terminology without diagnostic process skills leads to inaccurate clinical judgments. Similarly, diagnostic skill without terminology is akin to speaking ability without language. The two are inseparable. Nursing diagnosis is prerequisite to effective treatment planning and beyond this, to articulating the unique perspective of nursing.

Diagnostic categories are in a process of evolution. As recently as 1973, Kristine Gebbie and Mary Ann Lavin at St. Louis University called the first conference on classification of nursing diagnoses. This began the international effort to identify, standardize, and classify health problems treated by nurses. The relevance of this work to practice, education, and research has sustained enthusiasm for further development. Since the first edition of this book was published in 1982, use of nursing diagnosis in practice and education has grown considerably. Currently, most clinical textbooks used by students include diagnostic categories identified by the North American Nursing Diagnosis Association. Nursing process literature now emphasizes diagnosis as distinct from data gathering. In professional standards, policy statements, and many nurse practice acts diagnostic judgment is described as an essential component of professional practice. Although diagnostic categories are not sufficiently precise, conceptually consistent, or fully descriptive of the unique aspects of nursing, clinicians find the available categories useful in describing their clinical judgments, and many are studying ways to improve their validity and reliability. Students need to recognize that in any profession, concepts evolve as knowledge evolves.

In this second edition of *Nursing Diagnosis: Process and Application,* two chapters have been added, all have been updated, and most chapters have been revised. The major themes have been retained: what is a nursing diagnosis, how are diagnoses made, how are they used in nursing process and in care delivery. In this edition, outlines appear at the beginning of each chapter so that topics are more easily accessed by students and faculty. The typeface has also been changed to facilitate readability. Rather than placing questions and exercises at the end of chapters, these are incorporated into the text as a learning tool. Questions that students may raise, or should raise, are incorporated into the text. In some chapters the questions refer to actual problems informally solicited from undergraduate students learning nursing diagnosis. Questions also encourage students to be alert to the forthcoming topic and stimulate thinking as well as reading. This method teaches students to raise their own questions as they study and use nursing diagnosis. Exercises followed by a discussion of right and wrong answers are also incorporated into the text. This provides immediate feedback and permits learning to be applied before moving to the next topic. Within the text, salient points are italicized or listed for easier identification by the student. Summaries at the end of chapters provide a succinct outline of important points. Appendices include the most current information on diagnoses and their development, as well as simple to complex exercises in aspects of the diagnostic process.

Since publication of the first edition, the functional health pattern assessment format has been implemented in many health care settings and used in a number of textbooks and diagnostic manuals. A new chapter has been added on this format. Each functional pattern is defined and discussed, and screening questions are listed for initial assessment of an individual, family, or community. Two variations in format pertaining to assessment of infants and children and the critically ill are added. These include the different phrasing for infant and child assessment and the diagnoses to be selectively screened when assessing the critically ill for whom a full nursing history is not possible. The second edition also contains a new chapter on dysfunctional patterns described by current diagnostic categories. Each diagnosis is briefly discussed to provide the student with a beginning understanding of terms and their use. This is not intended to substitute for the detailed study of each condition.

To describe in writing a process as elusive as diagnostic reasoning and judgment is difficult. An attempt to overcome this difficulty has resulted in major changes in chapters related to this topic. The process of going from data to diagnosis is viewed as a search for the meaning of cues. Student and faculty reviewers have found that this method of organization makes the diagnostic process clearer and more easily grasped. Additional clinical examples have also been included.

This book goes beyond other textbooks that present current diagnostic terms and their use in nursing process. It is designed to offer the learner an in-depth understanding upon which further learning as a student and as a professional can be based. The approach to the discussion of nursing diagnosis is based on four assumptions.

The first and most important is that nursing diagnosis is an integral part of nursing process. Diagnoses are made for purposes of planning care, therefore, the student will find diagnosis discussed in this context. The second assumption is that nursing diagnoses are not made in isolation. Although *nursing* diagnosis is emphasized in this book, the student will gain a broad perspective on clinical diagnosis in the health professions. Many professionals interact in care delivery, and each has to appreciate the others' focus of practice.

A third underlying assumption is that understanding facilitates development of clinical reasoning and judgment. Being aware of the logical operations involved in processing assessment data facilitates development of diagnostic judgment. Thus, the student will find an emphasis on cognitive aspects of the diagnostic process. Logical relationships are clearly described among the following: (1) a nursing model and format for assessment, (2) strategies for collecting and processing information, (3) diagnostic statements, and (4) use of diagnoses in care planning and other nursing activities. Examples in these areas can be grasped by students who have completed pre-clinical arts and sciences.

The fourth assumption is that professional students will eventually assume professional responsibilities. An appreciation must be gained of the issues surrounding classification system development and issues in nursing practice to which nursing diagnosis applies. Therefore, the relevance of nursing diagnosis to quality assurance, prospective payment and reimbursement, staffing, and other care delivery issues is discussed. It may be that we emphasize collaboration more than independent thinking in nursing education. Based on this premise, an underlying theme in the text is responsibility and accountability for diagnosis. A small section is included on implementation in practice settings so that students will recognize opportunities to share their knowledge.

The last chapter of the text introduces the topics of classification system development and the activities of the North American Nursing Diagnosis Association. These areas will be of interest after nursing diagnosis has been mastered and when questions begin to arise about how diagnostic categories were identified.

This edition has been written with the expectation that the student will begin to use this book in the first course dealing with nursing process. As clinical experience with clients increases, it will be useful to again refer to the sections on process and application. In fact, development of diagnostic expertise requires a life-long commitment to learning.

Many individuals contributed to the development of this book. Early interest in the diagnostic process was stimulated by debate and deliberation with colleagues, especially Carol Soares-O'Hearn and Florence Milliot. Further work in cognitive theory was made possible by a 1970 National Institutes of Health Fellowship for doctoral study (grant number 1FO4-NU-27,282-01) and by two encouraging advisors, John Dacey and John Travers. Fourteen years' association with the North American Nursing Diagnosis Association sharpened ideas about diagnostic nomenclature. My association with the Massachusetts Conference Group on Classification of Nursing Diagnosis prompted consideration of specialties other than my own and broader issues of implementation. Thoughts generated from lively intellectual discussions about diagnosis with colleagues in this group are reflected in this book. For raising questions that needed answers, I thank graduate students; and for discussion of ideas, I am grateful to colleagues at Boston College. For raising my consciousness about ethical issues related to diagnosis and treatment, appreciation is extended to Catherine Murphy.

For all the times she listened, challenged, advised, read, and reread drafts of this book, I am particularly grateful to Ann McCourt and to her family who tolerated our long conversations and provided encouragement. Deep gratitude is extended to other friends for their support, particularly Ardra Taylor and Winifred Hickman who provided encouragement and understanding at critical times. I am also indebted to Maura Keane for sharing problems in using diagnosis from a student's perspective and for humor and much needed assistance in typing parts of the manuscript. Lastly, gratitude is extended to Sally Barhydt, nursing editor at McGraw-Hill, who deserves special thanks.

Marjory Gordon

THE CONCEPT OF
NURSING DIAGNOSIS

THE CONCEPT OF NURSING DIAGNOSIS

Nurses have always collected information through the process of assessment and used this information to make judgments about a client's[1] need for care. About three decades ago this process began to be called *nursing diagnosis.* The identification of a diagnostic language permitted labeling of clinical judgments and recognition of the health problems that are the unique focus of nursing. The implementation of nursing diagnosis in practice required that nurses sharpen their diagnostic judgment skills and assume responsibility and accountability for their nursing diagnoses.

As nursing diagnosis was implemented in practice settings, it became a focus for the assessment of quality nursing care delivery and a measure of accountability to the consumer. Directors of nursing departments in health care agencies began to appreciate that nursing diagnoses combined with medical diagnoses could offer a means for determining the number and competency of staff required to deliver care and the nursing cost component of care delivery. As client's records in hospital and community agencies became computerized, statistics on nursing diagnoses, treatments, and outcomes of care became available for practice, research, and educational purposes. Are all these developments in every health care agency? Not at this time, but there is strong evidence that these are the directions in which nursing is moving. For this reason it is important to grasp the concept and definition of nursing diagnosis, as well as its evolution in the profession and current definition.

An understanding of nursing diagnosis begins with its development. In this chapter the concept will be traced from its first appearance in the nursing

[1]The term *client* will be used to refer to individuals, families, and communities.

literature to its present definition within nursing process. The similarities and differences in nursing and medical diagnosis will be discussed while considering the place of nursing diagnosis in nursing process, nursing practice, and health care delivery. A broader view of the concept will be attained after studying Chapter 2 which contrasts and compares nursing diagnosis with other health professionals' use of diagnosis in their practice.

The next area of learning involves how to make a nursing diagnosis that will direct nursing treatment. The first step is to have a good comprehension of a nursing model for practice that guides assessment and diagnosis, as well as providing direction for developing nursing treatment plans. Chapter 3 will consider diagnosis from the perspective of various nursing models. Chapter 4 presents a *functional health pattern assessment format* compatible with these models. This format for assessment is currently used in a variety of health care settings and permits the nurse to move from data to diagnosis with the least cognitive strain. Chapter 5 contains an overview of nursing diagnoses or *dysfunctional patterns.* Having studied what to assess and common diagnoses, the reader will be guided through the diagnostic process starting with information collection in Chapter 6. How to arrive at a diagnostic judgment and problem formulation are the focus of Chapters 7 and 8.

A grasp of nursing diagnosis and the diagnostic process will prepare the reader to consider the use of diagnosis in direct care in Chapter 9. This chapter will also include discussion of written and computerized records. New views of somewhat old practice issues will be discussed in Chapter 10. These issues include how to implement nursing diagnosis and the relevance of nursing diagnosis to evaluation of care, staff allocation, legal and moral accountability, standards of care, prospective payment, and cost containment. Issues in developing a classification system for nursing diagnoses will be discussed in Chapter 11. A brief review of research, as well as methods for the clinical study of nursing diagnoses, is included in Chapter 11. The assumption is that the reader will be enthusiastic about the concept of diagnosis and wish to influence its development and direction. This chapter reviews methods for identifying and clinically testing diagnostic categories. In summary, this book will focus on the area of practice described by nursing diagnoses. It will deal with what a diagnosis is, diagnostic process, and application in nursing practice.

HISTORICAL TRACES

As a term, nursing diagnosis has had a relatively short history; as an act it goes back to the founding of modern nursing. Nightingale and her colleagues diagnosed nutritional deficits and other health problems exhibited by Crimean War casualties. On the basis of those nursing diagnoses, interventions were undertaken to correct the system of care in military hospitals. It was nearly a century later when nurses began to recapture the image Nightingale had portrayed as diagnostician, epidemiologist, and researcher.

In the 1950s the term nursing diagnosis appeared in the literature. At that time nursing leaders were faced with a need for regional planning for professional practice and education. Nursing was described as a set of tasks and valued as the "handmaiden" of the physician. Nursing care was disease-focused with an associated dearth of attention to individualized responses. Although most nurses were licensed to practice independently of the physician, the autonomy that characterizes a profession was lacking. Clarification of the nurse's functions was needed. This led to the first mention of nursing diagnosis in the literature and the first "standards" for professional practice that included nursing diagnosis. The functions of the professional nurse were stated as:

1 Identification or diagnosing of the nursing problem and the recognition of its interrelated aspects
2 Deciding upon a course of nursing action to be followed for the solution of the problem in light of immediate and long term objectives of nursing, with respect to prevention of illness, direct care, rehabilitation, and promotion of the highest standard of health possible for the individual (McManus, 1950, p. 54)

It is interesting to note, with the predicted future increase in chronic illness, that the first major clinical use of nursing diagnosis was in care of clients with chronic illness and disability. Bonney and Rothberg (1963) employed nursing diagnosis as a client evaluation instrument to predict needs for nursing care. The objective was to use the clients' nursing diagnoses as predictors of staffing needs in long-term care facilities, as well as a focus for nursing intervention. As one of the authors commented recently:

> We were determined to show that nursing was a cognitive process, that it wasn't just a simplistic laying on of hands, that it had a process that was logical and consistent, one that could predict outcomes . . . The crucial point underlying the entire movement [use of nursing diagnosis] is that nursing is a cognitive process (in addition to its intuitive and empathetic aspects) and good nursing care is the result of thoughtful analysis. (Rothberg, 1982)

As the term began to appear in the nursing literature, concern was expressed that diagnosis was the province of the physician. Levine (1965) suggested the word *trophicognosis* to more clearly express the idea of diagnosis in nursing. Others believed that *nursing diagnosis* was more easily understood and King (1967) dispelled the notion that only physicians use the cognitive process of diagnosis. Today the term is used widely in journals, textbooks, and manuals indicating its acceptance as a term to describe problem identification in nursing practice.

Many of the early writers on nursing diagnosis recognized the importance of clinical judgment and clear identification of health problems requiring nursing intervention (Fry, 1953; Abdellah, Beland, Martin, and Matheny, 1961; Komorita, 1963; Rothberg, 1967). Yet, until diagnostic terminology was developed no clear and consistent language was available for use in clinical settings. At the First National Conference on Classification of Nursing Diagnoses in 1973 a list of

34 diagnoses was developed by clinicians, educators, researchers, and theorists who attended (Gebbie and Lavin, 1975). Since that time six additional conferences have been held. Participants further developed and identified diagnostic terms to describe the actual and potential health problems amenable to nursing intervention. At present there are 61 diagnostic categories and subcategories accepted for clinical testing by NANDA,[2] the North American Nursing Diagnosis Association (Hurley, 1986).

Recognition of the concept as a useful, cognitive tool for practice by national associations influenced its implementation. Beginning in the 1970s the American Nurses' Association (ANA) included nursing diagnosis in generic and specialty standards of practice (1974, p. 2). Standard II states: "Nursing diagnoses are derived from health status data." The standards were followed by a Social Policy Statement which defined nursing as follows:

> Nursing is the diagnosis and treatment of human responses to actual or potential health problems. (ANA, 1980, p. 9)

Both the standards of practice and the policy statement make explicit nurses' responsibility to consumers. Even more important in the area of accountability is the gradual changes in licensing laws during the 1970s and 1980s. A number of state practice acts have been updated to reflect accountability for nursing diagnosis, or problem identification, in nursing practice.

In the last decade cost containment, quality assurance, and the desire of many consumers to obtain reimbursement for care by nonphysician providers have become important health care issues. It has been suggested that nursing diagnoses could be the basis for third-party (government and private insurers) reimbursement to consumers for nursing services in the community, in addition to the reimbursement for delegated medical activities (Joel, 1986). Quality assurance through peer review would be a mechanism for assuring accountability in reimbursement. Development of home health care reimbursement models based on nursing diagnosis was a resolution adopted by state delegates to the ANA convention in 1984. In addition, consensus was reached at a national conference in 1985 on reporting of nursing statistics by health care agencies. It was agreed that the Nursing Minimum Data Set to be proposed to the U.S. Department of Health and Human Services include nursing diagnosis and other data (Werley and Lang, 1987). If accepted, this eventually may influence government reimbursement for the cost of nursing care. National standards, policy statements, practice acts, reimbursement focus, and statistical reporting of nursing diagnosis suggest the importance of this concept in practice.

Comments on the usefulness of diagnosis in practice have appeared in the nursing literature since the early 1970s. In recent years its implementation has been discussed in such areas as acute care (Davidson, 1984), intensive care (Kim, 1983; Guzzetta and Dossey, 1983), long-term care (Leslie, 1981; Hardy,

---

[2]NANDA is composed of nurses actively involved in the identification and classification of nursing diagnoses. Until 1982 it was called the National Group for Classification of Nursing Diagnoses.

1983), community care (Simmons, 1980; Dalton, 1979), and ambulatory care (Clark, 1984; Steele, 1984). Use in specialty areas of practice has also been described: maternal-child (Barnard, 1983; Gordon, Sweeney, and McKeehan, 1983), psychiatric (Bruce, 1979; Loomis and Wood, 1983), occupational health (Lister, 1983), operating room (Mahomet, 1975), and cancer nursing (Moritz, 1978; Mundinger, 1978). (Other specialty-based literature may be found in the annotated bibliography at the end of this book.) In addition to direct care activities the usefulness of nursing diagnosis had been described in quality assurance (McCourt, 1986; Young and Ventura, 1980; Gordon, 1980; Westfall, 1984, 1986), staffing distribution (Halloran, 1983; Halloran, Kiley, and Nadzam, 1986), computerized information systems (Long Island Jewish-Hillside Medical Center, 1985; Gordon, 1985a), continuing care planning (McKeehan, 1979), teaching and curriculum (Suhayda and Kim, 1986; Fredette and O'Connor, 1979; Gaines and McFarland, 1984), and as a basis for theory development (Kritek, 1978; Meleis, 1985, pp. 89–90). The wealth of literature currently being published on nursing diagnosis should not suggest that there are no controversial issues. These issues will be explored in Chapter 11.

Most would agree that the listing of health problems diagnosed and treated by nurses is incomplete. Work continues on the identification, refinement, and classification of diagnoses. All scientific knowledge is tentative and this is particularly true with a classification system containing health problems that have neither been formally tested in clinical practice nor subjected to conceptual analysis. This is important to remember when using diagnostic categories. Although limitations exist, clinicians find the use of a diagnostic language facilitates their practice and clarifies what they have to offer clients.

DEFINITION OF NURSING DIAGNOSIS: CATEGORY AND PROCESS

Some words people use to communicate their ideas have two or more definitions. The way in which the word is used clarifies the meaning. So it is with the term *nursing diagnosis*. It refers not only to the process of diagnosing but also to the diagnostic judgment reached and expressed in a category name.

Separating diagnostic category labels and the diagnostic process is artificial; the two are actually interdependent. Yet it makes learning easier if initially they are considered separately.

DIAGNOSIS DEFINED AS A CATEGORY

When a nurse describes a client's condition as "impaired mobility (level II) related to decreased activity tolerance," a diagnostic category label is being used. To help the reader understand the meaning of nursing diagnosis as a category for naming a health problem, it will be defined from three perspectives. Its *conceptual definition* will deal with the focus and meaning of nursing diagnosis and the *structural definition* will describe what it "looks like." In the last section of this chapter a *contextual definition* will specify its relationship to nursing process and health care delivery.

Conceptual Definition

A conceptual definition communicates the meaning of an idea. The following definition of nursing diagnosis has been proposed:

> Nursing diagnoses, or clinical diagnoses made by professional nurses, describe actual or potential health problems which nurses by virtue of their education and experience are capable and licensed to treat. (Gordon, 1976, p. 1299)

According to this definition there are *two important characteristics* of nursing diagnoses:

1 Who is responsible for making diagnoses.
2 What diagnoses describe.

Diagnostic Responsibility   The definition states that diagnoses are made by professional nurses. National standards of practice, educational preparation, and licensing laws support the exclusive use of nursing diagnosis by professional nurses. Who are considered professional nurses? Currently, whoever is licensed by the state to practice as a registered nurse. Yet many would argue that the baccalaureate nursing curriculum best prepares clinicians to assume this responsibility. Other nursing personnel may contribute information or carry out specified care, but registered nurses make nursing diagnoses.

The belief that registered nurses are responsible for making nursing diagnoses was evident at the NANDA Business Meeting, 7th Conference on Classification of Nursing Diagnoses, St. Louis, Missouri, March 1986. The General Assembly passed a motion that NANDA support the concept that only registered, professional nurses be responsible and accountable for identifying the nursing diagnoses for their patient population.

Diagnostic Focus   The second characteristic of nursing diagnoses stated in the definition is that they describe actual or potential health problems. *An actual problem is an existing deviation from health.* Dysfunctional grieving is an example. A client may be unable to progress through the grieving process after a loss, and this may influence many life activities. Ineffective airway clearance is another example of a health deviation.

Nurses do more than treat conditions that have already occurred. Traditionally, a high value has been placed on preventing health problems. Risk factors are identified that predispose individuals, families, or communities to health problems. *When a set of risk factors is present, the condition is referred to as a potential problem.* Potential for injury and potential skin breakdown are examples. Any listing or definition of nursing diagnoses has to include both actual and potential health problems. These are included in the currently identified diagnostic categories (Appendix A).

Some believe that limiting the scope of nursing diagnosis to actual or potential health problems (prevention and treatment) is too restrictive (Gleit and Tatro, 1981). Nurses also deal with clients seeking enriched personal growth in areas such as parenting, health management, and self-development. As categories are identified in these areas, the definition of nursing diagnosis may expand beyond problematic or potentially problematic conditions.

Would you agree that the phrase *describes health problems* in the above definition is rather vague? Physicians and others also deal with health problems. What is needed is a conceptual focus to describe the scope of nursing diagnosis. For example, fruit is a broad concept. It includes apples, bananas, melons and more. What concept would include all the diagnoses in Appendix A? As will be seen in Chapter 11 this is a major point of discussion in nursing diagnosis because the conceptual focus guides identification of diagnostic categories.

Lacking a universally accepted focus for nursing diagnosis, the previous definition uses a qualifier. It states that nursing diagnoses describe:

> health problems that nurses, by virtue of their education and experience are capable and licensed to treat independently. To treat, or the provision of treatment refers to the initiation of accepted modes of therapy . . . This definition thereby excludes health problems for which the accepted mode of therapy is prescription drugs, surgery, radiation, and other treatments that are defined legally as the practice of medicine. (Gordon, 1976, p. 1299)

Some may argue that clarifying domains of practice by using the qualifier *competency to treat* is inadequate. They argue that nurses do participate in the treatment of diseases. Nurses do, indeed, report observations and judgments, carry out physicians' orders that clients cannot carry out for themselves, and diagnose and treat diseases under physician supervision or protocols.[3] These activities of disease-related care are, in a sense, under the cognitive control of the physician. The nurse must anticipate what the physician would think and do (Hammond, 1966, p. 29). This is not the case with nursing diagnoses.

The important point is that diagnosis is merely an intellectual exercise unless followed by nursing care designed to resolve the problem. If a nurse is not *capable* of treating the problem judged to be present (whether the diagnosis is a nursing diagnosis or not), the client should be referred.

Another way of clarifying the focus and domain is to state that nursing diagnoses "can be alleviated by nursing actions" (Soares, 1978, p. 276). Therefore, it follows that *nurses are independently accountable for the outcomes of nursing diagnoses* (Feild and Winslow, 1985). For example, nurses assume

---

[3]Protocols are guides for analyzing and treating a disease process or symptom complex. A protocol may be highly organized and directive or it may be general and flexible; this will depend on the situation, education, and experience of the users and the availability of physician supervision and support (Hudak, 1976).

accountability for knowledge deficit, anxiety, and independence-dependence conflict that may co-occur with a heart attack. Their education prepares them to treat these problems, which are also within the scope of their licensing laws.[4]

One method of specifying the domain of nursing diagnosis when territorial issues[5] arise with other care providers is to:

1 Demonstrate an understanding of these health problems and their resolution through clinical research
2 Demonstrate in practice settings that nurses assume accountability for assessment, diagnosis, and treatment of these problems

A review of the literature indicates that nursing is beginning to direct clinical research to the problems nurses diagnose and treat (Gordon, 1985b). This will establish nursing's unique domain of concern as well as benefit clients.

Saying that nursing diagnoses are treated by professional nurses does not mean that nonnursing consultants cannot be used. Aspects of treatment may require consultation with other specialized professions that emerged from nursing. These include occupational therapy, physical therapy, social work, and respiratory therapy. Each offers specialized skills related to parts of the client situation. Although aspects of a problem are referred, nurses are responsible for coordinating treatment of nursing diagnoses. Responsibility and accountability are important issues and will be considered further in other chapters.

Another widely used definition of nursing diagnosis stresses responsibility and accountability. In a national study of the meaning of nursing diagnosis, Shoemaker found that nurses agreed on the following essential features:

> Nursing diagnosis is a clinical judgment about an individual, family, or community that is derived through a deliberate, systematic process of data collection and analysis. It provides the basis for prescriptions for definitive therapy for which the nurse is accountable. It is expressed concisely and includes the etiology of the condition when known. (Shoemaker, 1984, p. 109)

This definition stresses the judgment process and the important role of diagnosis in intervention; both of these topics will be considered in detail in later chapters.

Comparison with Other Clinical Terms. There are a number of clinical terms used in nursing, both current and historical, that are sometimes confused with nursing diagnoses (Silver, Halfmann, McShane, Hunt, and Nowak, 1984). Consideration of these terms should help to avoid conceptual errors. In addition, *positive and negative examples are useful in clarifying a concept and drawing the boundaries.*

Positive examples of nursing diagnoses are contained in Appendix A. It is important to note that these diagnostic categories are not officially standardized, as

---

[4]State laws govern the practice of nursing; they are referred to as state nurse practice acts.
[5]Territorial issues are those conflicts and controversies that arise among care providers regarding domains and scope of practice. Underlying the issues are expertise and monetary concerns.

are the disease names used in medical diagnosis. To say these categories are *approved* means that they are sufficiently developed for clinical testing. As will be discussed later a few are marginal, given the previously discussed definitions.

The diagram in Figure 1-1 depicts entities that are not nursing diagnoses and are thus outside the boundary of the concept. Many are mentioned by Little and Carnevali (1976, p. 50).

The terms in Figure 1-1 deserve some comment. All are used in nursing practice, and it is not uncommon to confuse them with nursing diagnoses. *Remember that a nursing diagnosis describes a client's health problem.* It does not describe, for example, the "staff's problems in coping with clients" (Little and Carnevali, 1976, p. 50). That nurses and doctors react in stressful or frustrating situations has to be recognized, but *staff problems should not be labeled as diagnostic judgments about the client.*

Therapeutic needs are not nursing diagnoses; they do not describe health problems or health states. For example, "needs emotional support" or "needs suctioning" has been a common way of describing needs for nursing care. These are therapeutic needs; the question arises as to why the client has these needs. In other words, what is the underlying health problem, the nursing diagnosis? *Once a diagnosis is established, therapeutic goals and interventions can be determined, but not before.*

As an example of the contrast between "needs" and diagnoses, imagine that a nurse says a client "needs emotional support." The client was observed (1) pacing the room during the day before surgery, (2) commenting about being unable to sit still, and (3) stating the wish that surgery was over. A nurse could rush in with emotional support, a diffuse nursing response. Yet in actuality the client may be having difficulty coping with the thought of disability from surgery. Perhaps a neighbor had the same surgery and suffered paralysis 2 days later.

FIGURE 1-1
Concept of nursing diagnosis and terms excluded from the concept.

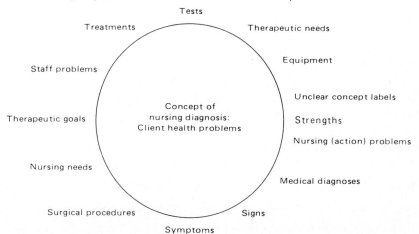

The client may be identifying with this situation although his risk for paralysis is extremely low. Diffuse emotional support would probably not assist this person in handling concerns; a problem-focused intervention is needed. *Using therapeutic needs as diagnoses bypasses the problem formulation step in care planning.*

The term *needs* is also commonly used in another context in nursing. When Maslow's needs hierarchy (Maslow, 1970), a nonnursing theory, is employed as a framework, physiological, safety, belonging, and other needs are stated. These are said to be needs of every human being. If unmet or conflicting, these needs are the basis for the development of health problems (Soares, 1978). To write "safety needs" on a chart communicates very little; everyone needs safety. So little information is contained in this statement that one is unable to infer what the problem may be.

Just as therapeutic need is not a nursing diagnosis, neither is a *therapeutic nursing goal,* such as "to maintain nutrition." Like "safety needs," this phrase transmits no information about the client's health problems. Everyone needs adequate nutrition. The question needs to be raised, Is there a potential or actual nutritional deficit?

The advantage of basing nursing intervention on a nursing diagnosis is the clear focus for care planning that the diagnosis provides. *When a plan is based only on therapeutic goals, there is no way of knowing the client's health problem.* In contrast, stating a nursing diagnosis clarifies the logical relationship that should exist between the client's problem and the proposed plan of care.

One *sign* or *symptom* is not a nursing diagnosis. For example, one sometimes sees "restlessness" as the nursing diagnosis. This could be a sign of pain, anxiety, or numerous other conditions. This sign is a totally inadequate base for planning treatment and may or may not be related to a problem nurses can treat. Similarly, a symptom, such as "fatigue," is not a nursing diagnosis. The presence of fatigue may be a predictor that the client will have a self-care deficit, impaired home-maintenance management, or other problems related to decreased energy. Isolated signs and symptoms do not identify the client's health problem. *A nursing diagnosis describes a cluster of signs and symptoms.*

The question sometimes arises, Is a nursing diagnosis the same as a *nursing problem?* The answer depends on how the term *nursing problem* is being used. If referring to a client's health problem that is amenable to nursing treatment, then *nursing problem* is synonymous with *nursing diagnosis*. *Nursing problem* or *medical problem* are terms used when care providers wish to specify who is treating a problem or wish to refer a client to the appropriate care provider.

The term *nursing problem* is not synonymous with a nursing diagnosis when used to refer to a therapeutic problem. How to promote healing may be a nursing *care* problem, but the health problem is *decubitus ulcer. A nursing diagnosis describes the client's problem, not the nurse's problem in designing and implementing care.*

Little and Carnevali (1976, pp. 48–49) take issue with the use of *concept labels* as nursing diagnoses. Just using a conceptual term, such as *stress* or *maternal attachment* does not indicate whether a problem exists. Yet not all signs and symptoms can be specified in the diagnostic label. If they were, the diagnosis would be lengthy and would not serve as a shorthand expression. The point Little and Carnevali (1976) make is that a diagnosis should adequately identify the problem for purposes of communication.

As seen in Figure 1-1 and as Little and Carnevali (1976) so clearly point out, nursing diagnoses do not describe *treatments, tests,* or *equipment.* For example, "catheter," "adrenalectomy," or "on heparin" are clearly not within the concept of nursing diagnosis. *Treatments and tests do not represent health problems, nor do they represent a cluster of signs and symptoms.* Possibly, further data collection will reveal a health problem and a need for nursing intervention.

The diagnosis of disease, or *medical diagnosis*, is not within the concept of nursing diagnosis. If a nurse makes a tentative judgment about a disease or a disease complication, this judgment is made for purposes of referral. These judgments are an important part of nursing practice but are not nursing diagnoses.

As previously mentioned, *pathophysiological manifestations of a diseased organ or system,* such as impaired gas exchange, are not nursing diagnoses. In the *collaborative* or *interdependent* area of practice (Feild and Winslow, 1985; Jacoby, 1985; Kim, 1985), nurses help clients to monitor these conditions and carry out medical treatment until the clients can do it by themselves. Traditionally, nurses have not assumed responsibility for treatment of and research on pathophysiological manifestations of disease. The current responsibility of the nurse is to identify and refer the problem to a physician and to prevent complications, if possible.

Some nurses argue that they are capable of making medical diagnoses, and indeed they are. It is not illegal to exercise one's intellectual capabilities. Yet if the diagnosis is communicated to the patient *and* if treatment, or lack of it, produces harm, it will probably be extremely difficult for the nurse who is responsible to present a substantive defense in court against a malpractice claim.

There are nursing roles in which additional educational preparation legally permits diagnosis and treatment of diseases under physician supervision or protocols. These roles are commonly practiced in ambulatory care or other community-based settings. The portion of the nurse's role that relates to medical diagnosis is similar to the performance of medical acts by a physician's assistant. Although not to the same extent as in ambulatory care, critical care nurses are also responsible for making disease-related judgments and providing treatment under protocols.

Judgments related to observations of disease manifestations or to treatments do not have to be labeled as nursing diagnoses. Disease terminology is perfectly adequate. It would seem ridiculous to relabel a disease with a nursing diagnosis when in fact it cannot be treated except under medical protocols. *Clearly, not everything a nurse does will be labeled with a nursing diagnosis.*

Although *medical diagnoses* are not referred to as nursing diagnoses, there is a connection: nursing diagnoses can co-occur with a disease. This important point will be considered later in sections dealing with medical and nursing diagnoses in practice.

Strengths of the client are areas of healthy or optimal functioning. Some authors refer to strengths as nursing diagnoses (Martens, 1986). They are not a focus of *treatment* so this appears to be a misnomer. Client strengths require important nursing judgments that arise out of health assessment; their importance lies in the *intervention phase* of care. Strengths can be mobilized to deal with problems or to move toward higher levels of human functioning.

States of health, well-being, or *optimal functioning* are not nursing diagnoses per se. They are goals of nursing. If a client is "healthy" and has no dysfunctional or potentially dysfunctional health patterns, it is unethical to diagnose a *problem* and charge for treatment. (Charges are appropriate for functional health assessment, health status evaluation, and periodic monitoring of health status.) Some clients desire help with further growth to realize their human potential. A number of nurses interested in this area are trying to develop terms for "health-related" nursing diagnoses (Gleit and Tatro, 1981; Gottleib, 1982). Currently clients cannot receive reimbursement for interventions directed toward only "desires" or "potential for growth" from government or private insurance in the United States. Health promotion and risk factor reduction are receiving great attention especially in occupational and primary care. Yet in most cases a potential problem (risk factors) is present, such as stress, sedentary life style, or nutritional excesses.

Appendix A and the previous discussion provide examples of what are and what are not nursing diagnoses. Try to apply the information in the following exercise containing correctly and incorrectly formulated diagnoses from hospital records. Which of these are examples of correctly formulated nursing diagnoses?

1 Needs suctioning
2 Inadequate insight
3 Self-bathing deficit (level II)
4 Backache
5 Alterations in parenting
6 Chronic lung disease
7 Difficulty taking medicine

It could be inferred that ineffective airway clearance is the problem in number 1, but we shall never know. The nurse has stated a need rather than a problem. Thus, needs suctioning is not a clinically useful diagnostic category. In number 2, the client's insight may be inadequate in some situations, but which ones and why? The modifier *inadequate* is too judgmental; what amount of insight is adequate? One would imagine there might be a health problem here, but it isn't well expressed. In contrast, number 3, self-bathing deficit, is a functional problem. It directs thinking about nursing care designed to help the client compensate for the deficit. (Level II means the person requires assistance or supervision.)

Backache, in number 4, is a symptom, not a diagnosis; it would cause the nurse to collect further information. Alterations in parenting, number 5, is an accepted diagnosis but is a rather broad category that requires further break-down and definition. Although useful for the time being because it describes an area of concern to nurses, this diagnosis encompasses a number of distinct problems.[6]

Chronic lung disease, number 6, is obviously a medical diagnosis. No doubt a client with this diagnosis has problems amenable to nursing therapy. Perhaps the nurse lacked the language to express nursing diagnoses, or chronic lung disease was the diagnosis used to organize the care ordered by the physician and was erroneously labeled as a nursing diagnosis. Number 7, difficulty taking medicine, is an observation, not a nursing diagnosis. It discloses nothing about the nature and cause of the difficulty. The trouble could be caused by the nurse's method of administration, the nature of the medication (pills versus liquid), or a number of other things.

In summarizing this discussion of the conceptual definition of nursing diag-nosis, it will be useful to keep in mind the following characteristics of a nursing diagnosis:

1 Conditions described by nursing diagnoses can be accurately identified by *nursing* assessment methods.

2 Nursing treatments, or methods of risk factor reduction, can resolve the condition described by a nursing diagnosis.

3 Because the necessary treatments to resolve nursing diagnoses are within the scope of nursing practice, nurses assume accountability for outcomes.

4 Nursing assumes responsibility for the research required to clearly identify the defining characteristics and etiological factors and to improve methods of treatment and treatment outcomes for conditions described by nursing diagnoses.

Now let us consider nursing diagnosis defined from a structural perspective.

Structural Definition

One of the simplest ways to grasp the concept of nursing diagnosis is to ask, How would I know if I saw one? To build on the ideas already discussed, consider how a nursing diagnosis may appear on various record forms. There are three essential components in a nursing diagnosis; they have been referred to as the *PES format* (Gordon, 1976). *The three components are the health problem (P), the etiological or related factors (E), and the defining characteristics or cluster of signs and symptoms (S).*

---

[6]Clinical testing will probably reveal two or more health problems (each of which is treated differently) within some of the current diagnostic categories. Alterations in parenting is an example.

Problem Statement   The first component of the structural definition is illustrated by the diagnoses listed in Appendix A. Each of these describes a problem, or health state, of the individual, family, or community. *The state of the client (problem) is expressed in clear, concise terms, preferably two or three words.* For example, *ineffective family coping* and *noncompliance (specify)* are concise terms that represent a cluster of signs and symptoms.

The term *specify* used in this manner directs the user of the category to state the area in which the problem occurs. For example, noncompliance may be in the area of medication regimen, dietary prescription, or any other health management practices that the client has previously expressed the intention to carry out.

Etiological or Related Factors   The second component of a nursing diagnosis is the probable factors causing or maintaining the client's health problem. These can be behaviors of the client, factors in the environment, or an interaction of both. As an example, impaired reality testing may be a factor contributing to nutritional deficit in a client with psychosis who thinks food is poisoned. Another example is decreased activity tolerance acting as a causative factor in impaired home-maintenance management. *Probable causes of a problem should be stated clearly and concisely, using a concise category name, if possible, to summarize the signs and symptoms observed.* Figure 1-2 contains some examples of factors that contribute to noncompliance.

Clients may have the same problem but exhibit signs and symptoms indicating different etiological factors. It is important to realize that a different diagnosis exists and different treatment is required when the causative factors are different. Consider the following four diagnoses, each of which requires different nursing intervention:

1 Self-care deficit, level IV, related to decreased activity tolerance
2 Self-care deficit, level IV, related to uncompensated sensorimotor loss
3 Self-care deficit, level IV, related to autism
4 Self-care deficit, level IV, related to impaired reality testing

FIGURE 1-2
Examples of diagnostic categories and possible etiological factors.

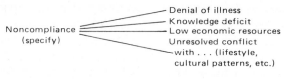

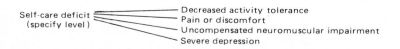

All four diagnoses share the common signs and symptoms of self-care deficit, level IV (level IV means the person is totally dependent and does not participate in self-care). Yet each has an additional set of signs and symptoms peculiar to the specified etiological factor.

When a self-care deficit, level IV, is judged to be present, a differentiation among possible reasons for the problem is required. This is an example of *differential diagnosis.* Differentiating among various contributing factors is critically important because interventions differ, as is clear from the above examples. Different modes of treatment obviously would be required. A person's ability to feed, bathe, dress, groom, and toilet is not going to improve with assistive devices if the cause is impaired reality testing. In fact, the problem may worsen if incorrect treatments are used.

Defining Characteristics   The third component of a nursing diagnosis is the set of defining characteristics (signs and symptoms) that appear in textbooks or manuals. These include the *critical defining characteristics* of the condition and *supporting data.*

Critical Defining Characteristics (Diagnostic Criteria)   Critical defining characteristics are the *major criteria* for diagnostic judgment. They *are found nearly always when the diagnosis is present and are absent when the diagnosis is absent.* Thus, critical characteristics of each category permit diagnosticians to make discriminations among diagnoses.

When a client manifests signs and symptoms that correspond to the critical defining characteristics, then the use of the diagnostic category is appropriate. For example, the critical defining characteristics of *fear (specify)* that all clients with the condition exhibit probably are:

1 Verbalized feelings of dread, nervousness or concern about a threatening event, person, or object
2 Verbalized expectation of danger to the self
3 Describes with or without assistance, the focus of perceived threat or danger (actual or imagined)

The above behaviors are criteria for making the diagnosis. The third behavior is used to identify the focus of fear and to design specific interventions. Note that for the category *fear* (specify), the critical data are verbal reports of the client in contrast to observations of the nurse. *Verbal reports are necessary whenever a nurse is diagnosing a subjective state or process.*

Supporting Characteristics   Usually nurses wish to check further to see if the client's report can be confirmed by their observations; they search for *supporting data.* Reports and observations are put together to increase confidence in the diagnosis. The remaining supporting characteristics (minor defining characteristics) of fear listed by NANDA describe *observable* reactions to fear:

4 Increased questioning, information seeking
5 Increased quantity and rate of verbalization

   6 Voice tremors, pitch changes
   7 Restlessness
   8 Narrowing focus of attention progressing to fixed
   9 Hand tremor
   10 Increased muscle tension
   11 Diaphoresis
   12 Increased heart rate
   13 Increased respiratory rate

The above characteristics *support* the judgment that fear is present but are *not* conclusive without the verbal reports described in 1–3 above. To test this idea, read characteristics 4–13 alone; think of other conditions besides fear that manifest the same signs. For example, restlessness or increased heart and respiratory rate can occur with discomfort, pain, and other conditions. Questioning and information-seeking also occurs with interest and intellectual curiousity. *To differentiate among conditions the diagnostician has to obtain information on the major, critical defining characteristics.* As with all "rules," this has an exception.

Consider the situation where the client is unable to speak? How would you know that a state of fear is present? A verbal report is not possible. Observations of a few of the above signs (7–13) and the context of the client's situation would have to be used. *One of the reasons that professional judgment is needed in nursing diagnosis is that client's conditions do not always match the "textbook picture."*

If each person who saw the same characteristics of a particular object called it by a different name, communication about the object would be impossible. As in medicine, or science in general, *terms used in nursing diagnosis have specific definitions.* The definition of the medical diagnostic category *myocardial infarction* is standardized internationally so that in journals or other types of communication no erroneous interpretation will occur. It is the responsibility of the person using diagnostic terms to use them correctly. Most nurses contributing to the identification of diagnostic categories believe that identification of the critical defining characteristics (signs and symptoms) of accepted diagnoses needs a great deal of attention. Yet this identification cannot be completed until diagnoses are used clinically and the signs and symptoms most frequently present are described.

In Chapter 8, when problem identification is discussed, more will be said about the nature and use of diagnostic categories; their development will be considered in Chapter 11.

DIAGNOSIS DEFINED AS A PROCESS

As previously stated, the word *diagnosis* has two meanings. It can refer to a name for a health problem found in a classification system of nursing diagnoses, the meaning explored in the previous section. The second meaning, *a process leading to a clinical judgment,* is the topic introduced in this section.

It is important to appreciate the various cognitive operations involved in acquiring and using clinical information. Equally important is the appreciation that clinical information is acquired through nurse-client interaction. The quality of this interaction directly affects what information is obtained and, subsequently, what diagnostic judgment is made. Let us first consider some general characteristics of the diagnostic process and its components.

The diagnostic process is, essentially, a way of determining a client's health state and evaluating the etiological factors influencing that state. Is it ever possible to truly know the state of another person, a family, or a community? Most philosophers who deal with questions such as this would say no. What the diagnostician seeks is sufficient understanding of clients and situations to evaluate health, predict future health, and provide assistance when needed. One definition of *diagnosis* is "an analysis of the nature of something" (Morris, 1978, p. 363). In clinical practice that "something" is a client's health status.

To diagnose is to distinguish or discriminate. As information is collected, the first discrimination that occurs is between indicators of a problem and indicators of health and well-being. This is a two-way discrimination task. If signs point toward a judgment of health, they are described and recognition is given to the client's health-promoting practices. Identifying and acknowledging healthful practices serves to support behavior that maintains health.

On the other hand, signs may point toward an actual or potential health problem. Search strategies are required to identify the problem clearly. Additionally, the cluster of signs and symptoms have to be labeled correctly with a diagnostic category. This process represents much more than a two-way differentiation between the presence and absence of health.

Diagnostic Process Components

Within the diagnostic process are actions, and within these are other, more specific operations involving reasoning and judgment. In its broadest sense, diagnosis involves four activities:

1 Collecting information
2 Interpreting the information
3 Clustering the information
4 Naming the cluster

From this list it would appear that the four activities are a sequence of steps and that the diagnostician has only to collect all information available, analyze and arrange it, and apply category names to the health problems identified. If diagnosis were this uncomplicated, any nurse's aide could be taught the steps.

Instead, *what occurs in the diagnostic process is a cycle of certain perceptual and cognitive activities.* Observations lead to inferences and inferences lead to further observation. This cycle continues until the diagnostician feels confident to name the problem.

Information Collection   The admission nursing history and examination begins the process of information collection, or assessment. (Actually, information collection never ends.) In adding a person, family, or community to his or her caseload, the nurse assumes the responsibility for collecting health-related information. Skillful collection of information, which is critically important in the diagnostic process, is influenced by clinical knowledge. One perceives what one expects to perceive (on the basis of stored knowledge). Clinical knowledge stored in memory provides the expectations that make one sensitive to cues.[7] Knowing how to frame a question or measure a pulse is a basic skill. *The judgment of when the question or measurement is appropriate is influenced by one's clinical knowledge.*

Information Interpretation   Collecting information is pointless if the meaning is not derived. Interpretation of cues to a client's health status allows one to predict or explain the findings. Two mental operations are involved, inferential reasoning and judgment.

Information Clustering   In clinical practice nurses collecting and interpreting information are heard to remark, "It fits the picture," "I'm getting a picture of . . . ," or "No, that doesn't fit the picture." What seems to be occurring is the clustering of information in a meaningful way based on its interpretation.

Nurses know "what goes with what." How do they know this? Probably, memory stores are searched for prevously learned, meaningful ways of clustering the clinical cues within diagnostic categories. The "picture" referred to is probably the memory cluster of defining signs and symptoms that defines a diagnostic category.

Naming the Cue Cluster   Information collection, interpretation, and clustering occur over and over during the diagnostic process. When observations seem to "fit" a diagnostic category, the category name is applied to the cluster of cues. For example, the client may (*a*) have excessive perspiration due to a fever, (*b*) be too weak to turn and reach for a drink of water, (*c*) express concern that her children are not getting good care during her hospitalization, and (*d*) have dry mouth. Cues *a, b,* and *d* fit the critical defining characteristics of the diagnostic category, potential fluid volume deficit. Thus, this name is given to the client's problem. The verbal report, *c,* does not fit but is possibly a cue to another problem; it requires further investigation. *Identification, or naming a health problem is an act of judgment that says "It is this and not that."* Diagnostic

---

[7]Cue is a word that will be used frequently in this text. It is a term borrowed from cognitive psychology meaning a signal to action, initially a cognitive action. A client behavior exists; it only becomes a cue if perceived and interpreted by the diagnostician.

reasoning and judgment are important because they are the basis for care planning.

The goal in health evaluation and diagnosis is correct and reliable judgments. Attaining this goal requires refinement of the commonsense approach that serves so well in everyday living. Refinement proceeds in a particular direction: *toward critical reflection and curiosity. These two abilities increase the reliability of diagnostic judgments and differentiate professional expertise from the layperson's commonsense approach.*

Thus far this chapter has provided information about nursing diagnosis as a category and a process. For implementation in practice it is important to know that:

1 Nursing diagnoses are made by professional nurses.

2 Nursing diagnoses describe actual or potential health problems that are amenable to *nursing* intervention.

3 Nursing diagnoses are *names* that refer to a cluster of cues indicating a health problem (see Appendix A).

4 Each nursing diagnosis has a small set of *critical defining characteristics* that represent the major signs and symptoms of the health problem. These characteristics represent the *diagnostic criteria* for making the diagnosis.

5 Each nursing diagnosis has *etiological or related factors* that contribute to, or maintain, the problem; their resolution or modification serve as a focus for nursing intervention. In the case of potential problems, *risk factors* are identified.

6 Within the diagnostic process there is *information collection, information interpretation, information clustering,* and *naming the cluster.*

7 Commonsense reasoning may be helpful in the diagnostic process, but a diagnostician's reliability depends on *critical reasoning (reflective analysis and the curiosity to ask "Why").*

8 Since 1973 there has been an international effort by NANDA to identify nursing diagnoses. All nurses have an opportunity to join in this work.

CONTEXTUAL DEFINITION OF DIAGNOSIS

Sometimes a concept becomes clearer if it is viewed in the context of related ideas rather than in isolation. In this section nursing diagnosis will be examined in its rightful place, within nursing process. *The important understanding to be gained is that the purpose of diagnosis is to provide a focus for nursing care planning and evaluation.*

Nursing process will be examined in its own right, then in the context of nursing practice that consists of more than just treating nursing diagnoses. Next, a look at the broader context of health care delivery will provide an understanding of the need for collaboration among health professionals, particularly in the treatment of the client's diagnoses. *The major appreciation to be gained is that nursing diagnoses are not made in isolation.*

Nursing Diagnosis in Nursing Process

Client care is the central focus of nursing. Caring for, about, and with clients are the scientific and humanistic elements. These elements of clinical practice describe a *helping relationship* actualized through nursing process.

Nursing process is a method of problem identification and problem solving.[8] Although derived from the supposedly objective scientific method, nursing process is not applied in an objective, value-free way. *Human values influence both problem identification and problem solving.*

The components of nursing process discussed in textbooks vary but generally include *assessment, diagnosis, outcome projection, planning, intervention, and outcome evaluation.* Having the key components spelled out encourages deliberation, organization, and thought as opposed to haphazard care planning. This is important when *human beings* are the recipients of care.

The six components named above only specify the activities to be done. How these activities are done requires a conceptual framework. A *conceptual framework* is a set of concepts that guide general decisions about *what* to assess and diagnose, *how* to intervene, and *what* to evaluate. In a later chapter a few selected frameworks will be discussed. The objective at this point is just to define diagnosis in the context of nursing process. The discussion here will be brief and introductory.

Nursing process begins with the *problem-identification phase.* In the first contact with a client a nursing history and examination are done. This information-collection process is referred to as *assessment.* During assessment actual or potential health problems may be revealed. Nursing diagnoses are used to describe these problems.

It is important to understand that problem identification contains *elements of uncertainty.* One rarely is 100 percent certain that a diagnosis is valid. This is not peculiar to nursing; all health care providers are faced with the same situation. In a later chapter, methods for dealing with this lack of certainty will be discussed.

When a cluster of signs and symptoms is categorized using a nursing diagnosis, clinical knowledge stored in memory can be retrieved. This knowledge facilitates problem solving or problem prevention. In the intervention phase of nursing process, diagnosis proves its worth. The diagnosis, or problem identified, provides a focus for *problem-solving activities.* These include outcome projection, care planning, intervention, and outcome evaluation.

The first step in helping a client solve or prevent a problem is to identify clearly the outcome desired. *An outcome is measurable behavior indicating problem resolution or progress toward resolution.* For example, if the diagnosis is potential skin breakdown, the desired outcome is intact skin. Did you notice what just occurred? *The diagnosis was used as a focus for projecting the outcome.*

---

[8]Most authors use the term *problem solving* to encompass both identification of the problem and its solution. To emphasize the two components, in this text they will be stated explicitly.

Having determined the desired health outcome, the nurse can now stop and think about what nursing care is needed to reach the specified outcome when the specified nursing diagnosis is present. Factors in the client's situation are also considered in decision making. Taking them into account serves to individualize care planning. During intervention there is continual assessment and evaluation of the problem, the effectiveness of care, and the progress toward outcome attainment.

This brief overview indicates how nursing diagnoses are used in nursing process. *Diagnoses provide a distinct focus for establishing desired outcomes of nursing care and for making decisions about what care is needed. A diagnosis also provides a focus for daily evaluation of a client's progress and for any necessary revision of the care plan.* For all these reasons nursing diagnoses make nursing care delivery easier. Further appreciation of this point will be gained when more specific guidelines and examples are provided in a later chapter.

Nursing Diagnosis in Nursing Practice

A broader view is necessary before nursing diagnosis can be thought of in the context of nursing practice. In this section we will see that nursing practice may include more than the treatment of nursing diagnoses. If clients have medical problems, nurses help them to carry out medical treatments (i.e., to follow their doctor's orders). It is important to grasp the difference. In one case, nursing diagnoses, the nurse is responsible for determining the care plan; in the other case, medical diagnoses, the responsibility is to see that the client is helped to carry out the care plan designed by the physician.

Aside from the issue of responsibility, in practice the separation is artificial. Clients have health problems. Physicians and nurses work together to help them overcome these problems. The issue that concerns many nurses is, *What is the essence of nursing in practice, and is sufficient emphasis given to this?*

The currently accepted diagnoses (Appendix A) occur in every specialty. Perhaps the incidence and the etiological factors are different, but the problems described by nursing diagnoses are the same. Self-care deficits, fear, disturbances in self-concept, potential for injury, and certain other problems seem to constitute a *core of nursing practice* irrespective of the setting and specialty.

Nursing diagnoses do not describe the whole of nursing practice. Clients have other health problems, as was previously stated, that are of concern to nurses. For a moment think of the whole of your practice as contained in a circle, such as that illustrated in Figure 1-3. Think of this whole as 100 percent of the time you spend in direct client care activities (ignore administrative tasks for the moment). Move the line to section off the circle in a 90:10 ratio of nursing diagnosis-related activities to medically delegated activities. This may describe time allocation in long-term care or rehabilitation where nursing diagnosis-related activities predominate. For ambulatory or clinic settings move the line to a 75:25 ratio of nursing diagnosis activities to delegated care activities.

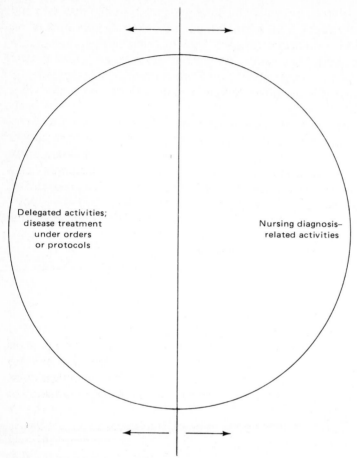

Delegated activities;
disease treatment
under orders
or protocols

Nursing diagnosis–
related activities

FIGURE 1-3
Time spent in direct care activities of nursing practice.

In home health care or extended care facilities, the distribution may be 60:40; with decreased length of stay in hospitals the acuity of the disease is greater in the home or community than previously seen. The increased acuity of hospitalized clients suggests a 30:70 ratio. Intensive care for problems of physiological instability may result in a 10:90 ratio for activities related to nursing diagnoses and to medical diagnoses, respectively. The line is movable, as is the emphasis nurses place on various aspects of practice.

The diagram is useful in conveying the information that nursing diagnosis is used in that aspect of practice unique to nursing. No one else is educated to perform this aspect of care. The diagram also helps clarify that nurses do not intend to ignore medical treatment orders or the client's disease; to do so would not be compatible with a holistic approach. It is important to notice also that disease-related nursing care is not considered "nonnursing" activity. The current emphasis on nursing diagnoses has come about because this aspect of practice (diagnosis) has not been described; the others have.

With a holistic approach to care, all problems are considered simultaneously. *Priorities are decided by the severity and significance of a health problem to the client's recovery and future health potential, irrespective of whether they are medical or nursing diagnoses.* In some instances the treatment of anxiety is more important than a routine dressing change if clients are treated as integrated human beings (as opposed to just physiological or psychosocial beings). In another case doing a medical treatment may be judged to be more important to the overall health of the client than treating anxiety. Nursing judgment about priorities is required in these instances. This type of judgment develops with experience.

It is important to point out that clinical judgments in nursing practice are not confined to nursing diagnoses. Judgment is required in reporting changes in the client's medical condition, the response to therapy, administration of drugs, carrying out medical treatments, and seeking nurse specialists' or others' consultation.

Nursing Diagnosis in Health Care Delivery

In this section we will take a broader view that encompasses nursing process and nursing practice. Health care delivery is the combined objective of many groups: physicians, nurses, administrators, agencies of the federal government, and others. Basic health services are delivered by two professions, nursing and medicine. These basic services to the consumer are supplemented as necessary by a number of other health care providers. For example, when clients' health problems warrant, referrals can be made to social workers, physical therapists, or psychologists.

Figure 1-4 symbolizes the components of coordinated care when only a nurse, a physician, and a consultant are involved in providing services. Although the interactions and outcome shown by the arrows do not always take place, coordination represented by arrows toward a central focus is a realistic goal.

Clients' contributions to the coordination of their health care management include (1) their personal perceptions of their health state, (2) their plans, and (3) their health practices. They have expectations that the "specialists" in health will offer information, recommendations, and the required care. Health professionals formalize clients' health concerns with diagnoses and treatment plans, as the diagram indicates. Thus the major elements are present for joint planning by the client, nurse, and physician.

Coordinated care as illustrated in Figure 1-4 is not a new idea; it can be found in textbooks dating back 30 or more years. Yet the challenge to implement this coordination is still present for the next generation of clinicians in the health professions.

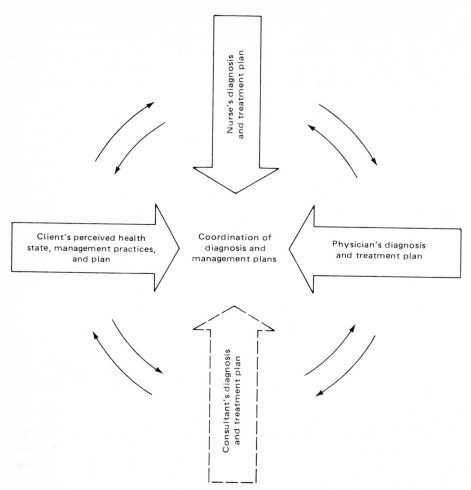

FIGURE 1-4
Components of coordinated health care delivery.

Figure 1-5 illustrates the current situation in many institutions devoted to health care, "part and parcel care delivery." The professions operate rather separately and each offers its own "parcel" to the consumer. Nursing has not clearly understood what its own contribution is, and consequently has not been able to clarify this matter for consumers. The language used in health care circles is not just one of actions and doing. It deals with what the problem is and what can be offered, a rather logical stance.

If health care is to go from the situation in Figure 1-5 to that in Figure 1-4, the *first* step is for nurses to share, in some clear and concise way, their conceptions of clients' current functional health status and nursing care needs. Nursing diagnoses provide a method for synthesizing and communicating nurses'

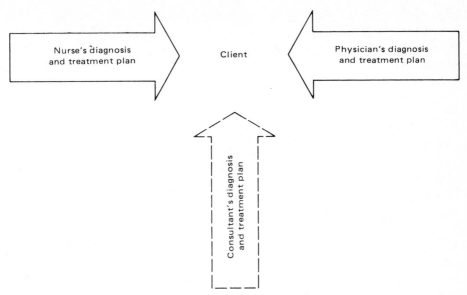

FIGURE 1-5
Independent (uncoordinated) components of current health care delivery.

observations. As later chapters will show, the ability to communicate health needs of clients can influence funding of preventive and comprehensive health care services.

It is predicted that chronic diseases will be the major medical problem as the twentieth century ends and the twenty-first century begins. Consistent with this, the main population using health services will be the "frail elderly." The need currently exists to delay the onset of chronic disease and disability. Underlying early onset are conditions such as obesity, stress management, accidental injuries, and drug abuse (nicotine, alcohol, and others). If functional health patterns of the population were surveyed, the nursing diagnosis *health management deficit* would probably outrank all other currently identified medical or nursing problems. Consumers are beginning to realize that they can control their health management. Guidance in health management and early detection of dysfunctional health patterns will contribute to delaying the onset of chronic disease and disability.

SUMMARY

Interest and enthusiasm about nursing diagnosis is widespread. Nurses in a number of countries recognize the implications for nursing practice, education, and research. In particular, those providing direct care to clients view nursing diagnosis as a way to improve care. As one nurse said, "It helps me to define what I do and to feel good about how I do it."

In this chapter, nursing diagnosis and the diagnostic process were introduced. It was noted that the term *diagnosis* is used to refer both to a *category name for a health problem* and *to a process of identifying health problems.* Diagnosis as a category was explained by contrasting what a diagnosis is with what it is not. Leaving other conceptual distinctions for a later chapter, *a nursing diagnosis was defined as an actual or potential health problem amenable to nursing intervention.*

In the description of diagnosis as a process of judgment the following points were emphasized:

1 The diagnostic process includes the collection, interpretation, and clustering of information. Then a name is given to the health problem.

2 Diagnosis as a process and diagnosis as a category can be separated for purposes of discussion, but they are inseparable when used in practice.

Nursing diagnosis was examined in the context of nursing process in order to establish its essential and practical meaning. Important points in that discussion were:

1 A diagnosis provides the focus for the helping relationship established with clients.

2 Nursing diagnosis is used in nursing process as a basis for projecting health outcomes and determining nursing interventions to reach the projected outcomes.

When the broader scope of nursing practice was considered, it was recognized that nurses make many types of clinical judgments. Nursing diagnostic judgments have a particular characteristic that distinguishes them from nursing judgments related to diagnosis and treatment of disease. The major points in this section were:

1 When nursing diagnoses are made, responsibility and accountability exist for determining the treatment plan, as opposed to implementing the plans of other care providers.

2 Nursing practice requires competency in three types of clinical judgment: diagnostic, therapeutic, and ethical. Moral reasoning and ethical judgment are involved in most diagnostic and therapeutic activities.

An examination of health care delivery demonstrated that a variety of professionals make diagnoses and develop treatment plans. Not to be overlooked are clients' perceptions of their health or their health management plans. Ideally, coordinated health care takes all of these into account. There were two important implications for nursing discussed. One was that *nursing diagnoses represent a clear focus for nursing participation in coordinated planning.* The second was that *nurses, physicians, consultants, and clients (insofar as their condition permits) have to pool their conceptions of health problems and treatment plans* in order to coordinate activities. It was suggested that *the incidence of chronic disease and disability in the population will rise unless there is early diagnosis and treatment of potential problems, such as health management deficits.* This is one area in which nurses can contribute to improving the health of the population.

Because nursing diagnoses are not made in isolation and because nurses need to increase their participation in joint planning, an appreciation of other professions is needed. When participating in a joint care planning conference it is important to know the perspectives of other professions (just as they need to understand the perspective of nursing). Chapter 2 will provide information on this subject. It will also provide an opportunity to see how nursing's perspective and the focus of diagnosis evolved.

BIBLIOGRAPHY

Abdellah, F. G., Beland, I., Martin, A., & Matheny, P. (1961). *Patient-centered approaches to nursing.* New York: Macmillan.

American Nurses' Association (1974). *Standards of nursing practice.* Kansas City, MO.

American Nurses' Association & American Association of Neuroscience Nurses (1985). *Neuroscience nursing practice: Process and outcome criteria for selected diagnoses.* Kansas City, MO.

Barnard, K. E. (1983). Nursing diagnosis: A descriptive method. *American Journal of Maternal/Child Nursing, 8:223.*

Bonney, V., & Rothberg, J. (1963). *Nursing diagnosis and therapy.* New York: National League for Nursing.

Bruce, J. A. (1979). Implementation of nursing diagnosis: A nursing administrator's perspective. *Nursing Clinics of North America, 14:509–516.*

Clark, S. R. (1984). Nursing diagnosis: Its application in an ambulatory care setting. *Topics in Clinical Nursing, 5:57–67.*

Crosley, J. (1986). Computerized nursing care planning using nursing diagnosis. In M. Hurley (Ed.). (1986), *Classification of nursing diagnoses: Proceedings of the sixth conference.* St. Louis: Mosby.

Dalton, J. M. (1979). Nursing diagnosis in a community health setting. *Nursing Clinics of North America, 14:525–532.*

Davidson, S. B. (1984). Nursing diagnosis: Its application to acute care settings. *Topics in Clinical Nursing, 5:50–56.*

Feild, L., & Winslow, E. H. (1985). Moving to a nursing model. *American Journal of Nursing, 85:1100–1101.*

Fredette, S., & O'Connor, K. (1979). Nursing diagnosis in teaching and curriculum planning. *Nursing Clinics of North America, 14:541–552.*

Fry, V. (1953). The creative approach to nursing. *American Journal of Nursing, 53:301–302.*

Gaines, B. C., & McFarland, M. B. (1984). Nursing diagnosis: Its relationship to and use in nursing education. *Topics in Clinical Nursing, 5:39–49.*

Gebbie, K. M., & Lavin, M. A. (1975). *Classification of nursing diagnoses: Proceedings of the first national conference.* St. Louis: Mosby.

Gleit, C. J., & Tatro, S. (1981). Nursing diagnosis for healthy individuals. *Nursing and Health Care, 2:456–457.*

Gordon, M. (1985*a*). Practice-based data set for a nursing information system. *Journal of Medical Systems, 9:43–55.*

Gordon, M. (1985*b*). Nursing diagnosis. *Annual Review of Nursing Research,* New York: Springer, vol. 3.

Gordon, M. (1980). Determining study topics. *Nursing Research,* 29:83–87.

Gordon, M. (1976). Nursing diagnosis and the diagnostic process. *American Journal of Nursing,* 76:1298–1300.

Gordon, M., Sweeney, M. A., & McKeehan, K. (1980). Nursing diagnosis: Looking at its use in the clinical area. *American Journal of Nursing,* 80:672–674.

Gottleib, L. N. (1982). Small steps toward the development of a health classification system for nursing. In M. J. Kim & D. A. Moritz (Eds.), *Classification of nursing diagnoses: Proceedings of the third and fourth national conferences.* New York: McGraw-Hill.

Guzzetta, C. E., & Dossey, B. M. (1983). Nursing diagnosis: Framework, process, and problems. *Heart and Lung,* 12:281–291.

Guzzetta, C. E., & Forsyth, G. L. (1979). Nursing diagnostic pilot study: Psychophysiological stress. *Advances in Nursing Science,* 2:27–44.

Halloran, E. (1983). RN staffing: More care—less cost. *Nursing Management,* 14:18–22.

Halloran, E. J., Kiley, M., & Nadzam, D. (1986). Nursing diagnosis for identification of severity of condition and resource use. In M. Hurley (Ed.), *Classification of nursing diagnoses: Proceedings of the sixth conference.* St. Louis: Mosby.

Hammond, K. R. (1966). Clinical inference in nursing: II. A psychologist's viewpoint. *Nursing Research,* 15:27–38.

Hardy, E. (1983). The diagnostic wheel: Identifying care that is unique to nursing. *Canadian Nurse,* 79:38–40.

Hudak, C. M. (1976). *Clinical protocols: A guide for nurses and physicians.* Philadelphia: Lippincott.

Hurley, M. (Ed.) (1986). *Classification of nursing diagnoses: Proceedings of the sixth conference.* St. Louis: Mosby.

Jacoby, M. K. (1985). The dilemma of physiological problems: Eliminating the double standard. *American Journal of Nursing,* 85:281, 284.

Joel, L. (1986). DRGs and nursing diagnosis. In Hurley, M. (Ed.), *Classification of nursing diagnoses: Proceedings of the sixth conference.* St. Louis: Mosby.

Kim, M. J. (1985). The dilemma of physiological problems: Without collaboration, what's left? *American Journal of Nursing,* 85:281, 284.

Kim, M. J. (1983). Nursing diagnosis in critical care. *Dimensions of Critical Care Nursing,* 2:5–6.

Kim, M. J., & Mortiz, D. A. (Eds.). (1981). *Classification of nursing diagnosis: Proceedings of the third and fourth national conferences.* New York: McGraw-Hill.

King, L. S. (1967). What is a diagnosis? *Journal of the American Medical Association,* 202:714–717.

Komorita, N. I. (1963). Nursing diagnosis. *American Journal of Nursing,* 63:83–86.

Kritek, P. B. (1978). Generation and classification of nursing diagnoses: Toward a theory of nursing. *Image,* 10:33–40.

Leslie, F. M. (1981). Nursing diagnoses: Use in long-term care. *American Journal of Nursing,* 81:1012–1014.

Levine, M. (1965). Trophocognosis: An alternative to nursing diagnosis. In American Nurses' Association, *Exploring progress in medical-surgical nursing practice.* In *Proceedings of ANA Regional Clinical Conference,* San Antonio, TX, 2:55–70.

Lister, D. W. (1983). The nursing diagnosis movement and the occupational health nurse. *Occupational Health Nursing,* 31:11–14.

Little, D., & Carnevali, D. (1976). The diagnostic statement: The problem defined. In B. Walter, P. Pardee, & D. M. Molbo (Eds.), *Dynamics of problem-oriented approaches: Patient care and documentation.* New York: Lippincott.

Long Island Jewish-Hillside Medical Center. (1985). *Computerized nursing care planning utilizing nursing diagnosis.* Washington, DC: Oryn Publications.

Loomis, M. E., & Wood, D. J. (1983). Cure: Potential outcome of nursing care. *Image,* 15:4–7.

Mahomet, A. D. (1975). Nursing diagnosis for the OR nurse. *AORN Journal,* 22: 709–711.

Martens, K. (1986). Let's diagnose strengths, not just problems. *American Journal of Nursing,* 86:192–193.

Maslow, A. (1970). *Motivation and personality.* New York, Harper & Row.

McCourt, A. (1986). Nursing diagnoses: Key to quality assurance. In Hurley, M. (Ed.), *Classification of nursing diagnoses: Proceedings of the sixth conference.* St. Louis: Mosby.

McKeehan, K. M. (1979). Nursing diagnosis in a discharge planning program. *Nursing Clinics of North America,* 14:517–524.

McManus, L. (1950). Assumption of functions of nursing. In Teachers College, Division of Nursing Education, *Regional planning for nursing and nursing education.* New York: Teachers College Press.

Meleis, A. (1985). *Theoretical nursing: Development and progress.* Philadelphia: Lippincott.

Moritz, D. A. (1978). Nursing diagnosis . . . what? *Oncology Nursing Forum,* 5:21.

Morris, W. (Ed.). (1978). *American heritage dictionary of the English language.* Boston: Houghton Mifflin.

Mundinger, M. O. (1978). Nursing diagnoses for cancer patients. *Cancer Nursing,* 1:221, 226.

Rothberg, J. S. (1982). *History of nursing diagnosis* (Audiotape Transcript). Paper presented at Conference on Nursing Diagnosis, Adelphi University.

Rothberg, J. S. (1967). Why nursing diagnosis? *American Journal of Nursing,* 67:1000–1042.

Shoemaker, J. (1984). Essential features of a nursing diagnosis. In M. J. Kim, G. McFarland, & A. McLane (Eds.), *Classification of nursing diagnoses: Proceedings of the fifth national conference,* St. Louis: Mosby.

Silver, S. M., Halfmann, T. M., McShane, R., Hunt, C., & Nowak, C. A. (1984). Identification of clinically recorded nursing diagnoses and indicators. In M. J. Kim, G. McFarland, & A. McLane. (Eds.), *Classification of nursing diagnoses: Proceedings of the fifth national conference.* St. Louis: Mosby.

Simmons, D. A. (1980). *Classification scheme for client problems in community health nursing.* (DHHS Publication No. HRA 80-16.) Washington, DC: U.S. Government Printing Office.

Soares, C. A. (1978). Nursing and medical diagnoses: Comparison of variant and essential features. In N. L. Chaska (Ed.), *The nursing profession: Views through the mist.* New York: McGraw-Hill.

Steele, J. E. (1984). The social policy statement: Assuring a positive future for nurse practitioners. *The Nurse Practitioner,* 9:15–16; 68.

Suhayda, R., & Kim, M. J. (1986). Implementing nursing diagnosis: Faculty perspective. In M. Hurley (Ed.). *Classification of nursing diagnoses: Proceedings of the sixth conference.* St. Louis, Mosby.

Sweeney, M. A., & Gordon, M. (1983). Nursing diagnosis: Implementation and incidence in an obstetrical-gynecological population. In N. L. Chaska (Ed.), *The nursing profession: A time to speak.* New York: McGraw-Hill.

Werley, H. H., & Lang, N. (Eds.) (1987). *Identification of nursing minimum data set.* New York: Springer.

Westfall, U. E. (1986). Outcome criteria generation: Process and product. In M. Hurley (Ed.), *Classification of nursing diagnoses: Proceedings of the sixth conference.* St. Louis: Mosby.

Westfall, U. E. (1984). Nursing diagnosis: its use in quality assurance. *Topics in Clinical Nursing,* 5:78–88.

Young, D. E., & Ventura, M. R. (1980). Application of nursing diagnosis in quality assessment research. *Quality Assurance Update* (American Nurses' Association), 4:1–4.

CLINICAL DIAGNOSIS IN THE HEALTH PROFESSIONS

CLINICAL DIAGNOSIS IN THE HEALTH PROFESSIONS

Placing the adjective *nursing* before the term *diagnosis* merely identifies the area of health care problems being addressed. Just as nurses use the term *nursing diagnosis* to refer to health problems within their scope of practice, physicians use the term *medical diagnosis* and social workers, *casework diagnosis.*

The client problems addressed by the various professions differ. Yet the overall method of identifying and using diagnostic categories is the same.[1] Appreciating these similarities and differences should enhance interprofessional communication as well as clarify some issues in nursing diagnosis. Usually, we can better understand our own domain of practice when it is viewed in the context of overall professional health care delivery. In this chapter clinical diagnosis in nursing, medicine, and social work will be examined according to five interrelated elements that are relevant to diagnosis:

1 *Professional focus* Describes the purpose or social mandate of a profession and influences its conceptual framework for practice.

2 *Conceptual framework* A set of general ideas, or concepts, that are logically interrelated. The one concept that will be examined here is the profession's conceptual model of the client that guides the naming of diagnostic categories (health problems).

3 *Concept of causality* The probable reasons for health problems. Etiological or related factors are commonly used to denote these reasons.

---

[1]In the profession of medicine, *clinical diagnosis* is used to refer to diagnosis based on a patient's history and examination. Supplementary laboratory or other types of tests are generally employed before a final judgment is reached.

4 *Classification systems* Names and classes of health problems that represent the phenomena of concern to the profession.

5 *Diagnostic process* The method for identifying client's problems.

The significance and meaning of each of these five terms will be discussed in the first section.

NURSING

Professions arise in order to fulfill a particular need of society. Having been created by society, they assume responsibility and accountability for that social need. The nursing profession arose out of needs associated with human suffering. First seen as a religious calling to care for the injured, ill, or infirm, nursing was practiced within religious orders. Today religious nursing orders exist, but the majority of practitioners are secular.

Nursing has passed through historical phases parallel to those of social or religious movements. Similar to western society in general, nursing had its "dark ages" coinciding with periods of general social neglect of human suffering. "Renaissance" periods paralleled periods of humanitarianism and social reform. In contemporary society nursing has taken an increasingly active role in health care policy formation and health care delivery.

Public attitudes and values sanctioned the nursing profession in its early days and are still favorable, even in the general atmosphere of criticism of health care that currently prevails. Sometimes, in striving for ideals, nurses are more critical of nursing than the public is. In a Maryland legal association's study of a representative sample of households, nursing was held in highest regard among eight established professions in society ("Maryland Public Rates Nursing High in Survey," 1979, p. 2094).[2] Society sanctions a profession through state licensing laws. In the last 10 years these laws have expanded or clarified nurses' social responsibility in health care. In many states, laws include statements about nursing diagnosis as a professional function. Delegated medical diagnosis and treatment is also permitted under some degree of supervision of the physician (V. C. Hall, 1975).

Nightingale's concept of nursing was formulated when she founded the profession; it is still current (1949). It emphasized helping both the sick and the well to perform activities that contribute to health and recovery. A definition of contemporary nursing is found in the American Nurses' Association (ANA) Model Practice Act:

> The practice of nursing means the performance for compensation of professional services requiring substantial specialized knowledge of the biological, physical, behavioral, psychological, and sociological sciences and nursing theory as the basis for assessment, diagnosis, planning, intervention, and evaluation in the promotion and maintenance of health; the casefinding and management of illness, injury, or

---

[2]The professions included dentistry, medicine, law, teaching, and others.

infirmity; the restoration of optimum function; or the achievement of a dignified death. Nursing practice includes but is not limited to administration, teaching, counseling, supervision, delegation, and evaluation of practice and execution of the medical regimen. . . . (ANA, 1980*a*)

As generalists or specialists, nurses are involved in all levels of health care. These levels include (1) primary care, focusing on health maintenance and preventive care in clinics or community settings; (2) secondary care, which may or may not require hospitalization for common illnesses; and (3) tertiary care, requiring the sophisticated technology of specialized units.[3] In each level the focus is on individuals and families. Primary care may also include the health of communities. Recognized areas in which nurses specialize include (1) settings, such as community health; (2) age groups, such as geriatrics and child health; and (3) health problems, or health states, such as maternal, medical-surgical, and psychiatric-mental-health specialties.

Some nurses have private practices. This is most common in the psychiatric-mental-health specialty. Reimbursement to clients through insurance payments may increase private practice in this and other specialties in the future. Most nurses are employees of health care institutions. This arrangement can sometimes present a dilemma to the practitioners because of conflicts between institutional and professional values. In fact, this conflict is experienced to some extent by members of all the health professions.

Professional Focus

All health professions are concerned with human behavior. Differences exist in the way health problems are conceptualized and labeled and the level of understanding sought. For example, medicine's predominant focus is on human biological phenomena, conceptualized as disease states. Understanding is sought at the cellular or subcellular level.

Historically, the focus of nursing has been individual, family, or community needs relevant to health and welfare. These needs have ranged broadly, from sanitation in a community to energy conservation in an individual. Generalizing across specialties and practice settings, the concern has consistently been human beings' optimal function in their environment.

Although expressed in various terms, the specific phenomena nursing addresses are potential or actual functional problems. Potential problems can result from health-related practices and may predictably contribute to future illness of an individual, family, or community. Actual problems occur in association with illness or with social, occupational, or maturational changes.

Each of the professions seeks a certain level of understanding of the phenomena with which it deals. As new knowledge becomes available, the level may change. For example, a few decades ago physicists sought to understand

---

[3]These are levels of care required by clients as opposed to primary, secondary, and tertiary *preventive intervention,* which is a model of intervention.

the nature of matter at the atomic level; today, as a result of advances in knowledge and theory, subatomic particles are the level of interest. Nurses seek to understand health-related behavior at the level of human organism–environment interaction. Clinical problems are viewed as holistic, or whole-person, expressions of this interaction, and diagnosis and intervention are performed within this holistic model. As we shall see in a later chapter, nursing theorists deal in different ways with the inherent complexity of this focus.

Underlying and supporting the focus of a profession is the art and science of practice. Theories, concepts, principles, and methods of treatment compose the *science of a profession.* The *art* is the way knowledge is used, especially in human interactions, and reflects attitudes, beliefs, and values. *Yet there can never be a clear separation of art and science.* Attitudes, beliefs, and values, whether internal or external to the profession, influence its science—particularly in the selection of methods, focus, and interpretations. Some interesting historical examples of the influence of changing beliefs and values on the naming and interpretation of diagnostic entities will be discussed in regard to medicine.

As would be expected in a profession with such a diverse practice focus and broad, holistic perspective, the body of clinical knowledge in nursing is extensive. Nursing science, as Rogers (1970) states, is only beginning to be identified. Currently the knowledge base for practice rests to a large extent on the application of biological, psychological, and social science theory. Extension of this knowledge in a way that is relevant to nursing concerns will develop the science of nursing.

The *body of knowledge* in a profession has to be *descriptive, explanatory, and predictive.* Increasing emphasis on clinical research in recent years has served to increase the science base of practice. Nursing diagnoses, because they isolate phenomena of concern to the profession, provide direction and focus for research and the development of nursing science.

Conceptual Frameworks for Practice

Each person views the world from some perspective, and this viewpoint affects the way the person explains and predicts events. Similarly, in the professions the *focus of concern* in practice is described and explained from a particular perspective or frame of reference.

A conceptual model is a simplification, a cognitive construction that ignores as irrelevant some aspects of the phenomenon being considered. It narrows attention to the area of concern and purpose. For example, some psychologists find a game theory model useful in describing interpersonal relations; the model helps explain and predict one phenomenon of concern—human interaction—although (perhaps *because*) it disregards some factors to focus on others. The conceptual models of the client to be discussed are merely approximations of reality. They currently provide practitioners with a useful way of thinking about clients. If knowledge, purpose, or values change in the profession, the models are subject to change.

One component of a framework is the conceptual model of the client which guides assessment and diagnosis. A brief consideration of the historical models of the client will help the reader understand the background of contemporary frameworks for nursing. Out of the belief that gods, demons, or evil spirits caused suffering arose the sanatoriums of ancient Greece. The priest-physicians and attendants of these temples of healing were the forerunners of the religious nursing orders that arose when Christianity spread through the world. From Kalisch and Kalisch's (1978) review of nursing history, it appears that nursing and Christian charity were interwoven. The "client" was seen as a "child of God," whether aged, infirm, orphaned, a casualty of war, or lacking relatives and friends to provide care. Devotion to religion motivated men and women of the Middle Ages to nurse the helpless in an evidently excellent manner (Tappert and Lehman, 1967, p. 296).

Industrialization and urbanization in the eighteenth and nineteenth centuries were accompanied by crowded living conditions, poverty, and devastating epidemics. The capacity of the religious hospitals and asylums was strained, and secular nursing began.

In the eighteenth and nineteenth centuries, both in America and Europe, the religious, devotional model of client care was lost in the public hospitals. Nurses were hired attendants who used alcohol and snuff as a means of psychological escape from the poor conditions. They were portrayed in all their depravity by Dickens's description of Sairy Gamp in mid-nineteenth–century England (Dickens, 1910, pp. 312–313). The physicians of that day were not much better. In America, "a common saying was that 'a boy who's unfit for anything else must become a doctor'" (Kalisch and Kalisch, 1978, p. 25). Interestingly, war provided the impetus for change.

The internationally recognized contributions of Florence Nightingale to the improvement of British military hospitals during the Crimean War and the postwar humanitarian concern in Europe combined to change these conditions. In America the Civil War brought about great changes in nursing. The changes of the late nineteenth and early twentieth centuries occurred in a social context: reform; women's rights; and advances in health care, particularly asepsis and beginning control of infectious disease. It must be remembered that these were the days where "common law and biblical tradition bound women to an inferior status" (Kalisch and Kalisch, 1978, p. 71).

When modern nursing began, illness was believed to be nature's *remedy* for removing the effects of conditions interfering with health. Neither nurses nor physicians "cured"; that was nature's realm. Out of Nightingale's experience with horrendous conditions in the Crimean hospitals, the idea began to be expressed that a person had to be considered in interaction with the environment (Nightingale, 1949, p. 26). Nature could not cure if sanitation, diet, and living conditions were not improved.

The emphasis within the client-environment model was clearly on the environment. The person was viewed from the perspective of a "dependency model." This perspective seemed logical when common practice dictated that the sick or injured were put to bed. The rationale was to conserve "vital power" (Nightingale, 1859, p. 6); rest and good living conditions were the major therapy for *all* illnesses. Ideally, the "rest cure" was provided at home. It was the poor and uneducated of the cities, the travelers, and the casualities from the battlefields who were brought to the hospital.

Clara Weeks Shaw, a contemporary of Nightingale, stressed the dependency model of the client and the complementary "maternity model of nursing": The "sick person is, for the time being, as a child and looks to his nurse for a mother's care" (Shaw, 1855, p. 19). This conception of nursing emphasized personal care, environmental comfort, and cleanliness.

Changes occurred in the first half of the present century. The dependency model was beginning to wane, influenced by society's focus on education of the masses, the mental hygiene movement, and advances in medical treatment. Nursing's participation and leadership in the public health movement of the late nineteenth century was also influential.

The nursing literature began to place stress on clients' regaining independence; this emphasis was reflected in discussions about learning hygienic practices, preventing illness, and using available community resources (Frederick and Northam, 1938, p. 3). This self-responsibility theme was further extended by Henderson (Harmer, 1955, p. 4; Henderson, 1966). She wrote of the individual's physical strength, will, or knowledge to perform activities related to health and recovery; nursing was required when these factors were *absent*.

From the textbooks of the time it appears that the biomedical model of the human being, used by medicine, was adopted by nursing. There were nurses who independently determined the nursing care needed, but generally the doctor was responsible for identifying problems (medical problems). Nurses were supposed to know how to provide comfort, observe for disease complications, and report observations. The frequent mention in the literature of "needs" and "needs-for-help" suggests that a human needs model of the client predominated around midcentury but focused on disease-related needs.

Orlando (1961) published a model of practice referred to as the dynamic nurse-patient relationship. Included was a distress-coping model of the client. Her method of assisting and of judging the client's need for help had a great impact and is still pertinent today. Orlando's model, and later Orem's self-care model (1959, pp. 5–6; 1971) emphasized self-direction and individual responsibility. Nursing was to do only what the person and his or her resources could not do unaided.

One can see the increased complexity of the nursing model for practice that was evolving in the twentieth century. If people were to learn responsibility for self-care and prevention of illness, nurses had to do more than carry out physicians' orders and administer routine personal care. They had to make judgments about what was needed and what was not.

Lydia Hall (1955, pp. 212–213) used the term *nursing process* in the early 1950s, and through the years her approach has evolved into the accepted method of delivering nursing care. The basic tenets of the Nightingale model—

client-environment interaction, religious traditions of wholeness, self-direction, and will—were retained in twentieth-century nursing (Orem, 1959, pp. 5–6; Harmer, 1955, p. 4).

At midcentury the term *nursing diagnosis* appeared in the literature (Mc-Manus, 1950). Bonney and Rothberg (1963) employed the term *nursing diagnosis* in a client evaluation instrument to predict needs for nursing service. The objective was to use clients' nursing diagnoses as predictors of nurse staffing needs in long-term care facilities. Their report defined diagnoses as a "listing of factors" which affected the client's condition. The list was divided into strengths and liabilities. Lists rather than problems were formulated, yet this contributed to shifting the focus of description from nursing actions to client conditions.

In 1980 the ANA published a *social policy statement* that identified the *phenomena of concern* to nurses as "human responses to actual or potential health problems" (1980*b,* p. 9). Human responses were viewed as:

> **1** reactions of individuals and groups to actual problems (health-restoring responses), such as the impact of illness-effects upon the self, family, and related self-care needs; and
>
> **2** concerns of individuals and groups about potential problems (health-supporting responses), such as monitoring and teaching in populations or communities at risk in which educative needs for information, skill development, health oriented attitudes, and related behavioral change arise. (ANA, 1980*b,* pp. 9–10)

These two areas of human responses are similar to the focus of nursing diagnosis previously identified in Chapter 1: problems in health management and problems secondary to illness, medical therapy, developmental changes, or life situations. The social policy statement reflects the current focus on clients' conditions (rather than nurses' actions) and social responsibility.

In the last two decades many nursing theorists have proposed conceptual frameworks to guide diagnosis and treatment. A few current conceptual frameworks will be reviewed in detail in Chapter 3. The basic tenets of the Nightingale model—client-environment interaction and religious traditions of wholeness, self-direction, and free will—were retained in twentieth century nursing frameworks. As the twenty-first century approaches consumers will assume more independence in personal health management, prevention of early onset of chronic disease and disability, and environmental control. The conceptual framework for nursing practice is consistent with the health services that will be needed. The degree to which nurses assume responsibility for health services will depend on choices by individual practitioners, resolution of "territorial" issues with physicians (Andrews, 1986), and consumer reimbursement for nursing services.

Concept of Causality

A profession's concept of causality is the way its members view the cause-and-effect relationships existing between health problems and the factors that interact to produce them. Some philosophers argue that the concept of causality should be abandoned; others say it is so implicit in human thinking that it cannot be discarded. The notion of causality in nursing practice is rarely addressed, although Field (1979) has provided a review of this concept in science. This is not to suggest that the idea is not used in nursing. Clinically, one hears explanations of the causes of clients' problems that range from single to multiple factors. Simple reasons and single causes may be valued for their noncomplexity. Yet when asked to explain the cause of a patient's clinical problem, nurses tend to respond with explanations that include complex, multifactor chains of events. In Chapters 5 and 8, causality and the concept of *etiology* will be considered further.

Classification Systems

Diagnosis and systems for classifying the health problems addressed by nurses did not receive widespread attention in nursing until the 1970s. Considering the way modern nursing evolved, this may be difficult to understand. During the Crimean War Florence Nightingale, 24 nuns, and 14 other women diagnosed and treated health problems so effectively that the mortality rate in British military hospitals showed an overall drop from 42 percent to 2.2 percent (Kalisch and Kalisch, 1978, p. 42). Well before this, in the twelfth century, when women studied nursing and obstetrics at the University of Salerno, the famous treatise *Tortula on the Cure of Diseases of Women* was written by a midwife (Kalisch and Kalisch,1978, p. 5).

At the end of the first century of modern nursing, concepts of practice emphasized procedures, tasks, and nursing functions. The first classification of nursing problems was for the purpose of education. A subcommittee of the National League for Nursing, while revising student record forms, perceived the need to describe generic nursing practice in terms of a client-centered, as opposed to task-centered, focus. From a survey of more than 40 schools of nursing, the first classification—of 21 problems—was completed (Abdellah, 1959, pp. 83–88). As Table 2-1 shows, these now-famous "problems" were therapeutic goals of nursing. This was consistent with the emphasis at the time on client needs (therapeutic needs) and nursing problems (therapeutic problems).

Nursing was commonly described as a set of functions. In fact the numerous studies of nurses and nurses' functions caused Abdellah to comment that "as valuable as such studies are, they portray what the nurse is doing, not why she is doing what she is, nor if she should be doing what she is" (Abdellah, 1959, p. 74). Fifteen years would elapse before a change in the focus of nursing diagnosis would begin to provide answers to the questions she posed.

In 1966 Henderson identified a list of 14 basic human needs that comprised the components, or functions, of nursing. This formulation further supported the functional needs approach. These basic needs, listed in Table 2-2, address not health problems of the client but areas in which actual or potential problems could occur. Both Abdellah's and Henderson's lists were widely used in education and practice. Their contributions stimulated nurses to go beyond routine

TABLE 2-1
NURSING PROBLEMS CLASSIFICATION ACCORDING TO ABDELLAH, 1959

Master List of Nursing Problems Presented by Clients

To facilitate the maintenance of oxygen to all body cells
To facilitate the maintenance of nutrition of all body cells
To facilitate the maintenance of elimination
To facilitate the maintenance of fluid and electrolyte balance
To promote safety through the prevention of accident, injury, or other trauma and through the
    prevention of the spread of infection
To facilitate the maintenance of regulatory mechanisms or functions
To facilitate the maintenance of sensory function
To promote optimal activity: exercise, rest, and sleep
To maintain good body mechanics and prevent and correct deformities
To maintain good hygiene and physical comfort
To recognize the physiological responses of the body to disease conditions—pathological and
    compensatory
To identify and accept interrelatedness of emotions and organic illness
To identify and accept positive and negative expressions, feelings, and reactions
To facilitate the maintenance of effective verbal and nonverbal communication
To promote the development of productive interpersonal relationships
To facilitate progress toward achievement of personal spiritual goals
To accept the optimum possible goals in the light of limitations, physical and emotional
To use community resources as an aid in resolving problems arising from illness
To create or maintain a therapeutic environment
To understand the role of social problems as influencing factors in the cause of illness
To facilitate awareness of self as an individual with varying physical, emotional, and
    developmental needs

Source: Abdellah (1959, pp. 83–88).

functions and tasks to identify therapeutic problems. This shift in focus set the stage for the next step—nursing diagnoses, or client problems, as the focus of care.

The shift from care organized around therapeutic problems, such as "to facilitate the maintenance of effective verbal communication," to care organized around client problems, such as "impaired verbal communication," began in the early 1970s. This change was facilitated by the First National Conference on Classification of Nursing Diagnoses in 1973. The conference provided a beginning language with which to express judgments and to organize nursing care.

National conferences have been held approximately every 2 years since 1973. Hundreds of nurses have participated in the conference objective, to develop diagnostic nomenclature (a system of category names) and classify nursing diagnosis. The evolution of the current classification system may be seen in Appendix B, which shows the changes, deletions, and additions that occurred in diagnostic categories in 1973, 1975, 1978, 1980, 1982, and 1986.

One could ask, What are nurses classifying? An examination of the category

TABLE 2-2
BASIC NEEDS CLASSIFICATION ACCORDING TO HENDERSON, 1966

Fourteen Basic Needs

Breathing normally
Eat and drink adequately
Eliminate body wastes
Move and maintain desirable postures
Sleep and rest
Suitable clothes—dress and undress
Maintain body temperature within normal range by adjusting clothing and modifying the
    environment
Keep body clean and well groomed and protect the integument
Avoid dangers in the environment and avoid injuring others
Communicate with others in expressing emotions, needs, fears, or opinions
Worship according to one's faith
Work in such a way that there is a sense of accomplishment
Play or participate in various forms of recreation
Learn, discover, or satisfy the curiosity that leads to normal development and health and use the
    available health facilities

Source: Henderson (1966, pp. 16–17).

names (Appendix A) would suggest that alterations in functions or functional patterns predominate. Ineffective, impaired, or altered human functions occur frequently in the listing. There is nearly a balance between physiological areas and psychosocial-spiritual areas. This division, of course, is invalid, since the signs and symptoms defining each category in many cases are biopsychosocial.

A developing classification system requires some *conceptual focus* to ensure consistency in classifying so that, for example, *apples, dogs,* and *chairs* do not get classified together. Consistency among the diagnoses classified is provided by this focus or framework. The development of a classification system will be addressed in a later chapter.

Diagnostic Process

The diagnostic process as such has not been widely discussed in the nursing literature. Basic textbooks rarely mentioned nursing diagnosis or the process of diagnosing to any great extent before the 1970s. Yet assessment, with emphasis on information collection, has had widespread attention in the literature of the last 25 years.

Nurses assumed responsibility for noticing the effects of illness and the needs it produced. As nursing practice became more clearly defined, assessment became important for determining clients' needs for nursing care. Today diagnostic process skills are recognized as critical if clinical practice is to be maintained at an acceptable professional level. Professional standards mandate that nursing diagnoses be derived from health status data (ANA, 1973).

Information collection and problem identification are viewed as components of the diagnostic process in nursing. Assessment for purposes of diagnosis requires history taking as well as examination of the client. Skill in observation and clinical interviewing are stressed as basic to adequate assessment. Carnavali and her colleagues (1984) have presented a good overview of problem formulation, including the need for logical reasoning. Gordon (1976) and Tanner (1984) have stressed the complexity of diagnostic judgments in nursing, error avoidance, and the probabilistic nature of judgments. Doona (1976) emphasizes the importance of the cognitive skill of judgment in nursing.

Little research has been done on the diagnostic process actually used by nurses, but it may be expected to adhere to general principles of cognition and problem identification. One major problem, noted by Bloch (1974), is the lack of agreement on definitions of crucial terms within the profession, such as *assessment* and *diagnosis.*

Nurses are just beginning to make conscious applications of conceptual models of the client in their clinical activities. As this application progresses, one should see a logical relationship among the conceptual model utilized, the assessment data collected, and the types of problems diagnosed. The diagnostic process can then be more systematically applied.

MEDICINE

Medicine's view of diagnosis is of interest here because of the many myths that surround disease and because of the interrelatedness of nursing and medical care, especially in acute care settings. Background information about the profession will provide a context for viewing physicians' assumptions, concepts, and practices in regard to diagnosis.

People naturally seek explanations for experiences that have an impact on their lives. So it has been with illness and disease. When people explained illness as being caused by evil spirits, they called upon the medicine man for therapy. When illness was viewed as the result of transgressions against the gods, the priest acted as physician; medicine and theology were one. When people themselves and the environment began to be implicated in disease and illness, medicine began to emerge as a science and healing became a profession.

Medicine has been a highly influential health profession during most of this century, although it also has had its "dark ages" (Duffy, 1967, p. 136). Although physicians are fewer in number than some other groups of health professionals, society has looked to physicians for direction in health care and related policies. As a result, they share both the adulation of society, for health care advances, and the scorn for current deficiencies in health care provision. Physicians traditionally have assumed responsibility and authority in health care matters. They have been protective of their professional boundaries and have been seen by many as pursuing a paternalistic role toward other health professionals.

Clinical medicine is concerned with the *diagnosis and treatment of disease.* Practice is based largely on knowledge from biomedical sciences. These sciences seek to describe, explain, predict, and control events associated with pathophysiology or psychopathology. Understanding of illness is sought at the *molecular level*. For example, medical researchers in the area of congestive heart failure are attempting to describe chemical and physical derangements in the metabolic process of failing myocardial cells, and biochemical changes in the brain are being studied as a means of understanding psychiatric disorders.

High value is placed on *scientific explanation* in medicine. Scientific generalizations about patterns of disease and general responses to treatments are being sought. These generalizations from medical research have to be applied to individuals so they may be used in the clinical care of patients; this is the task of the medical practitioner. The ideal practitioner is described as one who can combine the scientific aspects of medicine with compassion and understanding of the individuality of human beings (Tumulty, 1973, p. 66).

Diagnosis is an accepted part of the clinical practice of medicine. Both physicians and the public place high value on avoidance of diagnostic error. The consequences of error may be death, disability, or unwarranted expense. Society has high expectations of physicians, as is attested by the frequency of malpractice claims and the size of compensations awarded. When "injury," in the legal sense results form poor judgment, carelessness, or ignorance, society awards compensation through the judicial system (Cassell, 1977). Thus the physician, in making a diagnosis and determining treatment, is faced with a *moral and humanitarian concern* for the individual patient as well as concern about *personal legal liability*.

The value placed on diagnostic expertise within the medical profession is reflected in the clinical training of medical students. Repeated experiences are given in diagnosis and treatment planning, review of decisions, and case conferences. Practicing physicians are expected to expand their diagnostic skills continually. Opportunities are provided in hospital rounds and conferences for colleague review.

In medicine it is assumed that one never ceases being a student. This attitude is reflected in the following passage from a medical textbook:

> A fine method of continuing education is to place one's self in a situation where he will be continuously checked on, where his diagnoses are questioned daily and his treatments frequently modified. This is done best in a teaching hospital where young physicians and old mutually teach and learn. It takes courage and it takes humility for the established practitioner to do this, but it pays tremendous rewards. The physician who is afraid to have his opinions scrutinized is already out of date. (Keefer and Wilkins, 1970, p. 1051)

Professional Focus

The professional focus of medicine is diagnosis and treatment of disease. Since late in the eighteenth century physicians have studied and labeled pathophysiological and psychopathological phenomena. Disease has been conceptualized as a lesion. Predisposing factors, the historical course, morbidity, and mortality of disease have been studied extensively.

Challenges to the concept of disease as a lesion have arisen. Obesity is an example; it is a deviation from a statistical norm, not a disease per se. In fact, in many instances it is considered a behavioral problem similar to drug addiction or alcoholism. With medicine's professional focus on disease and its conception of disease as a lesion, what shall be done with these conditions?

Blaxter (1978) observes a contemporary trend toward widening the boundaries of medicine into social, psychological, and behavioral fields; she notes that this appears to be a return to the Hippocratic idea of "the whole person in his environment." Card and Good, medical educators, have broadened the definition of disease to "displacement from the normal state of dynamic, self-regulating system" (1974, p. 60).

The observations of these British authors possibly reflect the large and well-established family practice component of British medical care. Many of the health problems encountered by physicians in family practice are psychosocial. On the other hand, even American medical literature is beginning to reflect the need for a broader professional focus (Baron, 1985). It will be interesting to note whether this broader focus becomes a reality in practice. If medicine expands its current professional and diagnostic focus, will it be expanding into other professions such as nursing or social work? With the predicted future oversupply of physicians, practice boundaries will continue to be an issue in the next few decades.

Conceptual Frameworks for Practice

As was stated earlier, a conceptual model or framework for practice is a mental construction. It is used to derive meaning and understanding, that is, to make sense out of phenomena that are puzzling or disturbing. In addition, conceptual models of practice in the professions reflect the culture and milieu of the times. Early medicine, in particular, had strong ties to philosophy and theology.

Throughout history people have observed in themselves and others deviations that produce discomfort or disability. These deviations have been explained and treated in various ways. In primitive times few differences existed between medicine, magic, and religion (Rivers, 1927; R. L. Engle, Jr., 1963). Illness was thought to be produced by sorcery or a higher power such as a deity. Something was in the body that did not belong, or something had been removed! This simple dichotomous model was associated with a logical approach: The diagnostic problem was to find the seat of disease. The model guided the search for the demon possessing the person, the sin committed, or the witch involved.

Rational elements in thinking existed side by side with the magical in primitive times. The idea that symptoms occurred in combinations (anticipating the present-day notion of symptom clusters, or syndromes) was deduced from observations of people experiencing illness. However, it was thought that the symptoms, for example, fever, *were* the disease.

Scientific medicine began in ancient Greece. Hippocrates, who is considered the father of modern medicine, and his students and followers at Cos believed illness was due to a state of disequilibrium. Health was a condition of perfect equilibrium. The model for practice within the Hippocratic school emphasized the *wholeness of the person* as opposed to the mind-body dualism (separation) that arose later. Habits, lifestyle, pursuits, thoughts, sleep, and dreams were all of concern (Blaxter, 1978). This model was consistent with the philosophy of the times; the Greeks believed *equilibrium and harmony with nature were fundamental to life.*

The medical scholars of ancient Greece developed the *humoral model* to guide medical practice. Instead of a consequence of sin or demonic possession, illness was seen as a *disequilibrium in the humors:* blood, black bile, yellow bile, and phlegm. For example, in discussing convulsions (which were referred to as the "sacred disease" and associated with divine visitation), Hippocrates described the symptom cluster of inability to speak, choking, foaming at the mouth, clenching of the teeth, and convulsive movements. These symptoms, he thought, came about because the normal flow of phlegm from the brain to the mouth was blocked and phlegm consequently entered the blood vessels (King, 1971). Although this explanation of grand mal epilepsy sounds primitive today, it represented a dramatic departure from the previous explanatory model that combined theological and medical thought. One of the Hippocratic school's major influences on models for the practice of medicine was the idea that *disease could be explained by natural causes* such as the "humors" rather than supernatural or magical forces.

Building on the work of the Hippocratic school and influenced by Aristotelian philosophy, Galen introduced in the second century the idea that *nature was a dynamic, active process directed toward the restoration of health.* Interestingly, this is the root of the common sense notion of the "healing power of nature." The Galenic concept of vitalism was based on a model of purposeful, goal-directed activity inherent in humans and attributed to a psyche, soul, or life-force (King, 1971, p. 13; Ruesch, 1963). The search for the cause and cure of disease was beginning to move from a focus on outside influences to one on factors within the person and the environment.

In the fifth and sixth centuries there were few challenges to the accepted explanations of events or to models of disease and medical practice. Most medical care continued to be based largely on models of mysticism, magic, and a few scientific elements. Like other disciplines, the fledgling science of medicine almost disappeared during the Dark Ages.

In contrast to the marked influence of theology and philosophy in earlier times, after the Renaissance biological and physical science influenced medical thought and models of practice. Scientific investigation of disease processes predominated. Use of the scientific method led to rational rather than magical thinking about illness. The *alliance between medicine and the biological sciences* became firmly established and formed the basis for the biomedical model used in medical practice today. In part, this alliance was the result of theological influences.

The influential Christian church of the fifteenth century supported a mind-body dualism in regard to the study of humans. This position, in response to physicians' and scientists' anatomical dissections, mandated that the investigation of physical and mental processes should be undertaken by two different groups. The body was viewed as "a weak and imperfect vessel for the transfer of the soul from this world to the next" (G. L. Engel, 1977), and therefore, in Christian thought, it could be objectively studied as a machine and subjected to scientific and medical investigation. The mind and soul were left to the philosophers or theologians, who used noninvasive study techniques. The assumption was that the *whole human could be understood as a sum of the parts* (G. L. Engel, 1977, p. 131). An implicit agreement existed between the church and those wishing to perform dissection to increase medical and biological knowledge: The mind and the soul would be ignored. According to Engel's (1977) analysis, this agreement was largely responsible for the *anatomical and structural model* upon which western scientific medicine was to evolve.

Medicine is committed to advancing knowledge of disease and treatment. It employs the scientific method, which has procedural rules for concept formation, the conduct of experiments, and validation of hypotheses by observations and experimentation. The less manageable behavioral or psychosocial dimensions of disease are generally ignored (psychiatry is an exception) so that observations can meet the standards of objectivity required by the scientific method.

The current biomedical model combines this dualistic separation of mind and body with a mechanistic model. *Clients' diseases are viewed from the perspective of biophysical or biochemical processes.* Thus in the *biomedical model* the body is conceptualized as a machine; disease represents breakdown of the machine, and treatment consists of repair of the machine (G. L. Engel, 1977).

The reader may wonder whether a pure scientific approach to clinical care is possible, since physicians deal with people rather than inanimate objects or machines. What probably occurs is that the clinician considers the disease an entity in itself; in a sense, it is abstracted from the person with the disease. Other implicit models of psychosocial behavior are probably used to interpret the *behavior* of the person and to plan therapy.

The components, or subsystems, of the *biomedical systems model* are listed in Table 2-3. Except in psychiatry, the personal and social system is generally limited to structural factors such as the patient's place in the family network and the number of siblings. This segregation and limitation is typical of the dualistic framework employed during diagnosis, which separates the biological from the psychosocial.

Shortcomings of this conceptual focus on biological (physiological) systems have been described by G. L. Engel (1977, pp. 129–136), who argues that full understanding of the patient requires additional concepts and models. McWhinney (1972) has presented essentially the same arguments. He recommends a general systems theory approach which would deal with different levels of organization, such as molecular, organ, system, person, and family levels. This, he argues, would provide a more holistic way of viewing the phenomena of concern in medical practice.

TABLE 2-3
COMPONENTS OF THE BIOMEDICAL SYSTEMS MODEL

Cardiovascular system
Respiratory system
Gastrointestinal system
Genitourinary system
Neuromuscular system
Endocrine system
Reproductive system
Integumentary system
Personal and social system

The current biomedical model of the client narrows the body of knowledge with which the physician has to deal. This narrowing permits the clinician to focus on the already vast knowledge in biomedical diagnosis and therapy and to use a relatively commonsense approach to the psychosocial aspects of disease.

The secondary position given to human psychosocial behavior in medical diagnosis has produced controversy, particularly in medical specialties such as psychiatry and family practice. According to Lazare (1973), psychiatry in fact frequently uses a combination of conceptual models, although the combination remains implicit. Lazare describes the biomedical, psychological, behavioral, and social models. He concludes that all of medicine utilizes a multidimensional model of human behavior although not always in a conscious manner.

Concept of Causality

Various explanations of disease have dominated medical thinking down through the centuries. Ruesch comments that notions about what causes illness have remained relatively simple. Only *five origins of illness* are mentioned in the medical literature:

  1 Coercive intrusion into the organism of evil spirits, foreign objects, bacteria, or viruses.

  2 Deficient, excessive, or faulty intake of food, fluid, gases, poisons, or information.

  3 Deficient, excessive, or faulty output as it occurs in disordered elimination, excessive work and strain, inability to express feelings and thoughts, atrophy or hypertrophy of certain physical structures, or one-sided development of social and psychological functions.

  4 Loss of, or deficiency in, essential parts, for example, mental deficiency, castration, abortion, sensory defects, mutilation, loss of love objects, or loss of hope.

  5 Disintegration of orderly structures as in cancer, toxic states, senile psychoses, or breakdown of social relations and patterns of communication. (Ruesch, 1963, pp. 506–507)

The search for causation of disease has always been based on the need to understand, prevent, and treat. Indeed, there have been historical relationships between the prevailing notion of cause and the methods of treatment. A good example is the "removing" of disease by bleeding and purging the patient, which a generation later was supplanted by "building up" the patient with iron and diet (Berman, 1954).

In general the etiology of disease (the theory of causation) and the effect (disease state) have been viewed as having a linear, or direct, relationship. The doctrine has been that one basic main cause, known or unknown, existed for each disease. This *single-causation hypothesis* has dominated scientific medicine since the demonstration that a particular microorganism caused a particular infection. The goal has been to find the one cause for each disease entity. When cause is known, control can be instituted.

Science, in general, has moved to *multicausation (many interacting causal factors) hypotheses.* Multicausation is currently under discussion by physicians but not fully accepted in medical practice. Walter states that "the doctrine of one cause for one disease has certainly failed to be a profitable concept in the search for the etiology of many common diseases, such as cancer, arteriosclerosis, emphysema, and chronic bronchitis" (Walter, 1977, p. 3). According to Thomas (1978, p. 462), the multifactorial approach to the cause of human illness is now "in fashion"; infectious diseases are the exception. He groups current notions of causality into two classes, environment and lifestyle. Facetiously he describes the ultimate unified theory of causality that would appeal to the entire "political" spectrum:

> At the further right, it is attractive to hear that the individual, the good old freestanding, free-enterprising American citizen, is responsible for his own health and when things go wrong it is his own damn fault for smoking and drinking and living wrong (and he can jolly well pay for it). On the other hand, at the left, it is nice to be told that all our health problems, including dying, are caused by failure of the community to bring up its members to live properly, and if you really want to improve the health of the people, research is not the answer; you should upheave the present society and invent a better one. At either end you can't lose. (Thomas, 1978, p. 463)

In clinical practice, everyday thinking probably ignores the possibility of multifactorial causes. The simplified view prevails, that there is one cause of disease, whether that cause is known or unknown. Contributing or predisposing factors such as lifestyle may be considered but tend not to receive as much attention as metabolic derangements. Vaisrub describes the current divergent viewpoints this way:

> Suspended between the polarities of the known and completely unknown, multifactorial etiology can be interpreted in two ways. It can be regarded as a combination of factors, each contributing its share to the causation of a disease. Although one or more of these factors predominate in an individual case, none can be regarded as a single, specific cause. In fact, it can be assumed tacitly or explicitly that no single specific cause exists, and the pursuit of such cause would be futile.
>
> On the other hand, multifactorial etiology can be viewed as a temporary ad hoc concept, which will do until a specific cause, *the* cause, will be discovered. Presenting

this view, Thomas (1978) cites tuberculosis as an example of a disease that might have been easily consigned to a multifactorial etiology before the tubercle bacillus was identified as its cause. Like cancer, tuberculosis involves many organs and is influenced by environmental factors. Fortunately, the causative organism was discovered, and the disease escaped the multifactorial label before it was invented. (Vaisrub, 1979, p. 830)

Classification Systems

Discrimination among types of illnesses existed in primitive spiritual medicine; names were assigned to such conditions as loss of consciousness and convulsions. Many of the present labels for diseases are inherited from Greek and Roman civilizations (Fejos, 1963, pp. 52–53).

The beliefs and values of a society influence societal concepts of what shall be classified as health and illness. Leavitt and Numbers (1978, p. 13) comment, "Ideas, like individuals and institutions, have their own histories and concepts of sickness and health are no exception. What one generation of Americans may have considered an illness, another regarded as perfectly normal." *Normality, they point out, is socially defined and in part rests upon familiarity.* The more familiar a condition is, the less likely it is to be labeled abnormal. For example, childbirth and malaria, once considered normal, now are generally thought to require medical attention. On the basis of *social beliefs and values,* some conditions have shifted from sin to sickness and from sickness to normality.

Masturbation has had quite a history; once it was classified as sin, then it was considered a sickness, and now it is thought of as normal (Englehardt, 1978). Alcoholism, drug addiction, and obesity, at one time crimes and vices, are now considered illnesses (Leavitt and Numbers, 1978, p. 13). "Nervousness," hysteria, and other so-called self-indulgent female maladies were legitimized as illnesses when labeled *neurasthenia.* Neurasthenia also provided a reasonably respectable label to apply to the symptoms when they were experienced by men. The relabeling of neurasthenia served to establish a clientele for the new specialty of neurology in the early twentieth century (Sickerman, 1978).

Nosography, the systematic description and classification of diseases, began in the eighteenth century. Nosography arose because of a need to analyze the causes of death in the population. A model for classification existed; 100 years earlier botany had established its taxonomy (classification). By the year 1893, an international classification system for mortality statistics was developed. It had 161 diagnostic titles and was referred to as the *International Classification of Diseases* (ICD).

Today this classification contains 1040 categories and is the official international code for reporting morbidity and mortality statistics. Its periodic review is sponsored by the World Health Organization (1977). The *American Hospital Adaptation of International Classification of Diseases—Adapted* is the official code in the United States. It is used for discharge analysis of hospital records by the Committee for Professional and Hospital Activities of the Joint Committee on Accreditation of Hospitals.

In the specialty of psychiatry, mental disorders are classified in the *Diagnostic and Statistical Manual of Mental Disorders (DSM III)*, developed by the American Psychiatric Association. This manual "contains a multiaxial system emphasizing psychosocial factors" (Talbott, 1980, p. 25). The manual presents the first classification system that codes five client dimensions: mental disorders, personality and developmental disorders, physical disorders, psychosocial stress severity, and highest level of adaptive function in the last year. It is suggested that some axes will also be relevant to evaluations done by activity therapists, social workers, nurses, psychologists, and others.

A number of psychiatric classifications have been based on intensive study of single client cases in a prescientific era. This historical fact led to criticism of the American Psychiatric Association's *DSM II,* particularly because of the overlap in various diagnostic classifications. There is generally thought to be little support for specific clinical diagnoses, such as *paranoid schizophrenia* or *anxiety reaction,* and only general support for broad categories, such as *functional psychosis, psychoneurosis,* or *organic psychosis.* The recently published *DSM III* addresses some of the previous concerns.

Many other classification systems are in use in medicine and medical specialties. They vary depending on their purpose. As Engle and Davis have observed (1963, p. 517), *problems exist* because there is no unified concept of disease that could be used as an organizing principle. Disease and diagnosis may be based on "gross anatomical defects, microscopic changes, so-called specific etiological agents, specific deficiencies, genetic aberrations, physiologic or biochemical abnormalities, constellations of clinical symptoms and signs, organ and system involvement, and even just description of abnormalities" (Engle and Davis, 1963, p. 517). Another problem is that *diagnoses are not always well defined, often lacking specific etiologies.*

Vague definitions of diagnostic categories decrease accuracy and reliability. As understanding of diseases improves, the uncertainty about using categories decreases. Engle and Davis (1963, pp. 517–519) describe four levels of certainty associated with the use of various medical diagnoses. The levels of certainty are reflected in (1) category definition, (2) clarity of etiology, and (3) variances in the clinical picture (from person to person, or environment to environment). Sickle cell anemia (abnormal hemoglobin) is at the first level of certainty. The collagen diseases are ambiguous and are classed at the fifth, or lowest and most uncertain, level.

Diagnostic Process

In medicine, diagnostic skills are highly valued. Accordingly, much attention has been directed toward understanding and teaching the diagnostic process. Here it will suffice to consider briefly the elements of the process as it is used in clinical medicine.

The physician's purpose during diagnosis is to observe for any manifestations of illness and, secondly, to conceptualize the manifestations in terms of diagnostic categories. The *information* physicians collect during the medical history and physical examination is *standardized*. Each physician uses essentially the same format, which leads to consistency in the clinical data base and consistency among physicians.

Interpretation, analysis, and utilization of the information is facilitated because *classifications of diseases correspond to the history and examination categories*. For instance, one category of the history format relates to the gastrointestinal system. A physical examination of organs within this system is also done. Correspondingly, a set of gastrointestinal disease categories exist. From a cognitive perspective, clustering information according to an area of concern facilitates diagnosing disease of that area if such a disease is present.

Additionally, the basic information to be collected in each category is delineated in the standard data base. For instance, during the history a client is asked about the following gastrointestinal functions: appetite, digestion, nausea, vomiting, hematemesis, abdominal pain, food idiosyncrasies, jaundice, bowel habits, constipation, diarrhea, stools, hemorrhoids, hernia, and use of cathartics. These inquiries screen for the major diseases of the system. If the client's complaint suggests pathology, further review of symptoms is done. Laboratory tests may be used to supplement the clinical data.

This rather detailed description serves two purposes. First, it provides an *overview of the process of collecting information in medicine.* Second, it provides an example of *a system that conserves cognitive capacity* and *facilitates information processing.* We will return to these points in a later chapter.

Physicians use a hypothetico-deductive method in diagnosis (Elstein, Schulman, and Sprafka, 1978). This is an effective method, according to research findings about how human beings attain concepts. Hypothetico-deductive thinking involves careful observation and generation of diagnostic hypothesis about what early clinical data indicate. By deduction it is reasoned that if a hypothesis is true then certain cues should be present. Information is collected to test the hypothesis. On the basis of the information collected, diagnostic hypotheses are retained, discarded, or altered.

The emphasis placed on clinical reasoning and diagnosis in medicine has provided a fertile field for research by psychologists. Traditionally, "bedside diagnosis" has been considered an art involving a large component of clinical intuition. In recent years there as been more acceptance of *the fact that this "intuition" is a logical process that can be taught,* not a mysterious skill that is absorbed in apprenticeship training.

SOCIAL WORK

Social work, in comparison to medicine and nursing, has had a relatively short history. It arose out of the nineteenth-century Charitable Societies, which were designed to relieve poverty and suffering, reform the maladjusted, and, especially, relieve the community of the burden and unpleasantness of poverty (Robinson, 1978, p. 36).

The profession's traditions lie in social causes and a concern for the helpless of society. Its practitioners have been influential in the formulation of social policy at governmental levels by focusing attention on social conditions that influence the quality of life (Morris, 1977, p. 353). Social work has been referred to as the conscience of society, prodding it to recognize and deal with social problems (Cooper, 1977, p. 361). Through the social services it delivers, it is also the profession that reflects and implements contemporary social attitudes and values (Dean, 1977).

This twofold purpose can present a dilemma to the practitioner of social work, especially if he or she is employed by a public social welfare agency. In one sense the social worker is an *agent of society,* obliged to carry out its public programs and enforce conformity to the existing social environment, attitudes, and values. On the other hand the profession is committed to *improving social services,* the social environment, and the quality of life; these objectives may not always be consistent with current values or financial commitments.

As may be expected from the diversity of social problems within different age groups, social work deals with a variety of problems in a variety of settings. The unifying factor in the profession is its primary commitment to people, to society, and to the interrelationships between people and society. Differing viewpoints of *professional purposes* either emphasize the *individual in interaction with society* or focus upon the *society and its impact on people* (Simm, 1977, p. 394).

These viewpoints are reflected in the diverse areas of practice in which social workers engage. A large number are involved in social planning activities, but approximately 52 percent of social workers deliver direct care to individuals and families (Morales, 1977, p. 392). One example of practitioners who focus on the individual are the clinical caseworkers who provide psychotherapy through private practice or on mental health teams. Others who develop, modify, or administer social service programs focus on the society and its impact on people. Carroll (1977) has developed a three-dimensional model to encompass all the diverse areas of social work practice. As may be seen in Figure 2-1, the model incorporates the *phenomena that are of concern,* that is, *social problems;* the *units that are of concern, from individuals to societies;* and the technologies characteristic of social work practice, such as *family therapy* or *social planning* (Carroll, 1977, p. 431).

Currently, social workers are seeking licensure by the states in which they practice; a few states have licensure for clinical activities (nonmedical psychotherapy) (Morales, 1977, p. 390). A clear definition of social work practice is specified in the National Association of Social Workers Model Licensing Act. It defines social work practice as

> . . . service and action to effect changes in human behavior, a person's or persons' emotional responses, and the social conditions of individuals, families, groups, organizations, and communities, which are influenced by the interaction of social, cultural, political, and economic systems. (Morales, 1977, p. 390)

It is within these areas of practice that the *social caseworker,* who treats

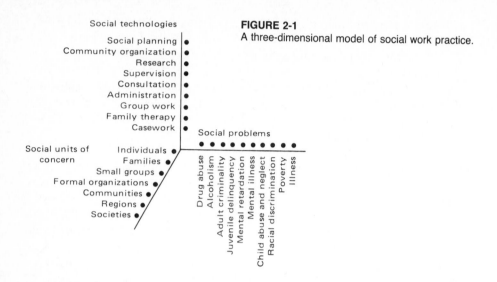

FIGURE 2-1

A three-dimensional model of social work practice.

individuals and families, interacts most frequently with physicians and nurses. Thus we will examine this area of practice most closely.

The typical pattern of casework practice in health care institutions (hospitals, clinics, and community health care agencies) is to assist clients and families with social problems referred by nurses or physicians. For example, a patient with a medical illness may have a problem, such as unsatisfactory living conditions, which contributes to the illness. Referral to the medical social worker in the social service department of the institution can bring assistance to the patient and specialized knowledge of community resources. If a team concept is employed in a health care setting (e.g., long-term or rehabilitative care) social workers participate with nurses and physicians in joint planning of a client's care.

In another situation, a multiproblem family may require coordination of social services in the community, such as child care, vocational counseling, and welfare. The social worker can coordinate these services on a long-term basis and help the family learn how to deal with their problems. Through client contacts, the need for programs may also become evident to a worker in the community and efforts may be made to engage the community in developing services, such as social programs for the elderly.

Professional Focus

In contrast to medicine, which seeks to understand clinical problems of clients at the molecular or physiochemical level, social casework emphasizes the intrapsychic, interpersonal, and social level of understanding. It draws heavily on psychological, psychiatric, and sociological theory in its practice.

The social problems addressed by the profession, according to Reid (1977, p. 374), are "social" in two senses:

1 The problematic behavior has social consequences for the individual or family.

2 The problem is troubling society.

Reid identifies broad problem areas, such as mental illness and emotional distress, difficulties in interpersonal relationships, dysfunctional and deviant behavior, and inadequate resources (unsuitable living arrangements, insufficient income, lack of health care, and the like).

Diagnosis was introduced into the practice of social work in its early years and influenced the development of casework. Also influential was an alliance with psychiatry and psychoanalytic thought (Germaine, 1970, p. 13). Today, consistent with the profession's modern focus, diagnoses describe problems, or social dilemmas, in the context of the client's interaction with the world.

Some schools of thought within the profession do not rely heavily on diagnostic categorization of clients' problems but do use a narrative type of problem identification as part of practice. Each of the four major approaches to casework (psychosocial, functional, problem-solving, and behavioral) defines the concept of *social problem* differently (Roberts and Nee, 1970, pp. 33–218). Some suggest that the diversity in practice negates a unified approach. Others argue that a uniform conceptualization of the problems addressed by social work is needed to clarify professional objectives (Reid, 1977, p. 374).

Conceptual Frameworks for Practice

It seems that as long as human beings form relationships in groups or societies, problems will arise. In noncomplex societies these problems are usually handled within families, tribal communities, or religious groups. When societies undergo rapid social and technological changes, as did western society with the advent of the Industrial Age, social problems arise that overtax the known ways of handling them. This was the situation in the nineteenth century when changes caused by industrialization produced stresses in the social order.

Charitable associations began to supplement the efforts of families and religious groups; "friendly visitors," the volunteers of these organizations, were dispatched to the homes of the poor. As an example, in Boston in 1884 there were 600 who visited "drunkards and their families and the poor widows with dependent children" (Robinson, 1978, p. 36). To relieve the conditions of poverty, they used advice, persuasion, and exhortation, as was dictated by the *Handbook for Friendly Visitors Among the Poor* (1883).

The *model for practice* at that time, if it can be called such, rested firmly on the society's belief that *hard work, thrift, and a belief in the Almighty would lead to individual success, thereby eliminating poverty and degradation* (Robinson, 1978, p. 36). In the early twentieth century the voluntary charity workers, as well as the associations for which they worked, became organized and the newly paid workers began to seek professional status. That was the beginning of the social work profession and the beginning of the development of conceptual models for practice. In order for these new workers to differentiate themselves from nurses in institutions, and in order to implement the scientific commitment inherited from the philanthropy movement, caseworkers adopted the medical process: study, diagnose, treat (Germaine, 1970, pp. 16–22).

Richmond greatly influenced this new profession with a book on *social diagnosis* (Richmond, 1917). It emphasized the "scientific" collection of information about the person as a basis for diagnosis. The approach to practice that utilized Richmond's ideas was referred to as the diagnostic school of thought.

Conceptual models were borrowed from medicine, particularly psychiatry, and from psychoanalytic theory, probably because of the events of that era. Caseworkers were needed to handle not only the demands of the poor in society but also the large numbers of emotional problems of veterans and their families after World War I. The birth of the mental health movement in the second decade of the twentieth century also influenced the practice models that developed in social casework (Germaine, 1970, p. 16).

The model for practice during the 1930s and beyond was derived from personality theory, particularly Freudian. Patients' conscious, preconscious, and unconscious thoughts were examined in order to understand problematic behavior (Germaine, 1970, p. 18). The use of the medical process model and psychoanalytic theory brought with it an emphasis on problems of the individual. This *focus on individuals represented a change from the earlier emphasis on social problems and social causes.* It produced controversy in the profession for many years, and the issue is still debated.

Today some conceptual models of social work practice emphasize the *service* aspect and focus upon the *therapeutic method of practice,* that is, what social workers do in handling clients' problems. In contrast, the diagnostic model (now referred to as the psychosocial model of practice) still strongly advocates the need for diagnostic classification, particularly clinical diagnosis (Hollis, 1970, p. 53).

With the increased development of knowledge in sociology, particularly role theory, the psychosocial model was broadened from the conception proposed by Richmond in 1917 and the personality focus. Theoretical constructs are derived from the behavioral sciences and include anthropological and cultural theories. The theories from these behavioral sciences in addition to theories developed in the profession are used to identify the problems of clients, such as character disorders, alcoholism, and drug addiction. Traditionally, medical and psychiatric caseworkers have used the *psychosocial model.*

Within this model of practice the client is viewed from a systems perspective and diagnosis is directed toward the "person-situation gestalt" (Hollis, 1970, pp. 33–76). This client model includes both the individual and the social environment as the entity of concern. Included in the concept of the social environment are social roles (family, work, social groups), the educational milieu, and other social systems.

Consistent with a systems theory approach, it is assumed that changes in one part of the mutual interaction between person and social environment, such as a role change, changes the entire system's equilibrium. In the use of this model, the phenomena of concern to the social caseworker are *interadaptational problems*. These include problems that arise in the subsystems of the client-situation complex, that is, the individual, the situation, or the interaction between individual and the social environment. These problems of equilibrium or adaptation of the person-situation complex are the focus for social intervention in the psychosocial approach to casework (Hollis, 1970, pp. 50–51).

Other conceptual models of social casework either bypass the diagnostic step in the clinical process or have a different conception and utilization of diagnosis. In some approaches diagnosis is seen as part of treatment, with treatment conceived as the client-therapist relationship process. This viewpoint results in an emphasis on diagnosis as a *process* for specifying the problem, rather than a basis for categorization prior to treatment. For example, the *functional approach to casework*,[4] as described by Smalley (1970, pp. 77–128), uses the term *diagnosis* but views it as an insight the client arrives at in relation to his or her problem. The "diagnosis" constantly changes as the client progresses during the relationship.

The *problem-solving model* of casework uses the term *diagnosis* to refer to the specification of the problem to be worked on at a particular time; diagnosis is an ongoing process as the client and caseworker together define the client's perception of the objective problem and subjective involvement in the problem. In this model the caseworker identifies the client's motivation and ability to solve the problem and the social means or resources available to the client (Perlman, 1970, pp. 129–180). As the name of the model implies, the focus is on guiding the client in problem solving. The social problem is not of maximum concern but, rather, the person's problem-solving motivation and ability.

All models for practice include a diagnostic statement although some do not label it as such. Due to the lack of agreed-upon nomenclature to summarize the clinical assessment, or due to the low value placed on specific problem identification and diagnostic classification, usually the caseworker writes a paragraph or more narrating the problem(s). There is *no generally accepted structure and format for the diagnostic statement*.

Concept of Causality

At the turn of the century, under the influence of the mechanistic physics of Newton, cause and effect were viewed as directly related. Each effect has one cause. It was believed that if the cause of a social problem could be found, the cure would be obvious (Germaine, 1970, pp. 10–11).

Today the high degree of complexity of social problems is recognized in the profession. Within the model of person-situation complex, the cause of a prob-

---

[4]The functional approach is characterized by its focus on objectives and function of the social agency, which are viewed as directly influencing the worker's role. The agency is seen as a system that may be the object of change as well as the instrument for social change (Germaine, 1970, p. 17).

lem can reside in the *person* or in the *situation.* Actually, it is more likely to be found in the *relationship pattern* or transaction between the two (Germaine, 1970, p. 29). Thus these three main elements have to be considered when determining causality, and multicausation is usually found.

In addition, all three aspects of the person-situation complex demonstrate growth, change, and potentiality. *Potentiality* refers to emergent capabilities such as new behaviors. Germaine suggests that to be "in accord with the modern scientific viewpoint, this requires that casework view and handle phenomena in terms of directions, flow, action and transaction, rather than in terms of cause" (Germaine, 1970, p. 29).

Classification Systems

In social work, as stated earlier, there is no generally accepted typology, or classification, of social problems. An attempt was made early in the history of the profession to specify the domain of problems addressed. With Richmond's concept of social diagnosis (Richmond, 1917) as a stimulus, in 1929 an alphabetical listing of casework problems was developed. The problems ranged from alcoholism to vagrancy (American Association of Social Workers, 1929).

Recent authors addressing the subject of a diagnostic classification system appear to agree with Reid's argument:

> The compelling advantage of formulating social work's objectives in terms of the problems it seeks to solve is that this formulation provides a clear basis for organizing and interpreting professional efforts, a basis that can be precisely explained and generally understood. (Reid, 1977, p. 376)

Classifications cited in the literature (Ackerman, 1958, p. 329; Ripple and Alexander, 1956, pp. 38–54) are specific for certain problem areas, for example, family therapy. Reid (1977, p. 374) proposes four areas of social work practice that could guide the conceptualization of specific problems: intrapersonal, interpersonal, personal-environmental, and environmental. Lowenberg (1977, pp. 53–54) specifies a set of three: interpersonal relationships, formal relationships, and role transaction. The examples given within these typologies range from symptoms to broad problem areas.

It is obvious from the literature in this field that a number of issues have to be resolved before a diagnostic classification system can be developed. The need for decisions about the domain of practice, a theoretical system to organize diagnostic categories, and determination of the unit of classification (individual, family, or community) are stressed by authors who advocated a classification system (Selby, 1958, pp. 341–349; Finestone, 1960, pp. 139–154).

Irrespective of whether the social work profession will undertake development of a classification system, the value of doing so has been recognized. Finestone (1960, p. 139) views this task as providing rich rewards for systematic theory building, for organizing knowledge for teaching, and for making practice more effective.

Diagnostic Process

As may be recalled from the discussion of other professions' diagnostic processes, information collection, analysis, and synthesis are broad common steps necessary to arrive at a concept of the state of the client and to label that state for purposes of treatment. In all the conceptual models of practice in social work, the collection of information is stressed as an important clinical activity. It is viewed as a means of understanding the client's problem and is an ongoing process. The information-collection process is referred to as casework assessment; it incorporates history taking.

All the models of practice emphasize the dual purpose served by information collection—the simultaneous establishment of a relationship with the client and acquisition of useful clinical information. Both of these purposes are probably of crucial importance in this profession, considering the focus of concern— social problems—and the psychosocial nature of the clinical data required. It is logical to expect that only after the caseworker has established trust and communicated empathic concern will the client share this type of personal information.

Some practice models stress to a great extent that treatment begins immediately. No doubt this is true. In the collection of psychosocial information, listening is required. Therapeutic outcomes may result as clients verbalize feelings and perceptions, the clinical data. In addition, clients may gain insights by relating a problem to another person. For all these reasons, social casework emphasizes the importance of the initial phase of interaction with the client in which assessment and problem identification occur.

Hollis (1970), who advocates the psychosocial approach to casework, states that the purpose of assessment is to deduce, from the information available and background knowledge of human behavior or social situations, the client's problem and what contributes to it. This deduction can then be used to determine the need and focus for change as well as the casework methods to be applied.

The data-collection method that is advocated is consistent with the psychosocial model. Hollis (1970, p. 51) states that assessment focuses on the client-situation complex, which "must be viewed repeatedly against a series of approximate norms of average expectancies 1) concerning behavior of the client and others, 2) concerning pertinent aspects of his social situation, and 3) concerning concrete realities."

The client-situation complex is viewed from sociological and psychological perspectives in order to collect information in problematic areas and to identify the scope of etiological factors involved (Hollis, 1970, p. 52). No one generally agreed upon systematic format (history form) for collecting a clinical data base is used in casework.

In social work, as in other professions, *analysis* of clinical data is emphasized. In order to make a decision about treatment, the caseworker must have an accurate and precise understanding of the problem(s). Hollis (1970, p. 52) recommends that alternative conceptions of the client and his or her situation be considered by examining the clinical data from various frames of reference.

Middleman and Goldberg (1974, pp. 88–89) suggest to social workers three areas for analysis: (1) patterns of interaction in the client's various social roles, (2) content themes that point to areas of concern, and (3) metamessages (usually nonverbal) underlying overt expression.

Caution is suggested in case analyses to avoid (1) stereotyping, which results from faulty deductive thinking; (2) overgeneralization from experiences that may not be representative; and (3) oversimplication of cause, such as single-focused explanations. The last two represent faulty inductive thinking (Lowenberg, 1977, p. 261). Any of these three practices can lead to diagnostic errors.

Concise diagnostic classification is not generally found in social work except when terms borrowed from psychiatry can be used. This situation exists even among caseworkers using the psychosocial (diagnostic) approach. Hollis, in her review of this model of practice, states that three types of diagnostic inferences are employed:

> These inferences will be mainly of three types: dynamic, etiological and classificatory. (1) In the *dynamic* diagnosis we examine, among other things, how different aspects of the client's personality interact to produce his total functioning. We look at the interplay between the client and other people and at other systems and the interactions within them to understand how change in one part of a system may affect another. The dynamics of family interaction are particularly important here and form a large part of what is often referred to as a family diagnosis. (2) *Etiological* factors are looked for, whether these lie in the current interactions or in preceding events which still actively affect the present and are among the causes of the client's dilemma. Usually, causation is seen as the convergence of a multiplicity of factors in the person-situation configuration. The dynamic and etiological aspects of the diagnosis together provide both a "linear" and an interactional or "transactional" view of causation. Where antecedents exist they are noted; they are usually seen as multiple. At the same time the continuous action between and among the various causative components in the transactional sense is an integral part of understanding the nature of the client-situation gestalt. (3) Effort is made to *classify* various aspects of the client's functioning, including, where pertinent and possible, a clinical diagnosis. (Hollis, 1970, p. 51–52)

SUMMARY

Neither nursing diagnosis nor client care is done in isolation. Nurses, physicians, social workers, and others have to collaborate if clients are to receive coordinated care. Understanding one's own and others' viewpoints is the first step toward collaborative practice. To take this first step was one of the purposes of this chapter.

The second purpose was to help the reader further define nursing diagnosis. Various concepts of diagnosis were compared and contrasted to promote understanding. The discussion pointed out that nursing traditionally has been concerned with individuals, families, and communities. Social work and medicine also have this broad area of concern. Actually, three professions evolved because of needs individuals, families, or society could not meet by themselves. Needs are expressed as societal mandates to the professions.

Although each profession follows essentially the same process for determining clients' needs, the information processed differs. Nurses, physicians, and social workers determine the need for professional services by collecting information and defining problems. Good judgment is valued in each profession and each sees itself as a helping profession. The three groups' distinctiveness lies in their social mandates and the models of practice developed from those.

Nursing, in contrast to the other two professions, has traditionally taken a holistic view of clients and their situations. Nurses are concerned with the broad range of human functional responses to life situations. Both physicians and social workers specialize in *areas* of the client's situation—disease and social problems, respectively.

Each profession uses conceptual frameworks for practice that are consistent with its mandate and concerns. If psychosocial problems are the focus of concern, then logically the model of the client should promote the collection of psychosocial information; if disease is the phenomenon of interest, then attention is directed toward pathophysiological or psychopathological manifestations. The focusing of attention leads to the naming and classification of conditions the profession can address. Thus there is consistency between a profession's focus and its classification systems.

Essentially the same cognitive processes are applied by each profession, but the focus for their application differs. The information collected, concepts used to interpret information, and the problems addressed vary. Generally, these differences are reflected in professional care.

The reader may not be sure that a clear understanding of *nursing's* focus has been attained. General aspects of a belief system have been emphasized but the topic of specific conceptual frameworks for diagnosis has been skirted. The next chapter will be devoted to this topic; as previously stated, a specific conceptual focus for diagnosis is crucial for its definition.

BIBLIOGRAPHY

Abdellah, F. G. (1959). Improving the teaching of nursing through research in patient care. In L. E. Heidgerken (Ed.), *Improvement of nursing through research.* Washington, DC: Catholic University of America Press.

Ackerman, N. W. (1958) *Psychodynamics of family life.* New York: Basic Books.

American Association of Social Workers. (1929). *The Milford conference report.* New York.

American Nurses' Association (1980a). *The nursing practice act.* Kansas City, MO.

American Nurses' Association. (1980b). *A social policy statement.* Kansas City, MO.

American Nurses' Association (1973). *Standards for nursing practice.* Kansas City, MO.

Andrews, L. (1986). Health care providers. *Journal of Professional Nursing,* 2:60–61.

Baron, R. J. (1985). An introduction to medical phenomenology: I can't hear you when I'm listening. *Annals of Internal Medicine,* 103:606–611.

Berman, A. (1954). The heroic approach in 19th century therapeutics. *Bulletin of the American Society of Hospital Pharmacists,* 11:320–327.

Blaxter, M. (1978). Diagnosis as category and process: The case of alcoholism. *Social Science and Medicine,* 12:10.

Bloch, D. (1974). Some crucial terms in nursing—What do they really mean? *Nursing Outlook*, 22:689–694.

Bonney, B., & Rothberg, J. (1963). *Nursing diagnosis and therapy.* New York: National League for Nursing.

Briar, S. (1976). Social work's function. *Social Work*, 21:90.

Card, W. I., & Good, I. J. (1974). A logical analysis of medicine. In R. Passamore (Ed.), *A companion to medical studies.* London: Blackwell, Scientific Publishers, vol. 3, sec. 60.

Carnavalli, D. L., Mitchell, P. H., Woods, N. F., & Tanner, C. A. (1984). *Diagnostic reasoning in nursing.* Philadelphia: Lippincott.

Carroll, N. K. (1977). Three dimensional model of social work practice. *Social work*, 22:428–432.

Cassell, E. J. (1977). Error in medicine. In H. T. Englehardt & D. Callahan (Eds.), *Knowledge, value and belief.* New York: The Hastings Center.

Cooper, S. (1977). Social work: A dissenting profession. *Social Work*, 22:361.

Dean, W. R. (1977). Back to activism. *Social Work*, 22:369–373.

Dickens, C. (1910). *Martin Chuzzlewit.* New York: Macmillan.

Doona, M. E. (1976). The judgement process in nursing. *Image*, 8:27–29.

Duffy, U. (1967). The changing image of the American physician. *Journal of the American Medical Association*, 200:136–140.

Elstein, A. S., Schulman, L. S., & Sprafka, S. A. (1978). *Medical problem solving: An analysis of clinical reasoning.* Cambridge, MA: Harvard University Press.

Engel, G. L. (1977). The need for a new medical model: A challenge for biomedicine. *Science*, 196:129–196.

Engle, R. L., Jr. (1963). Medical diagnosis: Present, past, and future: II. Philosophical foundations and historical development of our concepts of health, disease and diagnosis. *Archives of Internal Medicine*, 112:521–529.

Engle, R. L., Jr., & Davis, B. J. (1963). Medical diagnosis: present, past and future: I. Present concepts of the meaning and limitations of medical diagnosis. *Archives of Internal Medicine*, 112:512–519.

Englehardt, T., Jr. (1978). The disease of masturbation: Values and the concept of disease. In J. W. Leavitt & R. L. Numbers (Eds.), *Sickness and health in America* Madison: University of Wisconsin Press.

Fejos, P. (1963). Magic, witchcraft, and medical theory in primitive cultures. In I. Galdston (Ed.), *Man's image in medicine and anthropology.* New York: International Universities Press.

Field, M. (1979). Causal inferences in behavioral research. *Advances in Nursing Science*, 2:81–93.

Finestone, S. (1960). Issues involved in developing diagnostic classifications for casework. In *Casework papers, 1960. Papers presented at the 87th Annual Forum, National Conference on Social Welfare, Atlantic City, June 5–10, 1960.* New York: Family Service Association of America, pp. 139–154.

Frederick, H. K., & Northam, E. (1938). *A textbook of nursing practice.* (2d ed.). New York: Macmillan.

Germaine, C. (1970). Casework and science: A historical encounter. In R. W. Roberts & R. H. Nee (Eds.), *Theories of social casework.* Chicago: University of Chicago Press.

Gordon, M. (1976). Nursing diagnosis and the diagnostic process. *American Journal of Nursing*, 76:1300.

Hall, V. C. (1975). *Statutory regulation of the scope of nursing practice.* Chicago: National Joint Practice Commission.

Hall, L. E. (1955). Quality of nursing care. (Address at meeting of Department of Baccalaureate and Higher Degree Programs of the New Jersey League for Nursing, Newark, N.J., February 7, 1955). *Public Health News (New Jersey State Department of Health)*, 36:212–213 [Cited in H. Yura & M. B. Walsh. (1978). *The nursing process: Assessing, planning, implementing, evaluating* (3d ed.). New York: Appleton-Century-Crofts.]

Handbook for friendly visitors among the poor. (1883). Compiled by the Charity Organization Society of the City of New York.

Harmer, B. (1955). *Textbook of the principles and practice of nursing.* (5th ed.; revised by V. Henderson.) New York: Macmillan.

Henderson, V. (1966). *The nature of nursing.* New York: Macmillan.

Hollis, F. (1970). The psychosocial approach to casework. In R. W. Roberts and R. H. Nee (eds.), *Theories of social casework.* Chicago: University of Chicago Press.

Kalisch, P. A., & Kalisch, B. J. (1978). *The advance of American nursing.* Boston: Little, Brown.

Keefer, C. S., & Wilkins, R. W. (1970). *Medicine: Essentials of clinical practice.* Boston: Little, Brown.

King, L. S. (ed.). (1971). *A history of medicine: Selected readings.* Baltimore: Penguin Books.

Lazare, A. (1973). Hidden conceptual models in clinical psychiatry. *New England Journal of Medicine,* 288:346–353.

Leavitt, J. W., & Numbers, R. L. (eds.). (1978). *Sickness and health in America: Readings in the history of medicine and public health.* Madison: University of Wisconsin Press.

Lowenberg, F. M. (1977). *Fundamentals of social intervention.* New York: Columbia University Press.

Maryland public rates nursing high in survey (1979). *American Journal of Nursing,* 79:2094.

McManus, L. (1950). Assumptions of functions of nursing. In Teachers College Division of Nursing Education, *Regional planning for nursing and nursing education.* New York: Teachers College Press.

McWhinney, I. R. (1972). Beyond diagnosis: An approach to the integration of behavior science and clinical medicine. *New England Journal of Medicine,* 287:384–387.

Middleman, R. R., & Goldberg, G. (1974). *Social service delivery: A structural approach to social work practice.* New York: Columbia University Press.

Morales, A. (1977). Beyond traditional conceptual frameworks. *Social Work,* 22:390–392.

Morris, R. (1977). Caring for vs. caring about people. *Social Work,* 22:353.

Newman, M. (1979). *Theory development in nursing.* Philadelphia: Davis.

Nightingale, F. (1949). Sick nursing and health nursing. In I. Hampton (Ed.), *Nursing of the sick,* 1893. New York: McGraw-Hill.

Nightingale, F. (1859). *Notes on nursing: What it is and what it is not.* London: Harrison.

Nunehan, A., & Pincus, A. (1977). Conceptual framework for social work practice. *Social Work,* 22:346.

Orem, D. E. (1971). *Nursing: Concepts of practice.* New York: McGraw-Hill.

Orem, D. E. (1959). *Guides for developing curricula for the education of practical nurses.* Washington DC: Government Printing Office.

Orlando, I. J. (1961). *The dynamic nurse patient relationship.* New York: Putnam.

Perlman, H. H. (1970). The problem-solving model in casework practice. In R. W. Roberts & R. H. Nee (Eds.), *Theories of social casework.* Chicago: University of Chicago Press.

Reid, W. J. (1977) Social work for social problems. *Social Work,* 22:374.

Richmond, M. (1917). *Social diagnosis.* New York: Russell Sage.

Ripple, L., & Alexander, E. (1956). Motivation, capacity, and opportunity as related to the use of casework service: Nature of the client's problem. *Social Review,* 30:38–54.

Rivers, W. H. R. (1927). *Medicine, magic, and religion.* New York: Harcourt, Brace and World.

Roberts, R. W., & Nee, R. H. (1970). *Theories of social casework.* Chicago: University of Chicago Press.

Robinson, V. P. (1978). Changing psychology in social casework. In V. P. Robinson (Ed.), Development of a professional self. In *Teaching and learning in professional helping processes: Selected writings, 1930–1968.* New York: AMS Press.

Rogers, M. (1970). *Introduction to the theoretical basis of nursing.* New York: Davis.

Ruesch, J. (1963). The helping traditions: Some assumptions made by physicians. In I. Galdston (Ed.), *Man's image in medicine and anthropology.* New York: International Universities Press.

Selby, L. G. (1958). Typologies for caseworkers: Some considerations and problems. *Social Service Review,* 32:341–349.

Shaw, C. S. W. (1855). *A textbook of nursing.* New York: Appleton.

Sickerman, B. (1978). The uses of diagnosis: Doctors, patients and neurasthenia. In J. W. Leavitt & R. L. Numbers (Eds.), *Sickness and health in America,* Madison: University of Wisconsin Press.

Simm, B. K. (1977). Diversity and unity in the social work profession. *Social Work,* 22:394.

Smalley, R. E. (1970). The functional approach to casework practice. In R. W. Roberts & R. H. Nee (Eds.), *Theories of social casework.* Chicago: University of Chicago Press.

Subcommittee on the Working Definition of Social Work Practice for the Commission on Social Work Practice, National Association of Social Workers (1958). Working definition of social work practice. In H.R. Bartlett, Toward clarification and improvement of social work practice. *Social Work,* 3:3–9.

Talbott, J. (1980). An in-depth look at DSM-III: An interview with Robert Spitzer. *Hospital and Community Psychiatry,* 31:25–32.

Tappert, T. G., & Lehman, P. (Eds.) (1967). *Luther's works.* Philadelphia: Fortress Press.

Thomas, L. (1978). Notes of a biology watcher: On magic in medicine. *New England Journal of Medicine,* 299:462–463.

Tumulty, P.A. (1973). What is a clinician and what does he do? In R. T. Bulger (Ed.). *Hippocrates revisited: A search for meaning.* New York: Medcom Press.

Vaisrub, S. (1979). Groping for causation. *Journal of the American Medical Association,* 241:830.

Walter, J. B. (1977). *An introduction to the principles of disease.* Philadelphia: Saunders.

World Health Organization. (1977). *International classification of diseases.* Geneva.

FRAMEWORKS FOR THE DIAGNOSTIC PROCESS

FRAMEWORKS FOR THE DIAGNOSTIC PROCESS

The diagnostic process begins with the collection of information and ends with an evaluative judgment about a client's health status. To carry out this process in nursing, one must make decisions about *what information is important* and in *what areas responsibility exists for diagnosis.* A conceptual framework provides a basis for these decisions. As the term implies, a conceptual framework is a *set of interrelated concepts.* The concepts are abstract ways of looking at *client-environment interaction, nursing goal, and nursing intervention.* To be applicable in many diverse nursing situations, the concepts must be abstract and must provide a useful perspective for practice.

Concepts within a framework provide a focus for nursing process. In this chapter, four conceptual frameworks will be reviewed: *the life process, adaptation, self-care agency, and behavioral systems models.* Discussion will be limited to concepts related to the client environment, nursing goal, and the view of diagnosis within each framework.

One purpose for reviewing selected conceptual frameworks here is to find *what to assess and why.* One's conceptual perspective on clients and on nursing's goals strongly determines what kinds of things one assesses. Everyone has a perspective, whether in conscious awareness or not. Problems can arise if the perspective "in the head" is inconsistent with the actions taken during assessment. Information collection has to be logically related to one's view of nursing.

A *second purpose* for reviewing selected frameworks is to *further define nursing diagnosis.* Conceptual frameworks specify the focus of nursing and thus of nursing diagnosis. For example, one framework specifies that nursing diagnoses are actual or potential self-care deficits; another specifies ineffective adaptations as the problems of concern to nurses.

The two concepts in a framework that have relevance to the diagnostic phase of nursing process are the concept of the client and the concept of nursing goal. The concept of the client provides guidelines for logical deduction of what is to be assessed; the concept of goal describes a general idea of the health outcome that assessment, diagnosis, and care planning are to achieve.

During study of conceptual frameworks it is important to appreciate that *the frameworks cause you to see different things.* When looking at a client a nurse may pay attention to *self-care agency.* To this nurse, a body image disturbance would be viewed as a self-care agency deficit.[1] The nurse using an adaptation framework would view this disturbance as an ineffective adaptation to a leg amputation. All nursing frameworks specify optimal health as the goal of nursing, but ways of looking at health differ. Concepts of the client also differ, but they all focus on health-related behavior. The conceptual view of the client and of the goal of nursing are logically related;[2] a review of a few frameworks will demonstrate this.[3]

CONCEPTUAL FRAMEWORKS

There are a number of ways to arrive at a concept of nursing that provides guidelines for information collection (assessment) and for diagnostic judgments. One approach is to start with the abstract question, What is nursing?, and then *try to reason* "down" to the clinical level. A number of frameworks that have been proposed by nursing theoristis can be used to do this. A *deductive process* of reasoning is involved, beginning with assumptions and beliefs and ending with applications to specific situations.

A second way of deciding what is to be assessed is to *examine the assessment formats in current use.* In nursing there is no lack of proposed assessment tools; they are numerous in the literature. A review of these would show how items could be grouped into broad categories for guiding information collection. This would be an *inductive process* of reasoning, from particular to general areas. The assumptions of persons constructing these tools influence the end products—the assessment data—that result from use of the tools.

There is still another approach to determining what information to collect: *Why not look at the clients themselves?* What health problems amenable to nursing intervention do they have? A list of these problems could be turned into

---

[1]Self-care agency deficit should not be confused with self-care deficit, the diagnostic category (Appendix A). The former is an abstract way of thinking about *all* diagnoses and the latter is one diagnosis.

[2]This logical relationship between the goal and client focus (also intervention focus) is referred to as the *internal consistency* of a conceptual framework.

[3]Frameworks will not be comprehensively discussed; certain concepts have been selected because of their pertinence to diagnosis. The reader is encouraged to read the original work and the reviews listed in the bibliography at the end of this chapter.

broad assessment categories. Again it is true that the nurses doing the "looking" have assumptions that influence what they pay attention to in the situation. These assumptions influence the end product.

A related method is to ask clients one simple question: *Which health problems could nurses assist you with?* Asking this of many clients would provide items to categorize. What has been done is to shift the assumptions to the client. Now, clients' assumptions about nursing and what nurses do will influence the end product of the assessment process.

All these methods are encompassed to some extent in the conceptual frameworks of nursing that have appeared in the literature. Theorists who developed these frameworks are nurses, and their beliefs and experiences in nursing are incorporated. During the following discussion of selected frameworks (the life process model, the adaptation model, the behavioral systems model, and the self-care agency model), the reader may wonder why nursing has more than one way of viewing the client. We will return to this question; at this point the reader needs to know that philosophical differences exist, that there are strong vested interests, and that many are reticent to close off development of ideas at too early a point.

Life Process Model

A framework encompassing the whole of the life process is proposed by Martha Rogers (1970). Life is viewed as a creative, formative process. It is characterized by the human species' evolution toward greater diversity and innovation. Nursing promotes the attainment of these emerging potentialities by its focus on the means to this end of continuing development: maximum health potential. Individuals, families, and communities are conceptualized as energy fields that have pattern, organization, and openness to constant transaction with the environment.

The life process is a transaction between the human energy field and the environmental field. Both fields are characterized by wholeness of life pattern, and both are continuously and simultaneously repatterned as person and environment transact (Rogers, 1970, p. 53). This means that nursing focuses on the *whole person-environment complex,* not the sum of the psychological, biological, or social parts. Further, it means that the client and environment are continuously affecting each other.

With simultaneous and continuous client-environment interaction, new life patterns emerge. Nursing seeks to *help the client maintain a pattern of living that coordinates, rather than conflicts, with the emerging pattern.* Although assessment and diagnosis focus on the life process at a particular point in time, the probability that new behaviors will emerge has to be considered.

The ideas in this model need to be carefully considered from a broad, world-view perspective. For example, do you think new human and world patterns are developing? Is this happening sequentially, such that the human race is never what it was, only what it is becoming? Is emergence goal-directed? Is life pattern and organization getting more complex? Are the changes innovative and spiral (something like the Slinky toy with its cyclic spirals)? Is there order to evolutionary development?

If you answer yes to the above questions, you share the same *assumptions* about human beings as Rogers:

1 Man is a unified whole possessing his own integrity and manifesting characteristics that are more than and different from the sum of his parts.

2 Man and environment are continuously exchanging matter and energy with one another.

3 The life process evolves irreversibly and unidirectionally along the space-time continuum.

4 Pattern and organization identify man and reflect his innovative wholeness.

5 Man is characterized by the capacity for abstraction, imagery, language, thought, sensation, and emotion. (Rogers, 1970, pp. 43–77)

Nursing Goal Nursing can promote a client's progress toward his or her *maximum health potential* by (1) strengthening the mutual interaction of the human and environmental pattern, (2) recognizing the potentialities of the client and the environment, and (3) helping the client to use conscious personal choice in goal-seeking. Is change orderly? Yes. Is it predictable, that is, can we ever predict client health outcomes? Yes, but only in terms of probabilities and only by looking at the holistic, rhythmical pattern of the person and the environment (Rogers, 1970, pp. 89–102). Needless to say, highly probable predictions are few and far between unless the most influencing factors are identified. This, Rogers would say, requires research in nursing science.

Client Focus Rogers's conceptual model of the client focuses on *unitary man* and particularly the *life process* of human beings. The individual is thought of as an *energy field which extends into space.* Part of the field, the body, is visible. Pattern and organization of life (1) provide personal integrity, individuality, and wholeness and (2) reflect the life process, which is creative, formative, and evolving. The person and the environment affect each other's pattern, organization, and creative-formative evolution. The life process model, therefore, represents a holistic concept of the unity of person-environment. Neither the client nor the environment can be understood separately.

To understand the holistic life pattern, one must consider a *configuration of events* both within and external to the person's awareness. Examples would be client-other interactions (some of which are perceptible) or radiation levels in the environment (imperceptible) (Rogers, 1970).

In assessment of the client life pattern, the holistic concept must be at the forefront. At a point in time, the nurse describes the extent to which the client is emerging toward maximum health potential. This emergence is assessed by (1) observing the pattern and organization of the creative, formative process (life process) and (2) determining the degree to which the environment permits achievement of maximum health potential. More specifically, the nurse assesses the (1) client and environment pattern and organization and (2) preceding patterns (configuration of events) leading up to the present. *Patterns that do not permit movement toward maximum health potential require nursing attention.*

Behavioral manifestations of unified human functioning are the assessment data (Rogers, 1970, pp. 124–127). This is the extent to which Rogers's publications specify what to assess. Data are synthesized to reveal a view of the client's life process (creative, formative). The life process model does not include a set of categories for guiding assessment of behavior or of patterns; only principles are delineated (Rogers, 1970). Nurses using the life process model have the challenge of developing holistic assessment parameters.

Theorist's View of Diagnosis   Rogers states, "The total pattern of events at any given point in space-time provides the data for nursing diagnosis." She refers to *the* "diagnostic pattern" and adds that "nursing diagnosis encompasses the man-environment relationship and seeks to identify sequential cross sectional patterning in the life process" (Rogers, 1970, p. 125). Health problems have multiple causes, and relationships between cause and effect are always probabilistic rather than absolute.

In summary, (1) the concept of the client in Rogers's life process model is unitary man, (2) diagnosis focuses on the pattern of client-environment interaction, and (3) the goal of nursing is to help clients repattern toward healthful behaviors (maximum health potential) in order to realize their creative-formative potentialities.

Adaptation Model

Roy (1976) and her colleagues (Roy and Roberts, 1981; Andrews and Roy, 1986) have proposed that an adaptation model provides a useful way of thinking about nursing. Adaptation is seen as a process necessary to (1) maintain human integrity and (2) free energy for healing and for attaining higher levels of wellness. This conceptual framework utilizes Helson's model, which views adaptation as a state of dynamic equilibrium (Roy and Roberts, 1981, p. 84).

Nursing Goal   Within this framework the goal of nursing is to *promote responses that lead to adaptation.* In turn, *adaptation* is a "response to the environment which promotes the person's general goals including survival, growth, reproduction, self-mastery, and self-actualization" (Roy and Roberts, 1981, p. 53). Adaptation is a term that refers to both a process and a state: the client may be either in the process of effectively coping with stressors or in the adapted state that results from effective coping.

Client Focus   Consistent with the goal of nursing, the client is viewed as an *open, adaptive system.* The adaptation level reflects the system's ability to cope with environmental interaction. Coping may be adaptive or ineffective in maintaining human integrity. *Ineffective coping behaviors require nursing attention.*

Two coping mechanisms are identified: the *cognator and the regulator.* The cognator mechanism consists of (1) perceptual information processing, (2) learning, (3) judgment, and (4) emotion (Roy and Roberts, 1981, p. 60). Coping with stressors also occurs through the regulator mechanism, which has "1) neural, 2) endocrine and 3) perception-psychomotor" processes (Roy and Roberts, 1981, p. 60).

The processes of the cognator and regulator are manifested in *four modes of adaptive behavior:* the physiologic, self-concept, role function, and interdependence modes. These are defined in Table 3-1.

The *four adaptive modes* provide a format for nursing assessment. In each mode behaviors are assessed and any stressors in the client-environment interaction are identified. Behaviors may be judged to be "adaptive or ineffective" relative to (1) the client's goals and (2) the maintenance of human integrity (Roy and Roberts, 1981, p. 57).

Theorist's View of Diagnosis   In the adaptation framework, a nursing diagnosis is defined as a "judgment about ineffective or potentially ineffective behavior within a mode and indentification of the most relevent influencing factors" causing the behavior (Roy and Roberts, 1981, p. 286). It is suggested that influencing, or etiological, factors can be *focal stimuli* (stressors) or *ineffective cognator and regulator processes.* The latter is discussed in relation to cross-modal diagnoses (Roy and Roberts, 1981, pp. 286–287).

This notion of etiology raises the question of whether intervention is facilitated by (1) specifying the stressor producing ineffective adaptation or by (2) describing the client's ineffective, or maladaptive, response to the stressor. If the nursing goal is to promote adaptation, identification of ineffective adaptive responses appears more useful for directing intervention. It is important in diagnosis that it be clear whether (1) the coping response to the stimulus or (2) the stimulus itself is specified as the cause of the problem. The former would dictate a typology of maladaptive coping responses (cognator and regulator processes)

TABLE 3-1
FOUR ADAPTATION MODES IDENTIFIED BY ROY

Physiologic mode	**Role-function mode**
Exercise/rest	Expressive/instrumental
Nutrition	Role identify
Elimination	Role expectations
Fluids and electrolytes	Role interactions
Oxygen and circulation	**Interdependence mode**
Regulation of temperature	Cognitive/affective,
Regulation of senses	parameters in relation
Regulation of endocrine system	to independency-
Self-concept mode	dependency needs:
Physical self	Affection achievement
Personal self	(love, support)

Source: Adapted from Roy and Roberts (1981, pp. 71–283).

and the latter, a typology of stressors and the needs of deficits they produce. This issue may be resolved as the adaptation model is further developed and tested in practice.

In summary, in the adaptation model (1) four categories (Table 3-1) and two coping mechanisms (cognator and regulator) are provided as a framework for assessment, (2) diagnoses are viewed as problems in adaptation, (3) the probable cause, or etiology, of problems is stressors or responses to stressors occurring during client-environment interaction, and (4) the goal of nursing is to promote adaptive responses so that higher levels of wellness can be attained.

Behavioral Systems Model

The behavioral systems model was initially proposed by Johnson (1968). In recent years it has been extended by Grubbs (1980).[4] Although the framework contains the term *systems,* the focus is different from the focus of the biomedical systems framework used in medicine.

Nursing Goal   Health, the goal of nursing, in the behavioral systems framework is viewed as behavioral balance or stability. This stability is seen as the ability to adjust and change but still maintain purposeful, orderly, predictable behavior (Grubbs, 1980).

Client Focus   Using the behavioral systems model, the nurse would view the client as an *organized, interrelated complex of interacting subsystems.* Each subsystem, for example, affiliation, has a pattern. Patterns that the client develops determine and limit interaction with the environment (Grubbs, 1980).

Development of efficient and effective behavioral patterns requires the "sustenal imperatives" of protection, nurturance, and stimulation (Grubbs, 1980, pp. 231–234). Drives explain goal-directed behavior, choice, predispositions to act, and the repertoire of actions developed to sustain each subsystem. Interrelationships among the subsystems are monitored and controlled by biophysiologic, psychologic, and sociocultural mechanisms (Grubbs, 1980, p. 235).

Stress can disturb the client's patterns and lead to disequilibrium. Factors that cause distrubances in regularity and orderliness of behavior patterns threaten the integrity and function of the entire behavioral system. Disturbances may be due to (1) inadequate drive satisfaction, (2) inadequate fulfillment of the functional requirements of the subsystems, and (3) fluctuations in environmental conditions which exceed the system's capacity to adjust (Grubbs, 1980, p. 224). Stress can also result from changes in sustenal imperatives (protection, nurturance, stimulation). As may be obvious from deductive reasoning, if the client is viewed as a system with behavioral subsystems, then these are assessed in order to determine health status.

---

[4]This review relies mainly on the presentation and extension of Johnson's theory by Grubbs (1980).

Assessment focuses on (1) behavioral patterns, (2) interrelations, and (3) sustenal imperatives. Questions that direct the assessment of subsystems may be, Is there an actual or perceived threat to loss of pattern stability? Are there changes in behavioral patterns? Are there sufficient "sustenal imperatives"? What are the abilities of the client to adapt? Problematic subsystem behavior, if identified, is further assessed in order to plan intervention; nine areas of problem analysis have been identified and include client actions, predispositions, and choice (Grubbs, 1980, pp. 239–240). The behavioral subsystems that lend structure to assessment when this model is used are listed in Table 3-2. The goal is behavioral stability; therefore, present behavior is compared to past behavior so that one may judge whether change has occurred and evaluate the contribution of the change toward stability.

Theorist's View of Diagnosis   Within this model, the meaning of diagnosis is to determine "underlying dynamics of the patient's problematic behaviors in a situation" (Grubbs, 1980, p. 240). *A problem is defined as actual or potential instability in the system.* As will be discussed below, the problem may be either functional or structural. Problem, etiology, and problem source are all included in the statement of the diagnosis. Problem source is stated as an adjective that classifies the problem.

Diagnostically, a health problem originating in one subsystem is classified as an *insufficiency* or a *discrepancy* relative to the subsystem goal. *Incompatibility* and *dominance* are the two classifications for multisubsystem problems. These classes are defined in Table 3-3 and help identify intervention, according to Grubbs. Grief is an example of a problem or behavioral pattern instability. The problem source is classified as insufficiency in the affiliative

TABLE 3-2
EIGHT BEHAVIORAL SUBSYSTEMS OF JOHNSON'S FRAMEWORK

Achievement subsystem To master or control oneself or one's environment; to achieve mastery and control
Affiliative subsystem To relate or belong to something or someone other than oneself; to achieve intimacy and inclusion
Aggressive/protective subsystem To protect self or others from real or imagined threatening objects, persons, or ideas; to achieve self-protection and self-assertion
Dependency subsystem To maintain environmental resources needed for obtaining help, assistance, attention, permission, reassurance, and security; to gain trust and reliance
Eliminative subsystem To expel biologic wastes; to externalize the internal biologic environment
Ingestive subsystem To take in needed resources from the environment to maintain the integrity of the organism or to achieve a state of pleasure; to internalize the external environment
Restorative subsystem To relieve fatigue and/or achieve a state of equilibrium by reestablishing or replenishing the energy distribution among the other subsystems; to redistribute energy
Sexual subsystem To procreate, to gratify or attract, to fulfill expectations associated with one's sex; to care for others and be cared about by them

---

Source: Grubbs (1980, p. 228).

TABLE 3-3
DIAGNOSTIC CLASSIFICATIONS OF DISORDERS IN THE BEHAVIORAL SYSTEMS MODEL

Single-subsystem disorder	*Insufficiency* This exists when a particular subsystem is not functioning or developed to its fullest capacity due to inadequacy of functional requirements. *Discrepancy* This exists when a behavior does not meet the intended goal.
Multisubsystem disorder	*Incompatibility* The goals or behaviors of the two subsystems in the same situation conflict with each other to the detriment of the individual. *Dominance* The behavior in one subsystem is used more than any other subsystem regardless of the situation or to the detriment of the other subsystem.

Source: Adapted from Grubbs (1980, pp. 240–241).

subsystem. Cause, or etiology, of the instability in the subsystem pattern may be either internal or external stress. In addition, the client may be an active or passive participant in the etiology (Grubbs, 1980, p. 241). Etiological classification is done on the basis of two possible causes: *structural stress* and *functional stress.* These are defined in Table 3-4. Grubb's classification places the source of structural stress within the subsystems (client). Functional stress is most often caused by factors in the external environment.

The active or passive participation of the client, as the cause of stress, rests on the assumption in the model that the client has a choice of alternative behaviors. An example of an etiology of structural stress is given: "deliberate avoidance of achievement situations" (Grubbs, 1980, p. 241); the cause is within the person and, more specifically, within the achievement subsystem. The goal of the subsystem is to master and control, but the behavior chosen is not meeting this goal. Thus, the etiology lies in the client's behavior: choosing not to achieve.

Grubbs compares the above example to functional stress. The eiology could be "lack of achievement opportunities." Grubbs says that in this case "the patient is essentially a passive victim of his environmental situation" (Grubbs, 1980, p. 241). Note the dichotomous judgment the diagnostician has to make regarding internal or external stressors when using this classification. The dichotomy will

TABLE 3-4
ETIOLOGICAL CLASSIFICATION IN THE BEHAVIORAL SYSTEMS MODEL

Etiology of health problem	Definition of etiological type
Structural stress	Refers to that which occurs within the subsystems; involves internal control mechanisms and reflects inconsistencies between the goal, set, choice, or action
Functional stress	Refers to overload or insufficiency of any of the sustenal imperatives and results in functional disorders; usually arises externally from the environment

Source: Adapted from Grubbs (1980, p. 241).

not appeal to those who support the concept of multicausality or those believing that problems result from the *interaction* between the person and environment.

The author states that identifying whether the stress is structural or functional is helpful for diagnostic purposes. Even if this dichotomy of probable sources of stress is accepted, caution would be needed to avoid value-laden statements (with or without sufficient clinical data). In Grubbs's example, the term *deliberate avoidance* has a negative connotation. Secondly, it does not seem that with this level of formulation "the intervention course becomes clear" (Grubbs, 1980, p. 241). A nurse who *thinks* "avoidance" is "deliberate" when the clinical assessment data are analyzed surely needs to go on to further understand why this is so.

The specification of etiology requires an in-depth assessment. It also requires analysis of clinical data to gain an understanding of the probable factor(s) that precipitate or maintain the less-than-optimal state. Explanatory concepts (etiology) are helpful in care planning if they are formulated at a level that suggests nursing interventions. For diagnostic purposes, if one accepts the dichotomy implied in this concept of etiology, then Table 3-4 is useful as a structure to organize thinking. It may ensure that neither the client's behavior nor external circumstances and events are ignored in understanding the probable contributing, predisposing, or precipitating factors.

In summary, in the behavioral systems model (1) the client is viewed as having a set of interrelated behavioral systems which form the framework for assessment, (2) diagnoses are problems of instability and occur because of structural or functional stress, and (3) the goal of nursing is behavioral balance, as evidenced by the ability to adjust to change. A number of guidelines are offered for identifying problems and their etiologies.

Self-Care Agency Model

Client self-care abilities and operations are the phenomena of nursing concern in Orem's (1980) self-care model. Emphasis is placed on the capacities of clients to manage their own health and that of their dependents, such as children. Nurses help them to do this.

Nursing Goal   In discussing the goal of health care, Orem uses a comprehensive definition of health: "Health signifies human functional and structural integrity, absence of genetic defects, and progressive integrated development of a human being as an individual unity moving toward higher and higher levels of integration" (Orem, 1980, p. 121). Within the overall goal of the health professions, which is to bring about health, nursing defines its role. *The goal of nursing is independent, responsible self-care on the part of the clients.* Self-care is considered to be present when the client's actions (in regard to self and dependents) regulate "internal and external conditions necessary to maintain life processes and environmental conditions supportive of life processes, integrity of human structure and functioning, and human developmental processes" (Orem, 1980, p. 24).

As may be evident, Orem's underlying view of clients is that they are *responsible and engage in deliberate choice and action.* In accordance with this view, clients are expected to be socially responsible agents of their own self-care and the care of their dependents. *Deficits or limitations in self-care actions, relative to requisites, require nursing attention.*

Client Focus   People are viewed as having universal, developmental, and health deviation self-care requisites. The requisites are described as follows:

1 Universal self-care requisites are common to all human beings during all stages of life. They are associated with life processes and with the maintenance of the integrity of human structure and functioning. Universal self-care requisites include sufficient intake of air, water, and food; elimination; a balance between activity and rest and between solitude and social interaction; prevention of hazards; and the promotion of human functioning and development relative to potentialities.

2 *Developmental* self-care requisites vary with age or with condition, such as pregnancy. Two categories of developmental requisites are identified:

> The bringing about and maintenance of living conditions that support life processes and promote the processes of development, that is, human progress toward higher levels of the organization of human structures and functions and toward maturation . . . [and] provision of care either to prevent the occurrence of deleterious effects of conditions that can affect human development . . . or to mitigate or overcome these effects. (Orem, 1980, p. 47)

Like universal self-care requisites, these developmental needs are met either through one's own abilities (if one is an able adult) or by another (as in case of dependent children).

3 In the third area of clients' self-care needs, *health deviation* self-care requisites, Orem identifies six categories and summarizes them as follows:

> Health deviation self-care requisites are associated with genetic constitutional defects, human structural and functional deviations and their effects, and medical diagnosis and treatment. (Orem, 1980, p. 41)

From these areas the total "therapeutic self-care demand" of any individual can be determined. Also, self-care actions can be examined for their "therapeutic value" (Orem, 1980, pp. 39–40). If therapeutic, the person's actions contribute to "(1) support of life processes and promotion of normal functioning; (2) maintenance of normal growth, development, and maturation; (3) prevention, control, or cure of disease processes and injuries; and (4) prevention of, or compensation for, disability" (Orem, 1980, p. 40).

When self-care is not done or is done in a nontherapeutic manner, deficits exist. Self-care deficits are determined by examining (1) an individual's therapeutic demands (required actions) in the universal, developmental, and health deviation areas; (2) the self-care actions currently being done; and (3) the therapeutic value of current actions. In addition, potential decreases in self-care abilities or increases in demands can be predicted.

Theorist's View of Diagnosis   It clearly follows from this model of the client that the focus of nursing diagnosis is deficits in self-care agency (abilities). These may be due to the client's lack of knowledge or skill, limitations in capacity (transitory or permanent), or lack of resources (Orem, 1980, p. 141). The diagnostic judgment of deficits or limitations is related to (1) universal self-care requisites and the quality and type of present self-care activities and (2) actual or predicted abilities or actions. Essentially, *diagnosis involves a comparison of current actions and potential for action with actual or potential demands.* If deficiencies are found, a problem in self-care agency is diagnosed.

Orem does not discuss a concept of *etiology* explicitly. Comments are made about the underlying cause of inability to perform self-care actions, such as nonuse of a fractured leg. It is stated that limitations in self-care "may be caused by the effects of the disease process, the therapy used, the lack of necessary knowledge and skills, or a lack of resources" (Orem, 1980, p. 141). In addition, lack of motivation to alter self-care actions can also cause limitations in therapeutic self-care or care of dependents (Orem, 1980, p. 62).

In summary, Orem's framework views the client as a self-care agent. The goal of nursing is the client's independence in self-care actions. As a framework for the diagnostic process this model would direct assessment toward data related to self-care demands and self-care capabilities. *Self-care agency deficits, actual or potential, would be the focus of diagnosis.*

The models reviewed above provide a sampling of various conceptualizations of the client from a nursing perspective. Recall that the purpose of reviewing these was to demonstrate that there are answers to the question of what information to collect and in what areas responsibility exists for diagnostic judgments.

In this discussion of frameworks for the diagnostic phase of nursing process, concepts of the client, diagnostic focus, and causality were of interest. For the conceptual frameworks reviewed, these ideas are summarized in Table 3-5. Although some overlapping can be seen, these are essentially different views based on different assumptions about clients.

To implement any framework for nursing process, the nurse must understand the entire model and its philosophical assumptions. The reader is encouraged to review a number of models and their interrelated concepts of client, intervention (nurse-client interaction), and nursing's goal. The bibliography at the end of this chapter contains references that pertain to the conceptual frameworks just discussed. Other nursing conceptual frameworks focus on human needs (Yura and Walsh, 1978; Putt, 1978); needs, conservation, and adaptation (Levine, 1973, pp. 1–33); needs and distress (Orlando, 1961); needs and social systems (King, 1971; 1981); existential becoming (Patterson and Zderad, 1976);

TABLE 3-5
FOUR FRAMEWORKS FOR THE DIAGNOSTIC PROCESS

Framework	Assessment focus	Diagnostic focus	Causality
Rogers life process model	Behavioral manifestations of events in the human and environmental field Holistic patterns of functioning (total pattern of events at a given point in space-time)	Pattern and organization of the life process which does not support maximum health potential and the creative-formative process (No diagnostic classification)	Multicausality found in human and environmental field interaction
Roy adaptation model	Adaptive responses to need deficits or excesses: Physiological mode Rest/exercise Nutrition Elimination Fluids and electrolytes Oxygen and circulation Regulation of temperature Regulation of senses Regulation of endocrine system Self-concept mode Physical self Personal self Moral-ethical Self-consistency Self-ideal Self-esteem	Potential problems in adaptation; actual maladaptation problems (Diagnostic classification according to 4 adaptation modes: physiological, self-concept, role function, and interdependence modes)	Causality lies in need deficits or excesses produced by stressors (focal stimulus) or in coping mechanisms (cognator and regulator) Multicausality concept, but intervention focus is on primary cause

(continued)

TABLE 3-5
FOUR FRAMEWORKS FOR THE DIAGNOSTIC PROCESS (*continued*)

Framework	Assessment focus	Diagnostic focus	Causality

	Role function mode
	Primary/secondary/
	tertiary roles
	Expressive/instrumental:
	  Role identity
	  Role expectations
	  Role interactions
	
	Interdependence mode
	Cognitive/affective,
	parameters in relation
	to independency-
	dependency needs:
	  Affection achievement
	  (love, support)
	
	Influencing factors: focal,
	contextual, and residual
	stimuli		

Johnson (Grubbs) behavioral system model	Structural and functional level of behavioral system and the behavioral subsystem: Achievement Affiliative Aggressive/protective Dependency Eliminative Ingestive	Instability in the system; behavior at variance with the desired state; behavior that does not maintain equilibrium: Intrasubsystem insufficiency Intrasubsystem insufficiency Intersubsystem incompatibility Intersubsystem dominance Inadequate coping/adaptation	Etiological classification according to source of stress/ instability *Etiology* used in singular sense

Model			
	Restorative Sexual Coping effectiveness	(Diagnostic classification according to 8 subsystems, intrasubsystem or intersubsystem problem)	Cause may be disease process; therapy used; or lack of knowledge, skills, resources, interest, or motivation
Orem self-care agency model	Eight universal self-care requisites, 2 developmental self-care requisites, and 6 health deviation self-care requisites (as well as interrelationships among these)	Presence of a deficit between existing powers of self-care agency and the demands on it	
	Current repertoire of self-care practices (self and dependent): Degree of development	Actual or potential deficits in type and quality (therapeutic value) of self-care actions	
	Degree of operability	(Diagnostic classification according to self-care needs in relation to (1) development, (2) health deviation, and (3) universal	
	Adequacy relative to demand		

Source: Adapted form Rogers (1970); Roy (1976), Grubbs (1978), and Orem (1980).

and stress (Neuman, 1980, pp. 119–134). Some have suggested that the framework, developed for classification of nursing diagnoses by nursing theorists and the NANDA Taxonomy Committee, could be used to direct assessment. This evolving framework is discussed in Chapter 11.

ACQUIRING AND USING A CONCEPTUAL MODEL

Now the question arises as to how to choose a model that can give purpose and direction to nursing process and, particularly, to diagnosis. For students, the conceptual framework of the curriculum should provide guidance. The framework includes the faculty's concept of the client, nursing goal, and nursing intervention.[5] For example, Roy's adaptation framework can guide a student to assess adaptation modes. Using the concepts underlying the curriculum organization as a framework for nursing process provides consistency between classroom theory and clinical aspects and makes learning easier.

The reader who is currently practicing nursing is already assessing, diagnosing, intervening, and evaluating on the basis of some framework, possibly without full awareness of what that framework is. It can be an interesting experience to discover one's own professional point of view by reflecting on one's own practice. Examining personal assumptions about clients and about nursing will lead to consciousness raising.

Sometimes nurses find they are using a medical or social work model to guide *nursing* practice! Although this sounds illogical, it can occur. The aforementioned reviews and further reading about conceptual frameworks may assist in formulating a model for nursing practice.

Those who claim "I don't need all that theoretical stuff to give nursing care" or "I don't need that, I just look at what the patients need or tell me they need" are deluding themselves. All nurses, including these, act on some of their observations and make referrals on the basis of others. Beneath these actions and referrals is a personal concept of nursing and some idea of what "should" receive attention.

Even implicit, unrecognized models influence perception and judgment. In the second statement quoted above, the nurse has a model but doesn't know it. A human needs model is obviously being used and probably just requires some conscious organization.

Testing a Model in Practice

Conceptual models or frameworks of nursing can be elegant designs with logical relationships between the concepts specified. The crucial test, however, is whether

---

[5]The organizing framework of concepts serves to structure the body of professional knowledge, skills, attitudes, and values in a curriculum. Its importance is reflected in the fact that one standard for national accreditation by the National League for Nursing addresses this.

a framework is workable in clinical practice. Does it provide a useful way of viewing clients? Does it capture the essence of the special contribution nursing makes to health care delivery? Does the concept of what nurses should do with and for clients (intervention concepts) seem realistic?

The only way to answer these questions about a model is to try it in one's practice. The concept of the client has to be used in assessment and diagnosis. One has to try stating and then evaluating client outcomes that are developed from the framework's concept of nursing's goal. The concept of intervention in the model has to be used as a guide for planning and implementing nursing care. After a number of months of this testing, the strengths, weaknesses, and areas needing further development become apparent. Undoubtedly the nursing theorist who developed the model would welcome a thoughtful critique and ideas for further development. These critiques and comments could be published in the nursing literature or relayed through personal communication. That is how conceptual models become refined. Clinicians have to test them in practice and identify their clinical usefulness.

Why the emphasis on models of the client? To reiterate, because *nursing diagnosis* cannot be done without a *nursing model* that provides clear guidelines for the collection of clinical information. It is as simple as that.

THE SEARCH FOR A UNIFIED MODEL

At this point, if not well before, the reader may be asking why nurses don't agree on just one model of the client. Riehl and Roy (1974, pp. 293–294) state that the advantage of having a single model would be facilitation of communication, development of a body of knowledge, and one common nursing approach to practice. On the other hand, they cite disadvantages and barriers: basic philosophical differences exist, frameworks have not been sufficiently tested, and there are strong vested interests. These authors note that with unification the question would arise as to *which* model to select. They point out that such a selection might inhibit creativity and close off new and more productive conceptualizations.

Although most theorists today would agree with the above list of advantages and disadvantages, Riehl and Roy now advocate a unified model of the client and goal (1980, pp. 390–403). They argue that this would still allow diversity in concepts of and approaches to nursing intervention. They synthesize various theorists' concepts of the client and nursing's goal under a systems model and suggest diversity be retained in the concept of nursing intervention.

Riehl and Roy (1980) are correct in saying there are areas of agreement among the theorists. Although, as Zderad (1978) has suggested, these would be more explicit if when a new model was proposed, similarities and differences were addressed. When conceptual models are published, it is rare for theorists to compare their perspective with previously published models.

The idea of a unified model is not foreign to other disciplines. In the general scientific community theories have been proposed to unify the sciences. For example, Miller proposed a living systems theory (1978). This, he suggests, could integrate the separate bodies of knowledge in all the sciences. Yet Miller's idea that interrelations among subsystems, for example, biological, psychological, and social, lead to understanding human beings is contradictory to the holistic pattern in Rogers's life process model.

There is a problem in assuming that the search for unification of the sciences presupposes that nursing also move in this direction. Within many sciences, there is a great deal of knowledge from research that can be integrated by a unified model. Nursing science is just beginning. For all the reasons discussed, it is unlikely that a unified model (client, goal, intervention) will be accepted in the near future. It might be well to examine what problems this presents for nursing diagnosis and if there are potential solutions.

For nurses who each day confront clients, students, or research data, the issue of a unified model of the client to guide assessment and diagnosis is not just an "ivory tower" idea. It has implications for nursing care delivery, nursing education, and research—and critical implications for developing commonly agreed upon diagnostic nomenclature. For example, diversity now exists among nursing care delivery settings: clients may have different aspects of their health status assessed, depending on the hospital they go to, the level of care they receive (primary, secondary, or tertiary), and the particular nurse they happen to encounter.

From the nurse's own perspective, every time there is a change in employment settings there usually is a different format for assessment. Similarly, it is not unusual for a student to be exposed to a different assessment tool with each different clinical instructor or area of practice. This variation certainly does not facilitate learning or the development of nursing practice expertise. Lastly, it does not facilitate clinical nursing research.

How can continuity of nursing care in various settings and with various nurses be provided if there is not a basic clinical assessment data base? How can there be studies of common health problems nurses treat? There is no assurance that assessment and diagnosis are comprehensively done. Nor can a consumer of nursing care be reasonably assured that all his or her actual or potential health problems have a high probability of being detected.

Components of nursing practice have been agreed upon and standardized nationally. From the consumer's perspective, it can be expected that nurses do assessment, diagnosis, intervention, and evaluation. This is the familiar nursing process that is incorporated into the American Nurses' Associations' Standards for Nursing Practice and the social policy statement described in Chapter 2. Clinicians no doubt found that there was no framework to decide what to assess, diagnose, act upon, and evaluate. Pressuring for unification at the abstract level of the *models,* which could remain diverse, may not be the solution. Maybe what is needed for practice, education, and research is a unification at the concrete level of *assessment* (information collection). Then more abstract concepts of nursing could be applied to the basic data.

Unification of Assessment Structure

Could there be agreement, at a very concrete level, about the information needed for nursing assessment? Are there common *areas* of information about the client that are needed to implement *any* of the models of nursing? For example, irrespective of the model used in clinical practice, is every nursing clinician interested in information about dietary patterns? Remember that the focus of this discussion is on structural aspects of assessment, that is, *what* information to gather. Differences are expected in the way the information is interpreted and used.

Let us consider some of the models. Take, for example, the clinician who believes with Orem that the goal of nursing is to facilitate self-care agency. The nutritional pattern is decidedly an aspect of self-care, so nutritional patterns are assessed. The approach includes a nutritional pattern description, but emphasis is given to self-care actions underlying the pattern.

The nurse clinician who has adopted Roy's adaptation framework wants to know the basic nutritional pattern, also. This nurse will approach the analysis of clinical data by determining the person's or family's adaptation of nutritional patterns under certain situations.

The clinician concerned with patterns of living coordinated with environmental changes (Rogers's life process model) is interested in nutritional pattern changes related to other rhythm changes, for example, during hospitalization. Information about diet would be considered as (1) a behavioral manifestation and (2) specific data to be included in synthesizing a holistic view of the life process. The client's dietary pattern would be evaluated in terms of the goal of maximizing health for the creative-formative process of evolution (becoming).

Diversity in nursing models does not prevent standardization of assessment structure. Standardization does not imply a standardized interpersonal *approach* to assessment or to analysis and synthesis of clinical data. Neither does it suggest that the profession should have a standardized concept of the goal of nursing and of nurse-client interaction.

Although diversity is the watchword of western society, at a concrete level there has to be some uniformity in practice. Every client deserves to know that, minimally, certain health-related behavioral patterns will be assessed for potential or actual problems relative to the client's own or external norms. The idea is certainly not new. Dorothy Smith (1968) has been prodding the profession for at least 15 years.

Standardization of assessment areas will require thoughtful consideration of related issues and consequences. In addition, proposed formats for standardized assessment will have to be evaluated, both initially and periodically, in all settings and specialties of nursing practice.

It is this author's opinion that the profession must take action to delineate the basic areas of assessment applicable to all clients. The result would be that (1) the domain of responsibility and accountability would be clear, (2) the focus for clinical studies would be identified, and (3) the focus for development of expertise in assessment and diagnosis would be clearly delineated for teachers, students, and practitioners.

A typology of assessment categories proposed in Chapter 4 is viewed as a step in the direction of unification of *structural areas.* As stated previously, each nurse's *approach* to these areas is dictated by the conceptual framework utilized.

SUMMARY

This chapter contains important ideas for using nursing diagnosis and the diagnostic process. There is an ethical responsibility in diagnosis. One aspect of that responsibility is to have a consciously defined purpose and a systematic approach. Clients should not be subjected to an unorganized set of questions, and the reasons for collecting information should be clear. Hence a conceptual framework is necessary for using the diagnostic process.

A few current conceptual frameworks were described in order to demonstrate that they provide a nursing focus for diagnosis. Particular attention was given to concepts of the client and of nursing's goal. These concepts are particularly relevant to the focus of information collection for diagnosis. No unified framework for nursing, accepted by all, exists or can be predicted to exist in the near future. At a *basic level,* all frameworks require similar assessment data.

BIBLIOGRAPHY

American Nurses' Association (1973). *Standards for nursing practice.* Kansas City, MO.

Andrews, H. A., & Roy, C. (1986). *Essentials of the Roy adaptation model.* Norwalk, CT: Appleton-Century-Crofts.

Grubbs, J. (1980). The Johnson behavioral system model. In J. P. Riehl & C. Roy (Eds.), *Conceptual models for nursing practice* (2d ed.). New York: Appleton-Century-Crofts.

Johnson, D. (1968). *One conceptual model of nursing.* Unpublished paper presented April 25, 1968, at Vanderbilt University, Nashville, Tennessee.

King, I. (1981). *Theory for nursing: Systems, concepts, process.* New York: Wiley.

King, I. M. (1971). *Towards a theory for nursing: General concepts of human behavior.* New York: Wiley.

Levine, M. E. (1973). *Introduction to clinical nursing* (2d ed.). Philadelphia: Davis.

Miller, J. G. (1978). *Living systems.* New York: McGraw-Hill.

Neuman, B. (1980). The Betty Neuman health-care systems model: A total person approach to patient problems. In J. P. Riehl & C. Roy (Eds.), *Conceptual models for nursing practice* (2d ed.). New York: Appleton-Century-Crofts.

Orem, D. (1980). *Nursing: Concepts of practice.* New York: McGraw-Hill.

Orlando, I. J. (1961). *The dynamic nurse-patient relationship: Function, process and principles.* New York: Putnam.

Patterson, J. G., & Zderad, L. (1976). *Humanistic nursing.* New York: Wiley.

Putt, A. M. (1978). *General systems theory applied to nursing.* Boston: Little, Brown.

Riehl, J. P., & Roy, C. (1974). Discussion of a unified nursing model. In J. P. Riehl & C. Roy (Eds.), *Conceptual models for nursing practice.* New York: Appleton-Century-Crofts.

Rogers, M. (1970). *An introduction to the theoretical basis of nursing.* Philadelphia: Davis.

Roy, C. (1976). *Introduction to nursing: An adaptation model.* Englewood Cliffs, NJ: Prentice-Hall.

Roy, C., & Roberts, S. L. (1981). *Theory construction in nursing: An adaptation model.* Englewood Cliffs, NJ: Prentice-Hall.

Smith, D. M. (1968). A clinical nursing tool. *American Journal of Nursing, 68:*2384–2388.

Yura, H., & Walsh, M. (1978). *Human needs and the nursing process.* New York: Appleton-Century-Crofts.

Zderad, L. (1978). *Future directions in nursing theory.* Taped seminar paper presented at Nurse Educator Conference, New York, Dec. 4–7, 1978. (Cassette available from Nursing Resources, Inc., Wakefield, MA.)

ADDITIONAL REFERENCES

Chinn, P., & Jacobs, M. (1983). *Theory and nursing: A systematic approach.* St. Louis: Mosby.

Fawcett, J. (1984). *Analysis and evaluation of conceptual models of nursing.* Philadelphia: Davis.

Fawcett, J., & Downs, F. S. (1986). *Relationship of theory and research.* Norwalk, CT: Appleton-Century-Crofts.

Fitzpatrick, J., & Whall, A. (1983). *Conceptual models of nursing: Analysis and application.* Bowie, MD: Brady.

Meleis, A. (1985). *Theoretical nursing: Development and progress.* Philadelphia: Lippincott.

Parse, R. R. (1981). *Man-living-health: A theory of nursing.* New York: Wiley.

Torres, G. (1986). *Theoretical foundations of nursing.* Norwalk, CT: Appleton-Century-Crofts.

Walker, L., & Avant, K. (1983). *Strategies for theory construction in nursing.* Norwalk, CT: Appleton-Century-Crofts.

90

CHAPTER 4

STRUCTURE FOR ASSESSMENT: FUNCTIONAL HEALTH PATTERNS

In Chapter 3, various ways of thinking about nursing from various conceptual viewpoints were discussed. It was stated that frameworks that guide practice have to be abstract. Otherwise, they would not be useful in a variety of nursing care settings or with diverse client populations. Yet, specific guidelines for assessment are also necessary. This chapter will present a set of health patterns which specify areas of basic information that are collected no matter what framework is being used. The objectives of the chapter are to (1) discuss the concept of functional health patterns, (2) define the eleven patterns proposed, and (3) help the reader consider how these patterns can provide a structure for assessment and a basic data base for nursing diagnosis.

The term *assessment* means evaluation. In nursing the term is used to describe initial and continued health status evaluation of a person, family, or community. Deliberative and systematic assessment is an intentional process with a plan for collection and organization of information. The typology of functional health patterns proposed in the next section provides this. Information can be organized in a way that facilitates health status evaluation and nursing diagnosis. Health pattern areas could provide a standard assessment format for a basic data base, irrespective of age, level of care, or medical disease of the client. The pattern areas have the additional advantages of

1 Not having to be continually relearned (application is expanded as clinical knowledge accumulates)
2 Leading directly to nursing diagnoses (Appendix C)
3 Encompassing a holistic approach to human functional assessment in any setting and with any age group at any point in the health-illness continuum

FUNCTIONAL HEALTH PATTERNS

All human beings have in common certain functional patterns that contribute to their health, quality of life, and achievement of human potential. These common patterns are the focus of nursing assessment. Description and evaluation of health patterns permits the nurse to identify *functional patterns* (client strengths) and *dysfunctional patterns* (nursing diagnoses). Both traditional and contemporary ideas of nursing practice are represented in a *concise, easily learned set of category names.*

Before further discussion of functional health patterns, consider the abbreviated definitions contained in Table 4-1. In a later section the 11 patterns will be fully defined. At this point let us concentrate on the idea of functional health patterns as a basic data base for nursing assessment.

Health Patterns as an Assessment Focus

The above listing of assessment areas uses the term *pattern, which is defined as a sequence of behavior across time.* Sequences of behavior, rather than isolated events, are the data used for clinical inference and judgment. For example, a nurse observes that a hospitalized client has an argument with her husband. What does the nurse conclude? Nothing, one hopes! Is the quarrel a sign of the client's general pattern of relationships, martial included? Maybe or maybe not. Obviously, information about interactions across time is needed to determine whether relationships are problematic for the client. Suppose additional information about the couple just mentioned shows that the marital relationship is a problematic area. The nurse is still at an elementary level of understanding. Other relationships have to be assessed to see whether the problem is generalized or specific. These components of the total relationship pattern may include parent-child, work, social, and other interactions. When these data have been collected, the diagnostician can move toward understanding the overall role-relationship pattern and the client's perception of the pattern.

As information is collected, the nurse begins to understand the area being assessed. Gradually, the pattern emerges. It is very important to recognize that *what occurs during information collection is the construction of a pattern from a client's descriptions and the nurse's observations.* Recognizing this:

1 Prevents superficial data collection that can lead to errors in diagnosis.

2 Reminds the nurse that patterns are not observable. They are *constructed* by cognitive operations on the data from assessment and are always open to challenge by new information.

Consider some examples of assessment from which a pattern may be constructed. In the first example a 50-year-old construction worker has the following sleep pattern:

TABLE 4-1
TYPOLOGY OF ELEVEN FUNCTIONAL HEALTH PATTERNS*

Health-perception–health-management pattern Describes client's perceived pattern of health and well-being and how health is managed

Nutritional-metabolic pattern Describes pattern of food and fluid consumption relative to metabolic need and pattern indicators of local nutrient supply

Elimination pattern Describes patterns of excretory function (bowel, bladder, and skin)

Activity-exercise pattern Describes pattern of exercise, activity, leisure, and recreation

Cognitive-perceptual pattern Describes sensory-perceptual and cognitive pattern

Sleep-rest pattern Describes patterns of sleep, rest, and relaxation

Self-perception–self-concept pattern Describes self-concept pattern and perceptions of self (e.g., body comfort, body image, feeling state)

Role-relationship pattern Describes pattern of role-engagements and relationships

Sexuality-reproductive pattern Describes client's patterns of satisfaction and dissatisfaction with sexuality pattern; describes reproductive patterns

Coping–stress tolerance pattern Describes general coping pattern and effectiveness of the pattern in terms of stress tolerance

Value-belief pattern Describes patterns of values, beliefs (including spiritual), or goals that guide choices or decisions

*The pattern areas were identified by the author about 1974 for purposes of teaching assessment and diagnosis at Boston College School of Nursing. Colleagues have suggested some minor changes in labels and content. Faye E. McCain's (1965) and Dorothy Smith's (1968; Becknell and Smith, 1975) assessment concepts were particularly influential, as were the comments of clinical specialists and students who reviewed and tried out the categories in practice.

93

Sleep-rest pattern States he feels rested after 6–7 hours sleep; ready for day's work. No delay in sleep onset, interrupted sleep, early awakening, or use of sleep medications. Dreams occasionally; no report of nightmares.

The information above indicates an optimal adult sleep pattern. Notice how you can "see" the client's pattern indicated by the data: restful, undisturbed sleep without the use of medications. In contrast, what pattern is evident in this report for another client 1 day prior to heart surgery?

Sleep-rest pattern States she always was a "good sleeper"; regular 7–8 hours; well rested when awakening. Reports "insomnia," delayed sleep onset 2–3 hours in last 3 weeks. Lies awake "worrying" about the success of the heart surgery? Gets "scared" at night when there is "no one to talk to."

Most apparent is the change in sleep pattern. Historically, this client had a normal sleep pattern but change has occurred. The abrupt change combined with the scheduled heart surgery suggests the change may be due to fear or anxiety. If the underlying problem is not diagnosed and treated, her sleep pattern may not improve. In the next example, try to identify the client's pattern:

Sleep-rest pattern Has not slept well for last few months. Did not sleep first night in hospital. Sleeping pill ineffective. Uses three pillows.

The above assessment is superficial. There is information to support a dysfunctional sleep pattern but information is incomplete. For example, "three pillows" suggests a breathing problem. Is this why the client has not slept well? What does the vague statement, "not slept well" mean? We are left with these questions because the pattern was not evident in the minimal data recorded on the chart. This led to a *delay in diagnosis* and, most importantly, a *delay in treatment.*

Even with adequate information to describe a pattern, understanding may be elusive until all functional patterns are assessed. This is because the 11 functional patterns are an artificial division of integrated human functioning. (Our limited cognitive capacity cannot easily grasp the complexity of the whole with one glance.) *Patterns are interrelated, interactive, and interdependent.* Reasons for a dysfunctional pattern (etiological factors) may be found within this composite, as well as the *strengths* needed to solve problems. No one pattern can be understood in isolation.

An example may clarify the idea of interrelatedness of patterns. During a home visit a community health nurse collected the following information as part of a data base.

Husband, 65 years old, has recently retired after selling the grocery store that previously occupied his time from 8 a.m. until 6 p.m. States he has little to do now and gets into arguments with his wife: "She doesn't like me around the house; it interferes with what she wants to do; I just want to spend more time talking to her and doing things together." Wife states she has the house to keep up, meals to cook, and her volunteer activities at the day care center every afternoon. States she can't get things done because "he's in the way" and "he mopes around the house."

The nurse collected two types of data: previous patterns and current patterns. Change was inferred. Even with this minimal information it can be seen that the problem may be in the area of roles and relationships; perhaps family conflict is a tenable diagnostic hypothesis at this point.

Look again at the list of functional health patterns in Table 4-1. In which categories might the etiology of this problem reside? Isn't it probable that data about coping pattern, activity pattern, and value-belief pattern would help the nurse to identify etiological factors and perhaps also to refine the problem? For example, is the husband's activity tolerance low? Is that why he doesn't engage in activities within or outside the home? Are the wife's and husband's values, relative to their relationship, divergent? Is there a lack of resources for retired persons in this community or has a choice been made not to use them? Certainly, questions could be raised regarding the contribution of all other pattern areas to this problem.

This example points out two things. First, the categories provide a structure for analyzing a problem *within* a category, as in the example of husband-wife conflict within family role and relationships. Secondly, a structure is provided to focus the search for causal explanations, usually *outside* the problem category; in the example of the grocer, activities, values, and coping patterns would be explored.

To make information processing even easier, the current list of approved diagnoses (Appendix A) can be classified into the functional health pattern areas (Appendix C). As will be discussed in another chapter, a nurse can move horizontally from data in a pattern area to problem identification and then vertically through the patterns to identify etiological factors. Diagnosis is facilitated if information is gathered and organized in a way relevant to problem identification.

Does the process just described sound foreign? Consider that one usually is unable to make a judgment about data, such as heart rate or blood pressure, unless base-line data are available. Even one base-line measure and one current measure describe an elementary pattern across time, *if the nurse puts the data together.*

As another example, think of a friend's behavior that came to your attention recently. Did you expect or not expect the particular behavior? Why did you even have an expectation? Knowledge of your friend's previous behavioral patterns caused you to notice a difference. To understand the friend's behavior, information about the whole person and the situation (environmental events) was necessary. You have now been led to a synthesis. Many pieces of information have been put together to gain understanding.

The process is not foreign; human beings process information this way every day. When it is important for the life or comfort of another person that the correct synthesis and judgment occur, the process is done consciously and systematically.

Functional Patterns and Disease Patterns that are dysfunctional can lead to disease. Consider, as an example, heart disease. List the patterns in Figure 4-1 that increase a person's risk for heart disease. If nurses treated dysfunctional patterns there could be an impact on illness and death statistics for many disease conditions.

Pathology and its treatment can alter functional patterns; these alterations are the secondary functional effects of disease or treatment. Examples are changes in usual coping patterns and stress tolerance with disease, changes in elimination patterns and metabolism with bed rest, and the not uncommon readjustment of value-belief patterns after a life-threatening illness.

Figure 4-1 depicts secondary functional effects of disease. Consider a common case. A person is hospitalized for weight loss, frequent urination, thirst, and an elevated blood glucose level. Medical tests support a diagnosis of diabetes mellitus. Nurses familiar with the typical newly diagnosed client with diabetes will attest to the fact that secondary effects are widespread. The pathology, its treatment, the personal response of the client and family, and the

FIGURE 4-1
Effect of disease on functional patterns and of functional patterns on development of a disease.

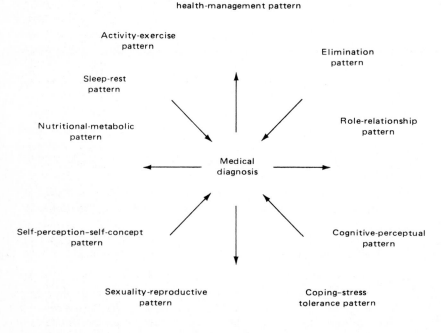

long-term management of the condition influence all functional patterns, as illustrated by the arrows in Figure 4-1 proceeding from medical diagnosis outward to pattern areas.

In addition to disturbances in functional patterns secondary to disease, dysfunctional patterns can occur when no evidence of disease is present. A client may be designated healthy from a medical perspective but still require nursing care. This phenomenon is also illustrated in Figure 4-1. Arrows proceeding from functional patterns to medical diagnosis represent the idea that unresolved dysfunctional patterns can increase susceptibility to various diseases, stressors, and microorganisms.

Few escape the media messages that life patterns can predispose to illness. One is told to walk or jog (exercise-activity pattern); cut down on saturated fats (nutritional-metabolic pattern); stop smoking, lose weight, and get regular checkups (health managagement pattern), learn to handle stress (role-relationship pattern), set priorities and ignore inconsequential annoyances (value-belief pattern), and remember "number one" (self-perception–self-concept pattern). This list is just to prevent cardiovascular disease.

Many people need help to work out productive health patterns. Nurses have always assumed responsibility for health promotion and health maintenance. Systematic, early identification and treatment of actual and potential problems (dysfunctional patterns) would probably have demonstrable effects on the health of the population.

Client-Environment Focus Interaction between the client and environment is an essential, common thread throughout all functional patterns. From this interaction, patterns develop. For example, patterns of role-relationships and self-concept are influenced by the environment, particularly people and culture. This influence begins at birth and is more pronounced as language and nonverbal behavior are learned. Taking and giving emotional support is another example of client-environment interaction; in this instance the interaction influences coping patterns.

Crop production, food additives, and environmental temperature all influence a nutritional-metabolic pattern. As another example, much has been said in news reports about human activities that negatively change the natural environment, such as industrial waste elimination patterns. This example illustrates a change in natural environmental patterns produced by human beings that then, in turn, influences human patterns. Client-environment interaction is an integral part of information collection in each pattern area.

Consider the example of environmental influences on the role-relationship pattern of an institutionalized elderly client confined to a wheelchair:

Role-relationship pattern States she is "last" of nine brothers and sisters; husband dead; no children; elderly friends not able to visit. Doctor (family friend) suggested she enter a nursing home one month ago after her stroke. Reports "what else could I do?" Prior to stroke was active socially. Currently is apathetic and withdrawn. States "everything is on schedule here; you're supposed to talk to people on schedule, go to this, go to that. Never before have I been told who I have to talk to. There is no way out; I can't do anything about it." States she asked to visit on another floor "where the clear-headed ones are" but "they're too busy or they come to take me when I'm tired sitting." States "They told me I had to live on this floor because I'm in a wheelchair." Appearance sad and withdrawn. Roommate and majority of other patients are confused.

The client's pattern of socialization and choices regarding socialization are dramatically influenced by her environment. Social isolation is evident. When combined with data in other pattern areas an underlying problem of powerlessness was diagnosed. Consideration of environmental influences on this functional pattern influenced care. Previously the patient had been considered "depressed," a superficial evaluation.

Developmental Focus   Nurses are concerned with human development of children and adults. Consequently any structure for information collection must include development. What is human development? Could it not be conceived as the development of the functional patterns? Human growth and development are reflected in each pattern area. Elimination patterns change, particularly in the area of control. Maturation toward adult norms occurs in role-relationship, cognitive-perceptual, and other patterns as years go by. The 11 functional patterns are judged, in part, against age norms, or developmental norms. Thus, a developmental focus is built into the functional typology.

Functional Focus   Questions may be raised about using the term *functional patterns*. Traditionally, "ways of living," or functional patterns, have been an important focus of nursing's health promotion, assistance, and rehabilitation activities. Yet *functional* is a term used in other professions also. It may be useful to consider differences and similarities. In medicine the word *function* is used to describe physiological function, such as respiratory function, cardiac function, or brain function. The diagnostic focus is on functions of organs and systems, not *integrative function of the whole individual.*

Another question is whether nurses are ever concerned *solely* with cardiac, neurological, or other systems assessment. In life-threatening situations, such as cardiac arrest, life saving takes priority. In caring for a patient who is unable to monitor his or her own heart rate or pupil dilation, nurses collect information for two purposes:

1 To understand or predict changes in functional health patterns
2 To report complications and disease progression to a physician when client lacks the expertise or ability to do this

The functional health patterns of clients represent human functioning at a higher and more complex level than the biological.

Usability in Practice   What makes an assessment format usable and useful in practice? *Usability* means that the format matches the competencies and time constraints of the users. *Usefulness* refers to the consistency between the format and the user's role.

Professional nurses are competent to assess the 11 functional health patterns. These are areas stressed in nursing textbooks and nursing education. In fact, the functional areas do not represent any new ideas, only a format for directing and organizing assessment in a systematic way. Higher levels of expertise develop with continued use.

The issue of an assessment tool's usability relative to the time available in clinical setting is important to nurses. As is often said, nurses never have enough time! This is not necessarily because they do not organize efficiently; sometimes clients' care needs exceed the staff time available. The length of time required to complete an admission assessment varies greatly. Time required depends partly on the ability of the nurse to zero in on the pertinent data and partly on the client. The *more health problems* a client has, the *more time* is needed to identify the underlying dysfunctional patterns.

It is hard to say which functional health patterns are not important to assess when a nurse is "too busy." Value-belief patterns? That one sounds abstract; can it be sacrificed? To do so is risky; later it may be found that all nursing care efforts have been in vain because the client's values or beliefs were ignored.

Is some information needed in all categories? It seems that an administrative problem exists if not every client entering the health care system can have a basic health assessment. If assessment is important, then it has to be done; if valued, then it will be done. Nurses have a difficult time depriving clients of something nurses feel is needed. When assessments are not done, usually it is because of the value-belief system of the nurse; when other valued activities cannot be carried out, the problem is referred to administration.

The practical response to the time dilemma can be problem screening in each pattern area. For example, a new client could be asked, "Most mornings when you wake up, do you feel rested and ready for the day's activities?" This screening question for the sleep-rest pattern may provide sufficient information to make a judgment about whether or not a problem exists. Other health problems, age, or observations can provide cues to help the nurse decide when the risk of screening, as opposed to full health assessment, can be taken.

In previous sections usefulness of the functional assessment has been discussed in regard to developmental and client-environment assessment. The usefulness for individual, family, and community assessment will become clearer in future sections of this chapter. If the central focus of nursing is human functioning, the format is useful in various specialties, such as psychiatric, gerontological, cardiac, and neurological nursing. From a nursing perspective, the client's disease or psychiatric disorder is just a variable influencing patterns, as is age and sex. Whether the nurse's framework is adaptation, self-care agency, life process or another model, functional patterns provide the *basic* data base. Perhaps the greatest argument for usefulness is that the format is being used. This is occurring in diverse settings and with diverse client populations and age groups.

Specific items that are assessed within each pattern are discussed in the next section. It will be clear that the functional pattern assessment format contains items required by most assessment tools. The format also screens for all current nursing diagnoses. *Functional health pattern assessment makes it easy to move from data to diagnosis.*

ASSESSMENT OF FUNCTIONAL HEALTH PATTERNS

An initial assessment of a client's functional health patterns is obtained through a nursing history and examination. Let us consider a brief overview of the history and examination so that the question "What to assess?" will be more meaningful.

Whenever a client is added to a nurse's caseload, an initial assessment is made of the 11 functional health patterns. This establishes the nursing data base. Initial assessments are referred to as a data base because (1) basic historical and current information about all health patterns is collected and (2) the information is used as base-line criteria against which any future changes are evaluated.

An admission assessment consists of a *nursing history* and an *examination.* The former is done by interviewing the client or others; the latter, by observation and other examination techniques. Generally, a comprehensive assessment is necessary. If a client's condition is critical (physiological or psychological instability exists), only very brief assessment of patterns may be warranted.

Information collection in the admission nursing *history* permits a systematic description of the 11 functional health patterns and the client's perception and explanation of any problems. Explanations clients provide for particular behaviors or situations are important. They can be diagnostic of knowledge deficits and health management deficits, among other things.

In primary care (ambulatory care) settings, a functional health pattern assessment and a biomedical systems assessment can be integrated. In these settings the history and examination are designed to detect dysfunctional health patterns *and* diseases. Tentative diagnoses of disease are referred to a physician or treated under protocols.

In home care a complete assessment is done when a family is initially visited. Similarly, community nurses responsible for program planning do a community assessment to reveal environmental and other problems influencing health patterns of groups. For example, in community assessment the *history* may include general dietary patterns of an elderly population; hazardous waste elimination patterns within a geographic area; the community's self-image pattern; and its level of activity as indicated by patterns of participation in work, political, or recreational activities. *Examination of the community* may include observations of people on busy streets or buses and observations of resources and facilities. (The local barber or bartender has a wealth of community information.)

Following the nursing history an *examination* is done. Observations are made of physical characteristics such as gait and mobility, skin integrity, heart rate, and range of joint movement. Cues obtained during history taking provide impressions of speech (tone, rate, and quality) and possibly interactions if another person is present (parent-child or client-other relationships). Assessment occurring in the home provides opportunities to observe living conditions, safety hazards, and the client's neighborhood.

At this point, it would be useful to review the nursing history and examination which appears in Appendix D. It will provide an overview of the "end-product." While reading the assessment in each of the 11 pattern areas notice the type of information collected in each area and the method of recording the admission interview. Underlying the history and examination is a structure for interviewing and observation. Screening questions and observations were planned in advance by the nurse, which helped the client describe his functional patterns and helped the nurse do a systematic assessment.

Let us now consider an assessment format for each functional health pattern. Depending on the practice setting, health screening may be limited to only one type of client: individuals, families, or communities. Yet, the identification and solution of a specific problem may require further information. The nurse may need to know about a *family* or *community* when identifying factors contributing to an *individual's* problems. Many times in family assessment, dysfunctional patterns of a particular member are detected; this may require use of the individual format. In *community assessment*, it may be necessary to interview a set of selected families if a high-risk group is detected. For these reasons it is important to be familiar with formats for assessing various types of clients.

While reviewing the following assessment formats,[1] note the following:

1 Each pattern is defined. The history (questions) and examination (observations) are derived from the definition.

2 Questions and observations are for *screening*. If the information obtained suggests problems are present (dysfunctional or potentially dysfunctional patterns), further questions and observations will be necessary. The critical defining characteristics of the diagnoses under consideration direct further assessment, as discussed in Chapters 6–8.

3 Questions in the history format are stated concisely. Individualize the interview by framing the question in your own way, and in a way suitable to the particular client and situation.

4 Combine information from the history and examination for *all* patterns to identify diagnoses and etiological or contributing factors.

1 Health-Perception–Health-Management Pattern

Definition   Describes the client's perceived pattern of health and well-being and how his or her health is managed. Includes the perception of health status

[1]Community assessment items are adapted from Gikow, F., & Kurcharski, P. Functional health pattern assessment of a community. Paper presented at American Public Health Association, 112th Annual Meeting, Anaheim, CA, November 13, 1984, which used the assessment to evaluate health-related needs of a community served by their agency.

and its relevance to current activities and future planning. Also included is the general level of health care behavior such as adherence to mental and physical preventive health practices, medical or nursing prescriptions, and follow-up care.

Discussion The goal of nursing is to promote health. Yet it is clients who actually perceive and manage their health. The clients' perceptions of their health status and the practices they use to maintain health can be assessed. This information may indicate a dysfunctional pattern or may influence decisions about interventions for other problems.

Clients may become despondent about changes in their health and believe they have no control over events. They may view "fate" rather than their behavior as the main determinant of health. Teaching health practices in these situations will be to no avail. Perceptions and beliefs have to be dealt with first.

The objective in assessing the health-perception-management pattern is to obtain data about general perceptions, general health management, and preventive practices. Specific details are explored in other relevant pattern areas. For example, if a client says laxatives are taken for constipation, this information is held and noted. The question that follows may be, "Do you find you can solve most of your health problems yourself?"

In this pattern area, cues to potential health hazards in client practices, potential or actual noncompliance, and unrealistic health or illness perception should not be missed.

Health-Perception–Health-Management Pattern: Individual Assessment
I History
  a How has *general* health been?
  b Any colds in past year? If appropriate: absences from work?
  c Most important things you do to keep healthy? Think these things make a difference to health? (Include family folk remedies, if appropriate.) Use of cigarettes, alcohol, drugs? Breast self-examination?
  d Accidents (home, work, driving)?
  e In past, been easy to find ways to follow things doctors or nurses suggest?
  f If appropriate: What do you think caused this illness? Actions taken when symptoms perceived? Results of action?
  g If appropriate: Things important to you while you're here? How can we be most helpful?
II Examination
  a General health appearance.

When asked, each of us can offer a generalization about our health pattern. Sometimes the reference is to recent years, for example, "I've really felt good these last few years." Other statements may refer to childhood, such as, "I was a sickly child and ever since . . ." or "I've never paid much attention to what I did; this illness has really taught me a lesson." The client's health perceptions can be used as a basis for understanding his or her past practices, including preventive measures, and for predicting future motivation toward health promotion.

Questions about health perceptions and health management may also elicit descriptions of illness. As the client talks about illness, *listen* for health perceptions and health management practices. For example, an adult client says, "After about a month of . . . (symptoms), I tried to find a doctor that would see me." Listening would cause the nurse to think, "Delay in seeking help? No established resource for health care? Knowledge of community resources? Routine check-ups?" Perceptions, meanings, responses, and practices are the nursing data.

Although examination is generally done after a history, general appearance can be observed during the interview. Observation of an individual's actual health practices is difficult. Usually a nurse has to rely on clients' reports unless information is available from home visits or a client in a hospital can be given responsibility for certain treatments.

Health-Perception–Health-Management Pattern: Family Assessment

I History

   a How has family's general health been (in last few years)?

   b Colds in past year? Absence from work/school?

   c Most important things you do to keep healthy? Think these make a difference to health? (Include family folk remedies, if appropriate.)

   d Members' use of cigarettes, alcohol, drugs?

   e Immunizations? Health care provider? Frequency of check-ups? Accidents (home, work, school, driving)? (If appropriate: Storage of drugs, cleaning products; scatter rugs, etc.)

   f In past, been easy to find ways to follow things doctors, nurses, social worker (if appropriate) suggest?

   g Things important in family's health that I could help with?

II Examination

   a General appearance of family members and home.

   b If appropriate: Storage of medicines; cribs, playpens, stove, scatter rugs, hazards, etc.

The family's perception of their health as a group usually is expressed in "we" statements such as "We've always been a healthy family because I see to it that. . . ." Usually one question phrased to obtain the group perception elicits both a perceived health pattern and explanations for the pattern. When individual members' health and health management (as perceived by the family representative speaking) are described, the nurse has to cluster data. A generalization about the family has to be made if each member's pattern and practices are described specifically. Listen to learn who seems to be the influential member in health-related decisions. This information may be useful if health practices need improving. Problems in the areas of general health management, risk factor control, use of health care system, and safety should not be missed.

Health-Perception–Health-Management Pattern: Community Assessment

I History (community representatives)

    a In general, what is the health/wellness level of the population on a scale of 1–5, with 5 being the highest level of health/wellness? Any major health problems?

    b Any strong cultural patterns influencing health practices?

    c People feel they have access to health services?

    d Demand for any particular health services or prevention programs?

    e People feel fire, police, safety programs sufficient?

II Examination (community records)

    a Morbidity, mortality, disability rates (by age group, if appropriate).

    b Accident rates (by district, if appropriate).

    c Currently operating health facilities (types).

    d On-going health promotion-prevention programs; utilization rates.

    e Ratio of health professionals to population.

    f Laws regarding drinking age.

    g Arrest statistics for drugs, drunk driving by age groups.

Listening to residents of a community, one may hear, "The drug problem here is terrible; this used to be a good community to raise children"; "We need a stop sign here for the children's crossing"; "They closed the clinic and now we have to go to the city"; or "Everybody's got the flu and it spreads through the schools; I can't remember a worse winter for sickness." Some of these statements provide cues to how people perceive the community's health pattern. Others provide cues about health management in the community. Sampling key groups can usually elicit historical patterns of "then and now" or "we've always been. . . ." The perceived reasons for patterns and practices usually are stated without prodding. If a problem is identified by a community group, the first step in health promotion is already accomplished. Other groups may have to be helped to gain insight into problems that exist.

Objective data on the health pattern of a community can be obtained from mortality and morbidity statistics, accident rates, and other data of public record. Assessing the use of health facilities and examining health legislation may also provide cues to a community's management pattern. Even more basic, do such services as home care, school health, and care of the aged exist?

2 Nutritional-Metabolic Pattern

Definition Describes pattern of food and fluid consumption relative to metabolic need and pattern indicators of local nutrient supply. Includes the individual's patterns of food and fluid consumption, daily eating times, the types and quantity of food and fluids consumed, particular food preferences, and the use of nutrient or vitamin supplements. Reports of any skin lesions and general ability to heal are included. The condition of skin, hair, nails, mucous membranes, and teeth and measures of body temperature, height, and weight are included.

Discussion   Clients' nutritional patterns and underlying dietary habits have always been a concern of nurses because of nurses' recognition that all life functions and well-being depend on adequate intake and the supply of nutrients to tissues. The focus of assessment in the nutritional-metabolic pattern area is food and fluid consumptions relative to metabolic need.

The assessment objective is to collect data about the typical pattern of food and fluid consumption. Additionally, gross indicators of metabolic need are assessed, such as growth states (child growth, pregnancy, and tissue healing). Subjective reports are obtained regarding food and fluid consumption, problems perceived by the client or others, the client's explanations of problems, actions taken to solve problems, and the perceived effect of those actions. Examination provides data on the observable effects of nutrient intake and supply relative to metabolic need.

Nutritional-Metabolic Pattern: Individual Assessment

I History
  a Typical daily food intake? (Describe.) Supplements (Vitamins, type of snacks)?
  b Typical daily fluid intake. (Describe.)
  c Weight loss/gain? (Amount.) Height loss/gain? (Amount.)
  d Appetite?
  e Food or eating: Discomfort? Swallowing? Diet restrictions?
  f Heal well or poorly?
  g Skin problems: Lesions, dryness?
  h Dental problems?
II Examination
  a Skin: bony prominences? Lesions? Color changes? Moistness?
  b Oral mucous membranes: color, moistness, lesions.
  c Teeth: General appearance and alignment. Dentures? Cavities? Missing teeth?
  d Actual weight, height?
  e Temperature.
  f Intravenous/parenteral feeding (specify).

The assessment of individual clients includes a typical daily intake of food, fluids, and nutrient supplements such as vitamins. Change in nutritional-metabolic patterns may be elicited through interview or observed during examination. Physical examination focuses on the skin, bony prominences, hair, oral mucous membranes, teeth, height and weight relative to age norms, and temperature. Physical indicators may provide validation of client reports regarding nutrient intake, nutrient supply to tissues, or metabolic need.

Assessment of the skin provides important data about quality of nutrient intake and supply of nutrients to this tissue. Indicators of nutritional pattern include tissue healing after injuries; skin integrity; and integrity of mucous membranes, hair, and nails. Skin and mucous membranes, in particular, are highly metabolic organs. Cell duplication is rapid and, accordingly, so is utilization of nutrients. Because of significant requirements, changes can be observed when problems exist in food or fluid consumption. Also, growth and physical development depend on nutrition and metabolism. As a minimum approach, the nurse should screen for patterns indicating nutritional and fluid deficits, excess intake, and skin alterations or breakdown.

Nutritional-Metabolic Pattern: Family Assessment
I History
  a Typical family meal pattern/food intake? (Describe.) Supplements (vitamins, types of snacks, etc.)?
  b Typical family fluid intake? (Describe.) Supplements: type available: fruit juices, soft drinks, coffee, etc.?
  c Appetites?
  d Dental problems? Dental care (frequency)?
  e Anyone have skin problems? Healing problems?
II Examination
  a If opportunity available: Refrigerator contents, meal preparation, contents of meal, etc.

Family or household patterns of food, fluid, and supplement consumption are especially important. Many of our habits, as well as likes and dislikes, are learned in the family setting. The family member who does the shopping and cooking is most important to the assessment (as well as to subsequent intervention); this may be the family member who makes the nutrition-related decisions. Again the aim is to obtain general patterns; if the need arises, a nurse may shift to individual assessment of one or more members.

Nutritional-Metabolic Pattern: Community Assessment
I History (community representatives)
  a In general, do most people seem well nourished? Children? Elderly?
  b Food supplement programs? Food stamps: rate of use?
  c Foods reasonable cost in this area relative to income?
  d Stores accessible for most? "Meals on Wheels" available?
  e Water supply and quality? Testing services (if most have own wells)? (If appropriate: Water usage cost? Any drought restrictions?)
  f Any concern that community growth will exceed good water supply?
  g Heating/cooling costs manageable for most? Programs?
II Examination
  a General appearance (nutritional appearance; teeth; clothing appropriate to climate)? Children? Adults? Elderly?

b Food purchases (Observations of food store check-out counters).
c "Junk" food (machines in schools, etc.).

There are nutritional-metabolic patterns for groups of people living in a geographic area. You've heard comments to substantiate this: "All these people are on food stamps, and you should see what they buy." "Look at the elderly in this place; they're all thin; never enough money for food." "Just sitting in the park you see all the pink-cheeked, healthy babies and kids; you know, our schools have thrown out all those junk food machines." By interview, observation of people, and checking community resources, a nurse can obtain an overview of qualitative and quantitative aspects of a community's pattern of food and fluid consumption.

3 Elimination Pattern

Definition   Describes patterns of excretory function (bowel, bladder, and skin) of individuals. Includes the individual's perceived regularity of excretory function, use of routines or laxatives for bowel elimination, and any changes or disturbances in time pattern, mode of excretion, quality, or quantity. Also included are any devices employed to control excretion. Includes family or community waste disposal pattern when appropriate.

Discussion   Regularity and control of elimination patterns are important in most people's lives. Perhaps culturally based toilet training and media commercials about body odor and waste disposal emphasize this functional health pattern. It is an important area in which to assess clients' concerns.

The assessment objective is to collect data about regularity and control of excretory patterns (bowel, bladder, skin, and wastes). Subjective descriptions, problems perceived by the client or others, the client's explanations of problems, remedial actions taken, and the perceived effects of those actions are the data of concern. Examination includes gross screening of specimens, inspection of prostheses (devices such as ostomy bags), noting any odors and observing family or community patterns of waste disposal.

Elimination Pattern: Individual Assessment
I History
   a Bowel elimination pattern. (Describe.) Frequency? Character? Discomfort? Problem in control? Laxatives, etc.?
   b Urinary elimination pattern. (Describe.) Frequency? Problem in control?
   c Excess perspiration? Odor problems?
   d Body cavity drainage, suction, etc. (Specify.)
II Examination
   a If indicated: Examine excreta or drainage color and consistency.

The individual client's descriptions of regularity, control, quantity, and other characteristics of bowel, bladder, and skin excretory patterns are assessed. If problems are perceived by the client or others, the nurse obtains explanations, finds out what remedial actions have been taken, and asks about the perceived effect of the actions.

The excretory pattern indicators (quantity, regularity, etc.) are applicable even if a client cannot utilize the normal route of excretion. There is still a bowel or urinary elimination pattern.

Laypeople have many misconceptions about regularity and control. Dependency on laxatives or enemas may mean that the client has a knowledge deficit regarding bowel regulation. This diagnosis should not be missed. Waste disposal, as discussed below, is also a component of excretory pattern that may be relevant to individual assessment during a home visit. Minimally, the nurse screens for patterns of incontinence and irregularity. Habits in regard to elimination, and data from other pattern areas (nutritional, for example), may explain a dysfunctional pattern.

Elimination Pattern: Family Assessment
I History
  a Family use of laxatives, other aids?
  b Problems in waste/garbage disposal?
  c Pet animals waste disposal (indoor/outdoor)?
  d If indicated: Problems with flies, roaches, rodents?
II Examination
  a If opportunity available: Examine toilet facilities, garbage disposal, pet waste disposal; indicators of risk for flies, roaches, rodents.

When asking about family excretory patterns, the nurse focuses on waste disposal and related hygienic practices. Thus in a home visit, the nurse may inquire whether garbage disposal is a problem. Observation should include sanitary practices related to waste disposal. These components of the excretory pattern would also be pertinent to an individual living alone.

Elimination Pattern: Community Assessment
I History (community representatives)
  a Major kinds of wastes (industrial, sewage, etc.)? Disposal systems? Recycling programs? Any problems perceived by community?
  b Pest control? Food service inspection (restaurants, street vendors, etc.)?
II Examination
  a Communicable disease statistics.
  b Air pollution statistics.

Communities are aggregates of individuals, households, and industries. Each of these social units has an excretory pattern of waste disposal that can influence the community. In recent years much attention has been given to hazardous waste disposal and air pollution. These topics, as well as common sanitation or disposal practices, are included in community assessment. Usually data can be collected from community leaders and from statistics on specific infections and diseases and radiation or pollution levels.

4 Activity-Exercise Pattern

Definition Describes pattern of exercise, activity, leisure, and recreation. Includes activities of daily living requiring energy expenditure, such as hygiene, cooking, shopping, eating, working, and home maintenance. Also included are the type, quantity, and quality of exercise, including sports, which describe the typical pattern. (Factors that interfere with the desired or expected pattern for the *individual*, such as neuromuscular deficits and compensations, dyspnea, angina, or muscle cramping on exertion, and, if appropriate, his or her cardiac/pulmonary classification, are included.) Leisure patterns are included and describe the recreational activities undertaken with others or alone. Emphasis is on activities of major importance to the client.

Discussion Movement is one of the most important functional patterns. It permits people to control their immediate physical environment. Assessment of activity patterns can lead to the detection of poor health practices, prevention of major functional losses, or helping to compensate for loss. The object of assessment is to determine the client's pattern of activities that require energy expenditure. Components reviewed are daily activities, exercise, and leisure activities. Subjective descriptions of these pattern components, problems perceived by the client or others, the client's perceived reasons for any existing problems, actions taken to solve the problems, and perceived effects of those actions are elicited. Observation is an important aspect of assessment in this pattern area.

Activity-Exercise Pattern: Individual Assessment

I History
  a Sufficient energy for desired/required activities?
  b Exercise pattern? Type? Regularity?
  c Spare time (leisure) activities? Child: play activities.
  d Perceived ability (code for level) for:

Feeding	_____	Grooming	_____
Bathing	_____	General mobility	_____
Toileting	_____	Cooking	_____
Bed mobility	_____	Home maintenance	_____
Dressing	_____	Shopping	_____

    Functional level codes:
      Level 0:   Full self-care

Level II: Requires use of equipment or device
Level III: Requires assistance or supervision from another
             person
Level IV: Is dependent and does not participate

II Examination

  a Demonstrated ability (code listed above) for:

Feeding ____   Dressing   ____   Cooking ____
Bathing ____   Grooming   ____   Shopping ____
Toileting ____   Bed mobility ____
General mobility ____   Home maintenance ____

  b Gait _____ Posture _____ Absent body part? (Specify) _____
  c Range of motion (joints) _____ Muscle firmness _____
  d Hand grip _____ Can pick up a pencil? _____
  e Pulse (rate) _____ (rhythm) _____ (strength) _____
  f Respirations (rate) _____ (rhythm) _____ Breath sounds _____
  g Blood pressure _____
  h General appearance (grooming, hygiene, energy level)

The nurse must assess the client's routine daily activities. These include the client's perceived capabilities for movement, self-care (feeding, bathing, dressing, grooming, and toileting) and, if relevant, home management. Each can be classified using the functional levels 0–IV. Classifications also exist for assessing activity tolerance of clients with cardiac or pulmonary problems.

Irrespective of the client's mobility level, some degree of either active or passive exercise is needed. During assessment the type, amount, and frequency of exercise should be elicited. People also need leisure activities. Assessment of the activity-exercise pattern includes the type of recreational activities and the amount of time spent pursuing them.

The screening examination of the client may be limited to gait, posture, muscle tone, absence of body part, and prostheses or assistive devices employed. If indicated, assessment of his or her range of motion in joints, hand grip, and ability to pick up a pencil will provide additional data. Pulse rate and rhythm and respiratory rate and depth may explain subjective reports about activity tolerance.

Minimally, screening assessment should reveal any actual or potential dysfunctional activity patterns. In particular, deficits in mobility, self-care, home management, and diversional activity should not be missed. The potential for joint contractures and ineffective airway clearance are also problems nurses have identified as within their scope of diagnostic judgment. These two conditions can predispose to activity pattern dysfunctions. In general, if a client has a cardiac, neurological, or respiratory disease, in-depth assessment is warranted. Also, developmental problems may be revealed by assessment of specific motor skills in children.

Activity-Exercise Pattern: Family Assessment

I History
  a In general, does family get a lot/little exercise? Type? Regularity?
  b Family leisure activities? Active/passive?
  c Problems in shopping (transportation), cooking, keeping up the house, budgeting for food, clothes, housekeeping, house costs?
II Examination
  a Pattern of general home maintenance, personal maintenance.

Families can exhibit activity patterns. Some households run at a hectic level, others seem almost lethargic. Pace of activities is a characteristic of family activity; it may or may not be related to the number of family members.

Other than clichés, such as "The family that plays [leisure pattern] together, stays together," minimal information exists in nursing about family activity patterns. Doing things together and sharing recreational interests would appear to increase family solidarity. No diagnoses have been identified in the area of family activity patterns. Problems in home maintenance, general self-care, and exercise or leisure patterns should not be missed.

Activity-Exercise Pattern: Community Assessment

I History (community representatives)
  a How do people find the transportation here? To work? To recreation? To health care?
  b People have/use community centers (seniors, others)? Recreation facilities for children? Adults? Seniors?
  c Is housing adequate (availability, cost)? Public housing?
II Examination
  a Recreation/cultural programs.
  b Aids for the disabled.
  c Residential centers, nursing homes, rehabilitation facilities relative to population needs.
  d External maintenance of homes, yards, apartment houses.
  e General activity level (e.g., bustling, quiet).

Communities have rhythmic activity patterns. Some "roll up the sidewalks" at 9 p.m. and other are bustling night and day. In communities, activity can be associated with noise and crowding and may elicit complaints from residents who wish for more peace and quiet. Community activity patterns are also often beneficial, such as scheduled recreation. These resources permit individuals and families to socialize and enjoy leisure. Any community could be described in terms of its diversional activities, both recreational and cultural.

Evidence that generalizations can be made at the community activity level include statements such as, "There is nothing to do in this town" or "I'm so busy since I retired, with all the senior citizen activities going on." Because political, recreational, and cultural activities fulfill the lives of people, community assessment should include this pattern area.

Communities also have mobility patterns—public transportation systems. Information in this area is important for understanding accessibility to facilities for health care, recreation, or socialization.

5 Sleep-Rest Pattern

Definition Describes patterns of sleep, rest, and relaxation. Includes patterns of sleep and rest-relaxation periods during the 24-hour day. Includes the perception of the quality and quantity of sleep and rest, and perception of energy level. Included also are aids to sleep such as medications or night-time routines that are employed.

Discussion Preoccupations with sleep arise only when it eludes us; otherwise it is something taken for granted. In today's busy world, rest and relaxation may also elude a lot of people.

The objective in assessing a sleep-rest pattern is to describe the effectiveness of the pattern from the client's perspective. Some are well rested after 4 hours of sleep; others need much more. Rest and relaxation are also assessed in regard to client perceptions. What may be relaxing to some is considered work by others. If problems are perceived by the client or others, explanations, previous actions taken, and perception of their effect are elicited.

Sleep-Rest Pattern: Individual Assessment
I History
    a Generally rested and ready for daily activities after sleep?
    b Sleep onset problems? Aids? Dreams (nightmares)? Early awakening?
    c Rest-relaxation periods?
II Examination
    a If appropriate: Observe sleep pattern.

The nurse screens the client's sleep-rest pattern by finding out about the person's general feeling of readiness for daily activities after sleep. If problems are perceived, the dysfunctional pattern is described. Rest and relaxation comprise a second component to be assessed in this pattern.

If problems are present, assessment should include sleep onset, sleep interruption (including dreams), or early awakening patterns. Sleep pattern reversal (day-night reversal) is another problem that should not be overlooked. Use of sleeping aids, both prescription and nonprescription, should be elicited during pattern assessment. As previously stated, the client's perception of a dysfunctional pattern provides valuable cues. Clients who appear to sleep but report sleep deprivation may not be getting sufficient deep sleep.

Sleep-Rest Pattern: Family Assessment

I History
  a Generally, family members seem to be well rested and ready for school/work?
  b Sufficient sleeping space and quiet?
  c Family find time to relax?
II Examination
  a If opportunity available: Observe sleeping space and arrangements.

There may be a general pattern of sleep within a family. Some adhere to "early to bed, early to rise." Rest and relaxation patterns also are frequently built into family patterns. These can be assessed. Sometimes the family pattern is disturbed because of one member's sleep problem. This situation may require a shift to individual assessment.

Sleep-Rest Pattern: Community Assessment

I History (community representatives)
  a Generally quiet at night in most neighborhoods?
  b Usual business hours? Industries round-the-clock?
II Examination
  a Activity-noise levels in business district. In residential district.

Communities usually have patterns of sleeping, resting, and relaxation. Some towns are described as "never shut down." Disturbances in the community sleep-rest pattern can be inferred from residents' comments about continuous highway noise or airplanes going over all night. Such disturbance produces health concerns and can increase levels of stress.

6 Cognitive-Perceptual Pattern

Definition   Describes sensory-perceptual and cognitive pattern. Includes the adequacy of sensory modes, such as vision, hearing, taste, touch, or smell, and the compensation or protheses utilized for disturbances. Reports of pain perception and how pain is managed are also included when appropriate. Also included are the cognitive functional abilities, such as language, memory, and decision making.

Discussion   To think, hear, see, smell, taste, and touch are human functions taken for granted until deficits arise. Prevention of deficits and helping clients to compensate for losses are important nursing activities.
    The objective of assessing the client's cognitive-perceptual pattern is to describe the adequacy of his or her language, cognitive skills, and perception relative to desired or required activities. Subjective descriptions, problems perceived by the client or others, compensations for deficits, and the effectiveness of efforts to compensate for them are elicited during the history.

During examination, observations are made of cognitive and sensory capabilities. Data in this pattern area are critical for future nursing intervention. For example, if judgment capabilities are inadequate, a client may need supervision. If the person is blind, safety may be a problem.

Cognitive-Perceptual Pattern: Individual Assessment

I History
  a Hearing difficulty? Aid?
  b Vision? Wear glasses? Last checked? When last changed?
  c Any change in memory lately?
  d Big decision easy/difficult to make?
  e Easiest way for you to learn things? Any difficulty?
  f Any discomfort? Pain? If appropriate: how do you manage it?
II Examination
  a Orientation.
  b Hears whisper?
  c Reads newsprint?
  d Grasps ideas and questions (abstract, concrete)?
  e Language spoken.
  f Vocabulary level. Attention span.

Cognitive and perceptual pattern components are assessed. Cognitive functions include language capability, memory, problem solving, and decision making. These are basic functions but should be evaluated relative to the complexity of environment chosen by the client. A mentally retarded person may function quite independently in a sheltered environment. An active business executive in the same type of environment may exhibit symptoms of sensory or cognitive deprivation.

Examination of cognitive patterns occurs during the history. The nurse observes the client's language skills, grasp of ideas and abstractions, attention span, level of consciousness, reality testing, and any aids required for communication. Some problem the client describes during assessment can be selected to measure problem solving and decision making. In fact, in each pattern area the client's perception of problems, reasons for problems, actions taken, and perceived effectiveness of actions provide a wealth on cognitive functions.

The subjective report of the client regarding patterns of vision, hearing, touch, taste, and smell can be supplemented by actual testing. For example, keep some newsprint in your pocket and use it to screen for visual difficulties. Don't forget to assess prostheses such as glasses or hearing aids.

The ability to feel pain or discomfort is another sensory capability of human beings. If pain is present, especially chronic pain, ask the client how he or she manages it. The answer may reveal deficits in pain management that require intervention. Nurses have many ways of helping people deal with pain.

In assessing cognitive functions and sensory modes, be alert to compensations clients may use that mask basic dysfunctions. Safety of the client may be jeopardized if problems are not detected. Remember that at times we all have memory lapses, make illogical statements, and fail to recognize a familiar object or person. It may be necessary to elicit impressions from family members to differentiate between common, temporary lapses and progressive deficits.

Cues to sensory deficits, sensory deprivation or overload, and pain management problems must not be overlooked. Impaired reasoning, knowledge deficits related to health practices, and memory deficits are additional problems that may exist and may even be the basis for other dysfunctional patterns. If problems are perceived by the client or others, explanations of previous actions taken to relieve the problem and perceptions of the effect of actions are elicited.

Cognitive-Perceptual Pattern: Family Assessment
I History
    a Visual or hearing problems? How managed?
    b Any big decisions family has had to make? How made?
II Examination
    a If indicated: Language spoken at home.
    b Grasp of ideas and questions (abstract/concrete).
    c Vocabulary level.

The cognitive-perceptual pattern of a family is evident in how family decisions are made, the concreteness or abstractness of thinking, and whether decisions are oriented to the future or present. Data in these areas may be the basis for understanding other problems such as family disorganization and stress. Nurses have a number of ways of helping families in the cognitive-perceptual area of health functioning.

Cognitive-Perceptual Pattern: Community Assessment
I History (community representatives)
    a Most groups speak English? Bilingual?
    b Educational level of population?
    c Schools seen as good/need improving? Adult education desired/available?
    d Types of problems that require community decisions? Decision making process? What's the best way to get things done/changed here?
II Examination
    a School facilities. Drop-out rate.
    b Community government structure; decision-making lines.

While assessing a community a nurse can obtain data on decision making, especially regarding health-related matters. Are the school board and parent-teacher association effective? How are community decisions made? Sitting in on meetings of committees dealing with health issues usually provides a wealth of information. Do all groups participate, and are their voices heard regarding health matters? Is future planning done, or are crisis reactions the pattern? These questions can elicit data about the cognitive processes operating in a community.

7 Self-Perception–Self-Concept Pattern

Definition   Describes self-concept pattern and perceptions of self. Includes the attitudes about self, perception of abilities (cognitive, affective, or physical), image, identity, general sense of worth, and general emotional pattern. Pattern of body posture and movement, eye contact, voice, and speech patterns are included.

Discussion   Many psychologists have tried to describe the consciousness of being, or awareness of existence, that all humans have. This sense of being is commonly referred to as the self. Clients have perceptions and concepts of themselves, such as body image, social self, self-competency, and subjective mood states. Negative evaluations of the self can produce personal discomfort and also can influence other functional patterns. Change, loss, and threat are common factors that may impinge on self-concept.

The objective of assessment in this pattern area is to describe the client's pattern of beliefs and evaluations regarding general self-worth and feeling states. Problems the clients or others identify, explanations or reasons they identify for the problem, actions taken to try to solve the problems, and effects of those actions are also described.

Assessment of self-concept and self-perception usually is not effective (accurate and thorough) unless the client has a sense of trust in the nurse. People tend not to share personal feelings unless the nurse has already established an empathic and nonjudgmental atmosphere. As Powell reminds us, "But, if I tell you who I am, you may not like who I am, and it is all that I have" (1969, p. 12).

Self-Perception–Self-Concept Pattern: Individual Assessment
I History
  a How describe self? Most of the time, feel good (not so good) about self?
  b Changes in body or things you can do? Problem to you?
  c Changes in way you feel about self or body (since illness started)
  d Things frequently make you angry? Annoyed? Fearful? Anxious? Depressed? Not being able to control things? What helps?
  e Ever feel you lose hope?
II Examination
  a Eye contact. Attention span (distraction).
  b Voice and speech pattern. Body posture.

c Nervous (5) or relaxed (1); rate from 1 to 5.
d Assertive (5) or passive (1); rate from 1 to 5.

A person's self-perception–self-concept pattern may be screened by obtaining data about (1) general feelings of self-worth and personal identity and (2) general emotional pattern. If cues or situations warrant, more in-depth assessment can be done.

Observation during an admission interview can reveal nonverbal cues about self-concept and self-perception. Body posture and movement, eye contact, and voice and speech pattern are important to observe. Cues to identity confusion, altered body image, lowered self-esteem, perceptions of powerlessness, situational depression, and fear should not be missed.

Self-Perception–Self-Concept Pattern: Family Assessment

I History
  a Most of time family feels good (not so good) about themselves as a family?
  b General mood of family? Happy? Anxious? Depressed? What helps family mood?
II Examination
  a General mood state: nervous (5) or relaxed (1); rate from 1 to 5.
  b Members generally assertive (5) or passive (1); rate from 1 to 5.

Families have perceptions and concepts about their image; their status in the community; and their competency, as a unit, to deal with life. Emotional patterns tend to be shared because of the close relationships in a family or household. Situations that affect one member usually produce an effect on the entire family group. To help a family realize its potential, the nurse needs to assess how the family members perceive their family.

Self-Perception–Self-Concept Pattern: Community Assessment

I History (community representatives)
  a Good community to live in? Going up in status, down, about same?
  b Old community? Fairly new?
  c Any age group predominate?
  d People's moods in general: Enjoying life, stressed, feeling "down"?
  e People generally have kind of abilities needed in this community?
  f Community/neighborhood functions? Parades?
II Examination
  a Racial, ethnic mix (if appropriate).
  b Socioeconomic level.
  c General observations of mood.

Just as families and individuals have patterns of self-worth and personal identity, so have communities. Image, status, and perceived competency to deal with problems are characteristics that can be assessed.

The image of a community may be reflected in housing conditions, buildings, and cleanliness. Community perception of self-worth may relate to school systems, crime rates, accidents, and whether residents and outsiders consider it "a good place to live." Competency in dealing with social and political issues and community spirit cause self-evaluation to be positive. Knowing the level of community "pride" may assist a nurse in innovative health programs. The emotional tone (fear, depression, or a generally positive emotional outlook) can usually be related to findings in other pattern areas. For example, tensions in the community relationship pattern may explain a general feeling of fear in the residents.

8 Role-Relationship Pattern

Definition Describes pattern of role engagements and relationships. Includes perception of the major roles and responsibilities in current life situation. Satisfaction or disturbances in family, work, or social relationships and responsibilities related to these roles are included.

Discussion Much has been written about relationships, including the human need for others and the influence of relationships on personal and group development. People engage in many levels of relationships. Some are very close, such as family relationships. Others are superficial and without any true sharing, as described in the lyrics of "The Sounds of Silence" by Paul Simon:

> And in the naked night I saw
> Ten thousand people, maybe more,
> People talking without speaking,
> People hearing without listening,
> People writing songs that voices never shared.
> No one dared
> Disturb the sounds of silence.[2]

The objective of role-relationship pattern assessment is to describe a client's pattern of family and social roles. The client's perception about his or her relationship patterns (satisfactions and dissatisfactions) is also a component of this pattern area. If problems are perceived by the client, the perceived cause, actions taken and effects of actions are elicited.

Role-Relationship Pattern: Individual Assessment
I History
   a Live alone? Family? Family structure (diagram)?
   b Any family problems you have difficulty handling (nuclear/extended)?
   c Family or others depend on you for things? How managing?
   d If appropriate: How family/others feel about illness/hospitalization?

[2]© 1964, 1965 by Paul Simon. Used by permission.

  e If appropriate: Problems with children? Difficulty handling?
  f Belong to social groups? Close friends? Feel lonely (frequency)?
  g Things generally go well at work? (School?)
  h If appropriate: Income sufficient for needs?
  i Feel part of (or isolated in) neighborhood where living?
II Examination
  a Interaction with family member(s) or others (if present).

The major role-taking and relationship patterns in a person's life situation are the components of the role-relationship pattern. Family roles, work or student roles, and social roles are some of the major aspects assessed. Clients' satisfactions and dissatisfactions with role responsibilities and relationships are elicited. If the client perceives problems in this pattern area, then perceived reasons for the problems, actions that have been taken to remedy the problems, and effects of those actions are assessed.

Family roles are usually particularly important in the individual's life. Discussion with a client in this area discloses how many are in the family group or household, including both children and adults, and whether there is a nuclear or extended family. Roles and relationships are usually reviewed before the sexuality-reproductive pattern. This sequence permits a natural transition in the discussion.

Loss, change, or threat produce the major problems in the role-relationship pattern. The cues that should not be missed are related to problems such as grieving, conflict, social isolation, impaired verbal communication, and potential for violence.

Working roles and relationships are an important area to assess. Statistics indicate that many people (nurses included) suffer occupational role stress (McLean, 1978). Assessment should include whether the client perceives the work environment to be safe and healthy. Does the work role leave time for rest and leisure? Because work has the potential to contribute to self-fulfillment, the client's satisfaction with work roles and organizations of work activities is assessed. Financial concerns, unemployment, and other issues related to work are identified. Assessment of the school-age client or college student should elicit any problems related to roles and relationships in these settings.

Role-Relationship Pattern: Family Assessment
I History
  a Family (or household) members? Member age and family structure (diagram).
  b Any family problems that are difficult to handle (nuclear/extended)? Child rearing?
  c Relationships good (not so good) among family members? Siblings? Support each other?
  d If appropriate: Income sufficient for needs?
  e Feel part of (or isolated) from community? Neighbors?

II Examination
   a Interaction among family members (if present).
   b Observed family leadership roles.

Roles and relationships of a particularly close kind are a fundamental aspect of family life. Relationships can be supportive and growth-producing. At the opposite extreme, violence and abuse can permeate relationships of families under stress.

As with individual assessment, structural aspects of the family are assessed. These include living space, number of members, their ages, and their various roles.

There are a number of ways the dynamics of family relationships can be assessed. One is in terms of interdependence, dependence, and independence. Another approach is based on the ways relationships influence the family's developmental tasks. Family developmental tasks, according to Duvall (1967), include (1) physical maintenance; (2) resource allocation; (3) division of labor; (4) socialization of members; (5) reproduction, recruitment, and release of members; (6) maintenance of order; and (7) maintenance of motivation and morale.

Role-Relationship Pattern: Community Assessment

I History (community representatives)
   a People seem to get along well together here? Places where people tend to go to socialize?
   b Do people feel they are heard by government? High/low participation in meetings?
   c Enough work/jobs for everybody? Wages good/fair? Do people seem to like kind of work available (happy in their jobs/job stress)?
   d Any problems with riots, violence in the neighborhoods? Family violence? Problems with child/spouse/elder abuse?
   e Get along with adjacent communities? Collaborate on any community projects?
   f Do neighbors seem to support each other?
   g Community get-togethers?
II Examination
   a Observation of interactions (generally or at specific meetings).
   b Statistics on interpersonal violence.
   c Statistics on employment, income/poverty.
   d Divorce rate.

The basic function of a community lies in its collaborative relationships and allocation of role responsibilities. Nursing assessment is particulary concerned with whether a community structure of roles and relationships permits residents to realize their health-related potentialities. Patterns of crime, racial incidents, and social networks are indexes of human relationships in a community.

9 Sexuality-Reproductive Pattern

Definition   Describes patterns of satisfaction or dissatisfaction with sexuality; describes reproductive pattern. Includes the perceived satisfaction or disturbances in sexuality or sexual relationships. Included also is the female's reproductive state, pre- or postmenopause, and any perceived problems.

Discussion   Sexuality is the behavioral expression of sexual identity. It may involve, but is not limited to, sexual relationships with a partner. Just as in other functional patterns, cultural norms regulate expression.

Currently in western society the norms for sexuality are in a state of flux. The distinction between what is masculine and what is feminine is sometimes blurred, and the scope of acceptable sexual expression is widening within some groups. Yet society imposes limits. Sexual abuse of children and incest is not tolerated. When clients choose modes of expression that are marginally acceptable, problems can arise. Individual problems may also arise when discrepancies exist between the expression of sexuality the person has attained and the expression he or she desires.

Reproductive patterns involve reproductive capacity and reproduction itself. The cultural norms that affect reproduction are also undergoing change. The number of children in families is smaller than in past generations and in many cases pregnancies and births are planned.

The objective of assessment in the sexuality-reproductive pattern is to describe perceived problems or potential problems. If problems exist the client is asked about contributing factors, actions taken, and the perceived effect of actions.

Sexuality-Reproductive Pattern: Individual Assessment

I History
   a If appropriate to age and situation: Sexual relationships satisfying? Changes? Problems?
   b If appropriate: Use of contraceptives? Problems?
   c Female: When menstruation started? Last menstrual period? Menstrual problems? Para? Gravida?

II Examination
   a None unless problem identified or pelvic exam is part of full physical assessment.

A screening assessment of an individual client's expression of sexuality is focused on developmental patterns and perceived satisfactions or dissatisfactions. If problems are perceived, the nurse obtains the client's explanation of the problem, a history of remedial action taken, and the client's opinion about the effectiveness of those actions. It is important not to miss problems related to expression of sexuality in clients of any age.

Assessment of reproductive patterns involves collecting information about the client's stage of reproductive development in relationship to developmental milestones such as menarche or climacteric. Number of pregnancies and live births provide information about a female client's reproductive pattern. Development of reproductive capacities (secondary sex characteristics and genital development) should be assessed in young clients. It is important not to miss problems associated with contraceptives, reproduction, menstruation, or climacteric.

Sexuality-Reproductive Pattern: Family Assessment
I History
  a If appropriate (sexual partner within household or situation): Sexual relations satisfying? Changes? Problems?
  b Use of family planning? Contraceptives? Problems?
  c If appropriate (to age of children): Feel comfortable in explaining/discussing sexual subjects?
II Examination: None

The information collected in assessment of a family's sexuality pattern includes a couple's level of satisfaction with their sexual relationship, any problems they perceive, how the problems are managed, and the results of actions taken to resolve the problems. When there are children in the household, the nurse would be interested in what information about sexual subjects is taught to children as well as when and how this is communicated. If the adults feel uninformed or uncomfortable in discussing sexual subjects with children, the nurse who is aware of the problem can provide important assistance. Although previously considered a very personal matter, sexual relationships and feelings related to sexual identity have become more openly discussed. This trend toward freer discussion may not affect all clients; thus the nurse obtains information in a sensitive manner.

The reproductive pattern assessment includes any problems the couple perceives, explanations they offer for the problems, actions they have taken to deal with the problems, and the result of the actions. The number and ages of children, number and outcomes of pregnancies, and birth control methods in use are included in the family data base.

Sexuality-Reproductive Pattern: Community Assessment
I History (community representatives)
  a Average family size?
  b Do people feel there are any problems with pornography, prostitution? Other?
  c Do people want/support sex education in schools/community?
II Examination
  a Family size and types of households.
  b Male/female ratio.
  c Average maternal age. Maternal mortality rate. Infant mortality rate.

d Teen pregnancy rate.
e Abortion rate.
f Sexual violence statistics.
g Laws/regulations regarding information on birth control.

Community attitudes toward sexuality are assessed. Do educational programs exist in schools or churches? Does the community desire such programs? If the residents view sex education as a function of the family, are there programs for parents?

Crime in general was assessed in the area of relationships. In the sexuality-reproductive pattern it is useful to note the incidence of sex-related crime or sexual abuse of children in the community. A high incidence may indicate the need for increased community awareness and action.

The reproductive pattern of a community is reflected in birth, miscarriage, and abortion rates. Maternal and fetal mortality rates are also very important indicators. The accessibility of health services as well as availability of childbirth education programs should be assessed. Access to family planning and abortion services is assessed in terms of the community's desire for such services. In areas with high rates of adolescent pregnancies, the availability of programs for continued schooling is assessed.

Compiling such information enables the nurse to evaluate community needs and available services. Problems are identified when needs and health services do not match. The sexuality-reproductive pattern of individuals, families, and communities can be viewed as a component of the role-relationship pattern. It is listed separately so that sexual and reproductive assessment are not neglected. An additional reason for separating the two is that sexuality and reproduction involve a different level of relationships than those established in social or work groups. The assessment interview should flow smoothly from self-concept pattern to relationships with others and then on to sexual relationships.

10 Coping–Stress Tolerance Pattern

Definition Describes general coping pattern and effectiveness of the pattern in terms of stress tolerance. Includes the reserve or capacity to resist challenges to self-integrity, modes of handling stress, family or other support systems, and perceived ability to control and manage situations.

Discussion Stress is a part of living for any person at any age. In fact, many say that without stress there would be no growth. For example, learning to walk places stress on bones, a factor necessary for their integrity and development. Separating from the security of home also produces stress but leads to social development.

Stressor, coping, and *stress tolerance* are three terms whose definitions are intertwined. A *stressor* is an event that threatens or challenges the integrity of the human being. It produces a psychophysiological response that can lead to growth and further development or to disorganization manifested as anxiety, fear, depression, and other changes in self-perception or roles and relationships.

People respond to events differently. To know if a particular event is stressful for a person, family, or community the nurse has to ascertain the *client's* perception or definition of the situation. Community disasters, loss of a family member, illness, or hospitalization are usually perceived as a threat to integrity or to the usual pattern of life activities; thus, these are stressors. The meaning of potentially stressful events and the perceived degree of control over the events influence the amount of stress induced.

The way in which people generally respond to events perceived as a threat is their *coping pattern.* Clients' general patterns of coping may or may not be effective in handling stressful situations. Some clients employ problem solving; others respond with denial or other mental mechanisms. All these are learned behaviors for dealing with stress. The more effective the coping pattern, the greater sense of control the client can exert over the threat to integrity.

Stress tolerance pattern describes the amount of stress the client has handled effectively. This, of course, is related to the amount of stress previously experienced and the effectiveness of coping patterns. A client's stress tolerance pattern predicts, to some extent, potential for effective coping; however, people can mobilize resources and withstand levels of stress that exceed their previous experience.

The objective of assessment in this pattern area is to describe the stress tolerance and coping pattern of a client. Not to be missed are changes in the effectiveness of a coping pattern, which can occur if a threat to integrity is perceived as beyond personal control (personal coping capacity). This type of situation should lead the nurse to make a more in-depth assessment of support systems available to the client.

Coping–Stress Tolerance Pattern: Individual Assessment
I History
  a   Any big changes in your life in the last year or two? Crisis?
  b   Who's most helpful in talking things over? Available to you now?
  c   Tense or relaxed most of the time? When tense what helps?
  d   Use any medicines, drugs, alcohol?
  e   When (if) have big problems (any problems) in your life, how do you handle them?
  f   Most of the time, is this (are these) way(s) successful?
II Examination: None

The nurse asks the client to recall stressful life events, briefly tell how they were managed, and evaluate the effectiveness with which he or she coped with those situations. This history provides information about stress tolerance and coping pattern.

Data from other pattern areas may indicate that the client perceives a current or an anticipated threat to integrity. If such a threat is perceived, assessment proceeds to an examination of perceived control; that is, the nurse inquires how the client plans to deal with the situation and has the client evaluate the likelihood that the proposed coping pattern will be effective.

Why the emphasis on the individual's perception of events? This is because, as Selye says, "It is not what happens to you, but the way you take it [that matters]" (1979). Surgical mortality rate may be less than 1 percent, a low probability of death, yet if the client perceives the threat of death as high, surgery will be a stressor. Clients' personal concepts, constructed from the knowledge they have, determine their reactions. In a sense it is irrelevant what reality is; reality "is" whatever the client perceives. This is why subjective data are so important. Intervention begins with the way the client views the situation.

Coping–Stress-Tolerance Pattern: Family Assessment
I History
  a Any big changes within family in last few years?
  b Family tense or relaxed most of time? When tense what helps? Anyone use medicines, drug, alcohol to decrease tension?
  c When (if) family problems, how handled?
  d Most of the time is this way(s) successful?
II Examination: None

Dimensions of family assessment in this pattern area are similar to those in individual assessment. It is well to remember that family life revolves around a set of interrelationships. These relationships can be the supportive structure of a coping pattern but also can be a source of stress.

Coping–Stress Tolerance Pattern: Community Assessment
I History (community representatives)
  a Any groups that seem to be under stress?
  b Need/availability of phone help-lines? Support groups (health related, other)?
II Examination
  a Delinquency, drug abuse, alcoholism, suicide, psychiatric illness, statistics.
  b Unemployment rate by race/ethnic/sex.

Stressors are sometimes experienced by a whole community. These are usually revealed in the data of previous pattern areas and may include such problems as unemployment, racial or ethnic tensions, drug problems, or accident rates. Natural disasters may threaten community integrity and require outside support for coping patterns.

A pattern of coping with community-wide stressors is usually revealed by interviews with community members. Leaders are quick to evaluate the effectiveness of community coping and "what works in our town." A community's stress tolerance depends upon supportive relationships between community groups.

11 Value-Belief Pattern

Definition   Describes patterns of values, goals, or beliefs (including spiritual) that guide choices or decisions. Includes what is perceived as important in life and any perceived conflicts in values, beliefs, or expectations that are health related.

Discussion   A pattern of valuing and believing is found at all ages. As people develop, the emerging pattern of values and beliefs becomes more complex and, generally, more conscious. Beliefs and values include opinions about what is correct, proper, meaningful, and good, in a personal sense. Collective value and belief patterns also exist within a society or culture. These group norms may or may not be consistent with the personal pattern of a particular client or health care provider. Conflicts can arise. When important alternatives present themselves, values help determine choices. Choices deal with what is right or wrong for the person. *Right and wrong* relate to action; *good and bad* refer to outcomes or goals (Steele and Harmon, 1979, pp. 1–4).

Belief patterns describe what people hold to be true on the basis of faith or conviction. They are arrived at by inference and form the basis for attitudes or predispositions. Beliefs are the philosophical and theological dimensions of personal knowing. They include explanations at a very abstract level, including explanations of life, existence, and why certain things are valued. Common, day-to-day actions may not require this level of thought and explanation. Illness and other significant events provide the time and motivation to review life, goals, and what is important.

Patterns of valuing describe the importance or worth accorded to goals, actions, people, objects, and other phenomena. The value pattern can influence a client's health-related decisions about personal practices, treatments, health priorities, and even life or death.

The objective in assessing clients' value-belief pattern is to understand the basis for health-related decisions and actions. This understanding increases sensitivity to value-belief conflicts that may arise if preventive action isn't taken.

Value-Belief Pattern: Individual Assessment
I History
  a Generally get things you want from life? Important plans for the future?
  b Religion important in life? If appropriate: Does this help when difficulties arise?
  c If appropriate: Will being here interfere with any religious practices?
II Examination: None

Life requires decisions. Thus, as human beings develop they construct a system of beliefs and values, in fact a philosophical system. This system provides guidelines for important decisions and ways of behaving. It may or may not be tied to theological and religious beliefs and values.

The assessment of value-belief patterns focuses on what is important to clients in their lives. Beliefs and values can be regarded as spiritual in the broadest sense of "human spirit." Usually nurses assess more specific areas, such as religious preference or religious practices. This broader view of "what is important" includes, but is not limited to, religious practices.

Understanding a client's personal value-belief pattern can increase sensitivity to potential conflicts and help clients examine ways their belief system can assist them in decision making. Clients' use of philosophical or theological values and beliefs as a predominant coping strategy has not been systematically studied in nursing. The nurse who understands the client's spiritual beliefs (including, but not limited to, religious beliefs) may be able to support coping strategies of this type.

Value-Belief Pattern: Family Assessment
I History
    a Generally, family get things they want out of life?
    b Important things for the future?
    c Any "rules" in the family that everyone believes are important?
    d Religion important in family? Does this help when difficulties arise?
II Examination: None

Families have value-belief patterns. Some say the sharing of values and beliefs is one of the important characteristics of a successful marriage. Dissimilar value-belief patterns within a marital or family relationship usually produce conflicts observed in other pattern areas, such as role-relationships. Conflicts also arise when members, such as teenagers, are in the process of developing a conscious awareness of values and beliefs. Because of the potential for family disorganization, value-belief pattern conflicts should not be missed during assessment.

Value-Belief Pattern: Community Assessment
I History (community representatives)
    a Community values: What seems to be the top four things that people living here see as important in their lives (note health-related values, priorities)?
    b Do people tend to get involved in causes/local fund raising campaigns (note if any are health related)?
    c Religious groups in community? Churches available?
    d Do people tend to tolerate/not tolerate differences/socially deviant behavior?

II Examination
  a Zoning laws.
  b Scan of community government health committee reports (goals, priorities).
  c Health budget relative to total budget.

Communities have values and beliefs, including health-related values; understanding these is critical in diagnosing conflicts when working with community groups. Value patterns underlie decisions about where tax money should be spent, and whether or not the community should have an abortion clinic, sex education in the schools, senior citizen centers, and special education for the handicapped. These and many other community issues that affect health ultimately rest on the predominant value-belief pattern of a community.

Other Concerns (Individual, Family, Community)

In individual, family, or community assessment it is important for the nurse to ask the client about other concerns when concluding the admission interview. There may be areas not previously discussed that the client wishes to mention or has questions about specific things. Further information may be elicited by asking the client the following:

  a Any other things that we haven't talked about that you'd like to mention?
  b Any questions?

The functional health pattern format guides the collection of a basic data base. If verbal responses to questions (history) or the nurse's observations (examination) signify a dysfunctional or potentially dysfunctional pattern, *collect further information to identify the problem. This is done by assessing behaviors that is characteristic of the diagnoses being considered.* As the client's problem becomes clear, assessment is guided by the *conceptual framework* of the nurse. Having considered each pattern, the reader may wish to refer to the *composite of assessment items* in Appendix E before considering special cases of functional assessment.

ADAPTATION OF ASSESSMENT FORMAT

Infant and Child Assessment

The functional health pattern format for assessment requires adaptation of questions to and observations of infants, children, and early adolescents. Also, their patterns have to be judged according to *developmental norms.* For example, nocturnal bedwetting is expected in an infant but not older children. Items assessed during a nursing history and examination reflect developmental considerations. Examples of questions and observations for infancy and early childhood are contained in Appendix F. A nursing history is obtained from (1) a parent (or guardian) or (2) the child *and* a parent or guardian. As communication skills develop, it is important to include the child's viewpoint. Adolescents usually can provide information for individual assessment (see format in previous section).

A further consideration in infant, child, and early adolescent assessment is environmental influences on development. In particular, parents and the family's functional patterns greatly influence child development. These should be briefly assessed using previously discussed formats for adult assessment. If problems are present, a further assessment of environmental factors is necessary (home, school, etc.).

Assessment of the Critically Ill

Clients who are critically ill, such as those with *severe* respiratory, cardiac, neurological, or psychological instability, are unable to respond to a full functional health pattern assessment. It is also not appropriate to obtain a full history in a recovery room, operating room, and emergency room. (Some clients come to an emergency room with a nonemergent problem; nursing judgment dictates the extent of assessment that is needed prior to clinic referral or discharge to home.)

During the critical phase of an illness the major objectives of nursing and medical care are to stabilize physiological or psychological processes and to prevent further complications, injury, and emotional distress. *Examination and observation are the major data collection methods used during the critical phase of an illness when the client does not have the energy, capacity, or attention span to provide a health history.* Family or close friends, if present, can supply historical information that may be appropriate to critical care. (When the client is transferred from intensive-care nursing, a full assessment should be completed.)

Upon the client's admission to intensive care, assessment should include screening for high-incidence nursing diagnoses and pathophysiological or psychiatric (in psychiatric intensive care) cues related to the disease and its complications. Anticipation of family responses to the crisis and attention to cues is also necessary. Any of the following conditions may be present during the critical phase of care; thus it is important that the nurse be sensitive to cues to these conditions:

Health-Perception–Health-Management Pattern

1 *Potential for infection* Risk factors should be assessed frequently, especially in clients with a depressed immunological system, trauma, general debilitation, or a surgical incision.

2 *Potential for physical injury or suffocation* Risk factors for this condition should be assessed if the client is confused or disoriented. Any client who demonstrates the capacity and intention to get out of bed or remove tubes and equipment should also be evaluated for these diagnoses. The risk of suffocation in an infant or child is important to evaluate.

Nutritional-Metabolic Pattern

3 *Potential nutritional or fluid volume deficit* This condition may occur in psychiatric intensive care. Even in medical-surgical intensive care, prevention of these problems may not be integrated into treatment of the medical problem.

4 *Potential skin breakdown* Risk factors should be observed closely in clients immobilized by equipment (including casts or traction), on bed rest, and immobilized with restraint. Attention to risk factors will serve to prevent decubitus or other pressure ulcers.

Elimination Pattern

5 *Potential for constipation leading to impaction* Daily observations are required to prevent this condition, especially when clients spend a number of days in intensive care. Certain drugs used in psychiatric intensive care may predispose clients to this problem.

Activity-Exercise Pattern

6 *Potential activity intolerance* Most clients receiving intensive care manifest activity intolerance; assessment is directed toward those who have risk factors for low tolerance but are beginning to assume some independent self-care.

7 *Total self-care deficit (Levels III–IV)* During severe physiological or psychological instability and immobility, assessment is directed toward the capacity of the client to participate in some aspects of self-care (except, of course, children who have not attained these skills). Depending on staffing and reimbursement procedures, this diagnosis (1) may be recorded for every client in intensive care or (2) because all have this problem, it may be *understood* that nursing time is spent in compensating for self-care deficits and no recording of the diagnosis is required.

8 *Potential joint contractures* Risk factors are usually present in clients with immobility for more than 2 days.

9 *Ineffective airway clearance* This is a common condition that should be assessed especially with illnesses affecting the respiratory system and in clients who are comatose or semicomatose.

Sleep-Rest Pattern

10 *Sleep pattern disturbance* Sleep-wake cycles should be assessed in all clients in critical care units. Sleep onset disturbances and sleep pattern interruption are two conditions that occur frequently.

Cognitive-Perceptual Pattern

11 *Uncompensated sensory deficit (specify)* Assessment of vision and hearing disturbances is essential. These conditions can percipitate anxiety or cognitive disturbances in critical care units.

12 *Sensory deprivation or overload; potential for cognitive impairment* Verbal reports or cues to hallucinatory experiences or nightmares are important to assess.

13 *Decisional conflict* Assessment for cues to this condition is important when clients or families are faced with certain treatment decisions.

Self-Perception–Self-Concept Pattern

14 *Fear (specify); anxiety* Cues to these conditions should not be missed in clients or families. Fear (death) is common during the crisis phase of an illness.

15 *Powerlessness* This condition may occur with clients who are conscious but have minimal control of their body and treatment decisions.

16 *Self-concept disturbance* If a client is conscious, disturbances in self-esteem or body image may be noted, especially following extensive, disfiguring surgery, trauma, burns, or debilitating medical illnesses.

Role-Relationship Pattern

17 *Anticipatory grieving* Perception of the future consequences of an illness may cause grieving as clients begin to regain consciousness after an injury, surgery, or a disease.

18 *Unresolved independence-dependence conflict* As the crisis of illness begins to resolve, cues to conflict over dependency may be manifested verbally or by independent activities which are contrary to the treatment regimen.

19 *Alteration in family process* Guilt, anxiety, or role disturbances that are associated with a client's illness may be manifested in family conflict or disorganization.

20 *Weak parent-infant attachment* Cues to this condition should not be missed in neonatal intensive care units where parents and infants are separated for long periods of time.

21 *Impaired communication* This condition should not be missed as it may be the etiology of anxiety, fear, or powerlessness.

Coping-Stress Tolerance Pattern

22 *Avoidance coping* Psychological abandonment of a dying client may be a cue to ineffective family coping strategies. Avoidance coping can be *beneficial* during a crisis and should not be diagnosed as a condition requiring treatment; denial in the early stages of a crisis may be used by either clients or families to provide the time necessary to integrate the event.

Value-Belief Pattern

23 *Spiritual distress* Distress about the meaning of suffering or death may be manifested by some clients during the crisis period of an illness.

The above conditions represent a sample of the health problems amenable to nursing intervention during the intensive-care phase of a life-threatening illness. Alterations in cardiac output, impaired gas exchange, alterations in tissue perfusion, excess fluid volume deficit, and many other disease-related conditions may also be present. These are treated collaboratively by physicians and nurses. During a physiological crisis the physician has primary responsibility for treatment decisions. Implementation of the medical plan, 24-hour observation, and reporting are collaborative areas of nursing practice that require high levels of clinical judgment. These collaborative activities are combined with nursing-diagnosis–based care during the crisis phase of an illness.

SUMMARY

The purpose of this chapter has been to present a *structural format for assessment* of clients who are considered healthy or have various diseases or types of mental illness. The usefulness of this assessment format extends through all phases of the health-illness continuum and all settings where nursing is practiced. Use in practice has supported its broad applicability to human beings of any age.

The assessment categories are not new to nurses; however, the format's major contribution is to organization of assessment data for purposes of identifying nursing diagnoses. The categories also provide a useful format for those nurses wishing to switch from a purely medical model to a nursing model for practice. Diseases influence functional patterns; therefore, it is logical to assume that assessment of pathophysiological processes would be incorporated into the examination phase of assessment. *What physiological processes should be assessed?* That depends on the disturbances anticipated from knowledge of the disease. *What developmental processes should be assessed?* That depends on the client's developmental phase. *What cultural patterns should be assessed?* Clearly, culture influences all functional patterns; assessment data should be evaluated in the cultural, developmental, and illness context of the client situation and further data should be collected when needed.

The discussion in this chapter focused on the description and use of functional health pattern assessment in clinical situations. Assessment items, or parameters, were presented that can be used to assess individuals, families, or communities. *How extensive should the assessment be when a new client is added to a nurse's case load?* The answer has two parts:

1 The nurse must decide how much of personal resources (time) can be allocated to the client and this decision has to be balanced with the amount of risk that can be tolerated. The risk involves missing diagnoses or a misdiagnosis because of insufficient information and the potential for the client to suffer discomfort, distress, or harm. In many instances when the professional staffing of units is low, the decision becomes a moral dilemma and even a legal (malpractice) concern for nurses.

2 Consideration of the client-situation helps to determine the extent of assessment on admission. Clients having surgery or delivering a baby in the next hours or day may not be able to focus their attention on topics they perceive to be unrelated to the impending experience. Critically ill clients may have neither the energy nor level of consciousness to provide a history. Obviously, "rules" regarding the extent of an admission assessment cannot be set; the decision involves professional judgment in the particular situation.

Having considered *what* information is useful to collect when screening for nursing diagnoses, let us now move to an overview of current diagnoses, or dysfunctional patterns, in Chapter 5. *The functional health pattern assessment format is designed to screen for these diagnoses.* The information from Chapters 4 and 5 will then be used in examining the process of diagnosis: information collection, interpretation, and clustering and the naming of the client's health problem or potential problem.

BIBLIOGRAPHY

Becknell, E., & Smith, D. (1975). *System of nursing practice.* New York: Davis.

Duvall, E. (1967). *Family development.* Philadelphia: Lippincott.

Gikow, F., & Kacharski, P. (1985). *Functional health pattern assessment of a community.* Paper presented at the American Public Health Association, 112th Annual Meeting, Anaheim, CA, Nov. 13, 1984.

Gordon, M., & Jones, D. A. (In progress). Validity of information units in the functional health pattern assessment format. Chestnut Hill, MA: Boston College School of Nursing.

Mc Cain, F. (1965). Nursing by assessment—not intuition. *American Journal of Nursing,* 65:82–84.

Mc Lean, A. (Ed.). (1977). *Reducing occupational stress: Proceedings of a conference.* Westchester Division, New York Hospital-Cornell Medical Center, May 10–12, 1977.

Miller, J. G. (1978). *Living systems.* New York: McGraw-Hill.

Powell, J. (1969). *Why am I afraid to tell you who I am?* Chicago: Argus Communications.

Selye, H. (1979). Stress without distress. In C. A. Garfield (Ed.), *Stress and survival.* St. Louis: Mosby.

Smith, D. M. (1968). A clinical nursing tool. *American Journal of Nursing,* 68:2384–2388.

Steele, S., & Harmon, V. (1979). *Values clarification in nursing.* New York: Appleton-Century-Crofts.

RECOGNIZING DYSFUNCTIONAL HEALTH PATTERNS
  Etiological or Related Factors
RECOGNIZING POTENTIALLY DYSFUNCTIONAL PATTERNS
DIAGNOSTIC CATEGORIES
  Health-Perception–Health-Management Pattern
  Nutritional-Metabolic Pattern
  Elimination Pattern
  Activity-Exercise Pattern
  Sleep-Rest Pattern
  Cognitive-Perceptual Pattern
  Self-Perception–Self-Concept Pattern
  Role-Relationship Pattern
  Sexuality-Reproductive Pattern
  Coping-Stress Tolerance Pattern
  Value-Belief Pattern
SUMMARY
BIBLIOGRAPHY

134

CHAPTER 5

DYSFUNCTIONAL HEALTH PATTERNS

Health patterns can be functional, dysfunctional, or potentially dysfunctional. As discussed in Chapter 4, when health patterns are functional they signify health and wellness, provide a basis for continued development of human potentialities, and are *strengths* to be recognized and mobilized in dealing with health problems. In contrast, *dysfunctional* or *potentially dysfunctional health patterns* do not meet expected norms and are defined as *health problems. A dysfunctional pattern generates therapeutic concern on the part of the client, family or friends, or the nurse.* In other words, the situation is viewed as a problem requiring therapeutic measures.[1] Diagnostic categories are currently being developed to describe these health problems (Appendix A).

To be clear about terms in current use, remember that there are two types of health problems described by diagnostic categories:

1 Actual health problems or dysfunctional health patterns
2 Potential health problems or potentially dysfunctional health patterns (high risk conditions)

The distinction is important because each type of health problem requires a different kind of nursing intervention. Treatment for dysfunctional patterns (actual problems) is directed toward factors that are contributing to, or maintaining, the problem, whereas for potentially dysfunctional patterns (potential problems), the objective is to prevent the problem by reducing risk factors.

---

[1]*Therapeutic concern* is a term used by Taylor (1971) to refer to a client's desire to receive treatment or a professional's desire to provide it.

RECOGNIZING DYSFUNCTIONAL HEALTH PATTERNS

A dysfunctional pattern is defined as a set of behaviors that do not meet norms for age, sex, or culture of the client and negatively influence the client's overall functioning. Patterns can change or development can be delayed leading to the following three types of dysfunctional pattern observed in clinical practice:

1 *Change from a functional to dysfunctional pattern* Is the change unhealthful when considering the whole client situation? Is it an acute, or recent change?

2 *Stabilized dysfunctional pattern* Is there a long-term history of a dysfunctional pattern? Chronic change over time?

3 *Stabilized, dysfunctional developmental pattern* Is development (of child, adult, elder) delayed or interrupted?

The first pattern may come to the nurse's attention when a change from the client's functional baseline occurs. An example of a recent change in activity pattern would be:

Client reports that he has had to "slow down in the last month." Cleaning his apartment used to be easy but now causes shortness of breath and greater fatigue. "Cleaning is too much for me since my heart can't be improved."

The judgment that change has occurred is based on the historical data, "used to be easy," and current data, "now causes shortness of breath and fatigue." *The judgment that a change has occurred is made by comparing historical and current data about the state of the client. Consideration of the client situation as a whole determines whether the change is functional or dysfunctional.*

A second type of health problem is a stabilized dysfunctional pattern. No recent change has occurred but the pattern is unhealthful for the client's developmental level. Historical and current data provide support for this diagnostic judgment as illustrated in the following example:

A geriatric clinical specialist found that her clients, elderly residents of an inner city housing complex, restricted their outdoor activities. Many confined themselves to their own building, except for arranged bus trips, because of a high incidence of violent crime in their neighborhood.

Although adaptive in the environment, their activity-exercise pattern was judged dysfunctional. *The judgment of a chronic dysfunctional pattern is made by comparing historical and current data with developmental norms.*

When assessing patterns of functional development be aware of a third type of dysfunctional pattern, chronic developmental lag. There are a number of theories and milestones (norms) of development that can be used in evaluation. Underdeveloped potential can exist in individuals, families, and even in regions of the world. Nurses are concerned when underdevelopment results from, or leads to, health problems. The following is an example:

A child in a school situation had not developed self-care abilities consistent with his age, such as tying shoe laces or dressing independently. His parents did not want him to "strain" in case his asthma might get worse. Some of the other children referred to him as the "baby" and gradually he became sullen and withdrew from play activities at home and in school.

The diagnosis of a dysfunctional developmental pattern is based on a comparison of developmental norms with current developmental achievements. In the above situation the child's developmental lag may be due to the parents' fear and misunderstanding of activity tolerance; the social isolation is secondary. The problem would be described as *developmental delay* to distinguish it from the loss of the ability, as occurs in the adult. A useful and concise way of stating this in the problem/etiology format would be: Developmental Delay/Parental Fear-Misunderstanding (Activity Tolerance). This diagnosis would be a subcategory of altered growth and development.

The purpose of discussing the various types of dysfunctional patterns is not to make diagnosis more difficult. Rather, it is to provide some concrete guidelines. When clients describe their functional patterns (what is eaten, how they cope with stress, perceptions of their health state, and so forth), obtain data to evaluate if change has occurred in a pattern area, when it occurred, and if the change has led to higher levels of functioning or overall dysfunctioning.

Etiological or Related Factors

When a dysfunctional health pattern is identified and labeled with a diagnostic category, related questions to raise are: *Why* does the problem exist? What factors have contributed to the development of the problem? What factors are maintaining the problem? *The factors that are probable causes of a health problem and which contribute to, or maintain, the problem are called etiological factors.* When they can be identified they are the focus of nursing intervention. *Related factors are associated with the problem.*

In practice settings reasons for a problem are referred to as "the etiology." This expression should not convey that only one factor is necessarily involved. Recognize that many factors influence the client situation. However, *nurses may select from multiple contributing factors the most probable etiological or related factor that can be influenced by nursing intervention at a particular time.* Explanations of *why* a problem exists require reasoning based on clinical data and theory stored in memory (causal reasoning and explanation will be discussed in later chapters). At this point let us consider how the functional health patterns are used to identify these factors.

It may be recalled that functional health patterns are interdependent and interactive. Human beings function as a whole within their environment and behavior is a product of the person-situation complex. Thus explanations, reasons, or probable causes of a health problem usually lie in one or more functional health patterns. For example, a dysfunctional sleep-rest pattern, delayed sleep onset, may be primarily caused by a dysfunctional self-perception–self-concept pattern, fear of surgical anesthesia. In addition, assessment of one client may reveal anxiety/sleep deprivation and another client's assessment may reveal sleep deprivation/anxiety. In the problem/etiology format the etiology represents the focus for nursing care activities. Formulation of problems from assessment data will be discussed in Chapter 8. To summarize the points discussed here:

1 Look for the etiological or related factors underlying a dysfunctional pattern within the functional areas.

2 Assessment data and the use of clinical reasoning determine what the problem is and what the etiological or related factors in particular situations are; use diagnostic category labels (Appendix A) to describe either a problem or etiological factors.

RECOGNIZING POTENTIALLY DYSFUNCTIONAL PATTERNS

Since modern nursing began, health promotion and preventive intervention have been an integral part of clinical practice. Thus, the identification of potentially dysfunctional patterns (potential problems) is equally important as diagnosing patterns of dysfunction. Similar to actual problems, potential problems can occur in the absence of a medical disease or be secondary to disease, surgery, or treatment. *A potential problem is a nursing diagnosis that describes a set of risk factors for a dysfunctional pattern. The focus of nursing intervention for potential problems is risk factor reduction.* During assessment be aware of two types of potential problems:

1 *High risk for change from a functional to dysfunctional pattern*   Diagnoses in this area describe a high risk for change toward a less functional pattern. This means there are risk factors in the client's behavior, the situation, or both that *predispose* to an actual problem. Examples would be: Potential Fluid Volume Deficit or Potential Health Management Deficit (Medication Regimen).

2 *High risk for a dysfunctional pattern of growth/development*   Diagnoses in this area describe a high risk for problems related to biopsychosocial growth of an individual or family. When entering a new phase of human development a child, adult, or family may not have the developmental background or situational resources for continued personal growth and development. Examples are: Potential for Developmental Delay (Social Skills) or Potential Family Conflict (Child-Rearing Practices).

To say that a client is susceptible to (or at risk for) a health problem requires the presence of risk factors. Usually the *historical or current data include a combination of signs in one or more patterns.* For example, the Surgeon General's report on health promotion and disease prevention (U.S. Department of Health, Education, and Welfare, 1979) states that 40 percent of American children ages 11 to 14 are estimated to have one or more risk factors associated with heart disease: overweight, high blood pressure, high blood cholesterol, cigarette smoking, lack of exercise, or diabetes. If children in a particular community are found to be similar to these national figures, this finding represents a set of potential problems, or potential dysfunctional patterns, requiring parent and child health education.

Potential for injury is another example of a risk state. Forty percent of hospital admissions for burns are due to scalding from excessively hot water in showers or bathtubs; 56 percent of fatal residential fires are cigarette-related, many due to smoking in bed, according to the Surgeon General's report. An example of a potential problem secondary to disease and its treatment is potential non-compliance. Multiple prescriptions and other factors increase the risk that a client may not follow the treatment regime even when desire and intention were initially present.

The diagnosis of potential problems is limited to individuals who have a greater number of risk factors than the population as a whole. For example, everyone has a potential for injury while crossing a city street, cutting vegetables in the kitchen, or shaving. Most clients are not at any more risk than the rest of the so-called normal population doing everyday activities. But those in the particular subpopulations with sensory-perceptual problems, a mobility deficit, or a bleeding tendency may be substantially at risk while performing these everyday activities.

Perhaps comparing two groups within a population of clients on a surgical service will clarify this idea. A client who is of normal body weight, doesn't smoke, has no chronic lung disease, and has been reasonably active is going to have surgery to remove the gallbladder. Compare this client to another, scheduled for the same operation, who smokes heavily, has chronic bronchitis, is 60 pounds overweight, and has relatively poor muscle tone because of a sedentary activity pattern. Which client has a potential for, or is at risk for, atelectasis postoperatively? Stated differently, which client should have intensive nursing treatment to prevent this pulmonary complication after surgery? Clearly, the second client is at high risk for atelectasis. (Postoperatively the risk increases if neither of these clients carry out deep breathing and coughing exercises due to incisional pain.)

This comparison illustrates the idea of *population at risk.* The first person represents the normal population having a cholecystectomy (gallbladder removal). The second client having this surgery comes from a different population whose characteristics of heavy smoking, chronic bronchitis, and weak muscle tone greatly predispose to atelectasis after upper abdominal surgery.

When formulating the etiology of an actual problem, one may ask, for example, why a particular client has a potential for atelectasis. However, such a question does not apply here. The *reason* for the risk state is already determined; risk factors have been identified. *All that is needed for formulating a potential problem are a cluster of risk factors and the diagnostic label to describe them.* Specifying causal factors would require restating the risk factors that are *already specified* as signs of the high-risk state. In addition, how can there be a probable cause for something that is *potential* but does not yet exist?

To diagnose a high-risk state consider the historical and current data in one or more functional patterns.

In clinical settings where diagnosis is just beginning to be used, clinicians may wish to call attention to the risk factors. This can be done by recording the diagnosis as *potential for atelectasis* and stating, in parentheses, *see risk factors.* This statement is more concise and less repetitive when risk factors have already been recorded. Ultimately, when risk factor specification is standardized, all nurses will have learned the signs of potential- or high-risk states.

To conclude this section, it may be said that a problem, from a nursing perspective, is a dysfunctional health pattern. A problem represents a dysfunctional change in a pattern or an unhealthful pattern that has stabilized. Developmental problems exist when development is stabilized at a dysfunctional level relative to the client's potential.

A potential problem is a risk state. It indicates the presence of factors that predispose a client to a dysfunctional health pattern. Potential fluid volume deficit, potential alterations in parenting, and potential noncompliance are examples that describe dysfunctional nutritional-metabolic, role-relationship, and health-perception–health-management patterns, respectively.

A potential state is a predicted state, not an actual state with an actual cause; thus, etiology is not specified. Intervention in this case is directed toward reducing risk factors.

DIAGNOSTIC CATEGORIES

In the previous section, dysfunctional and potentially dysfunctional health patterns were defined and some examples of diagnostic category labels were given. Now let us briefly review some diagnostic concepts and their category labels developed by nurses in the United States and Canada. Initially, diagnostic categories are learned in the same manner that one learns the concepts and category labels that describe signs and symptoms of medical conditions, such as hemorrhagic shock, congestive heart failure, or tetralogy of Fallot. *This review will provide only an introduction to the phenomena in clinical practice that are of particular concern to nurses; in-depth study of these diagnoses continues throughout a nurse's professional career.*

Most concepts and their category labels currently identified by the North American Nursing Diagnosis Association (NANDA) are in an early stage of development, as will be discussed in Chapter 11. Their evolution to scientific concepts within the professional discipline of nursing rests with the practitioners, theorists, and researchers who are working toward validating the phenomena and improving the precision of diagnostic categories. Continued development is a characteristic of any classification system. It is not too long ago that "dropsy" was a medical diagnosis, diabetes was a single entity, and acute immune deficiency syndrome (AIDS) was not labeled.

Further research is needed to determine if the currently identified diagnostic categories are valid descriptions of the realities encountered in practice. In addition, studies of the incidence of nursing diagnoses in particular age, sex, cultural, or medical disease populations are needed. There is one analysis of eight published studies (Gordon, 1985). Within the 25,895 diagnoses made by nurses, 36 diagnoses occurred with a frequency greater than 100. Table 5-1

TABLE 5-1
RANKINGS OF THE 10 MOST FREQUENTLY REPORTED NURSING DIAGNOSES IN
PUBLISHED CLINICAL RESEARCH REPORTS

Nursing diagnosis	Reported cases	Number of studies
Anxiety (Mild, $N = 2182$; Moderate, $N = 911$; Severe, $N = 169$; Panic, $N = 45$)	3586	5
Discomfort	2259	2
Self-Care Deficit (Altered Ability to Perform Self-Care Activities $N = 972$; Hygiene Self-Care Impaired, N $=179$)	1817	6
Alteration in Comfort: Pain	1479	6
Impaired Mobility (Mobility Deficit; Immobility)	1445	6
Potential Impairment in Skin Integrity	992	2
Nutritional Deficit (Less Nutrition than Required, $N = 901$)	976	2
Impaired Skin Integrity	948	2
Alteration in Self-Concept (Body Image, $N = 748$; Self-Esteem, $N = 44$)	828	2
Sleep-Pattern Disturbance (Dysrhythmia of Sleep-Rest, $N = 722$, Impaired Sleep-Rest, $N = 73$)	807	3

Source: Excerpted from Gordon (1985).

includes the ten diagnoses with the highest frequency (800 or more reported cases).[2]

When the frequency of diagnoses within health patterns were summed, the top ranking patterns were: activity-exercise (7051), nutritional-metabolic (5426), self-perception–self-concept (5187), and cognitive-perceptual (4874). Eighty-seven percent of the reported diagnoses were within these patterns. This is the only review that is available to give some indication of what diagnoses occur most frequently and what patterns are most frequently dysfunctional. Let us now consider the current categories for labeling dysfunctional and potentially dysfunctional patterns listed in Appendix B. (An asterisk signifies the category is *not* currently on the NANDA-approved list.)

Health-Perception–Health-Management Pattern

Health-perception–health-management patterns are influential in moving individuals, families, and communities toward their optimal level of human functioning. The two dimensions of this pattern interact; the way clients perceive their general health and health goals influences their health management practices.

Diagnostic categories grouped within this pattern describe dysfunctional health

---

[2]Caution must be exercised in attempting to draw conclusions from these data because they represent *only eight studies, six of which involved extremely small samples,* and *diagnoses were mainly drawn from nurses caring for hospitalized, medical-surgical clients.*

management practices and person-environment factors that place a client at risk for infection, injury, and other conditions. Four actual and five potential problems have been identified in this pattern area:

*Health Management Deficit (Total)
*Health Management Deficit (Specify)
Health Maintenance Alteration
Noncompliance (Specify)
*Potential Noncompliance (Specify)
Potential for Infection
Potential for Injury (Trauma)
Potential for Poisoning
Potential for Suffocation

The diagnoses in this pattern area may be used as a basis for designing nursing interventions to improve clients' health promotion and health management practices. Few differences exist between the *definitions* of *health management deficit* and *alteration in health maintenance.* An alteration in health maintenance results from a deficit in health management; thus management practices should be of primary concern in diagnosis. The broad category *alteration* is very general; specific kinds of alterations are not named. Also, this category should not be used indiscriminately to label all disease and illness states, a practice sometimes reflected in hospital charts. The term *specify* in health management deficit and noncompliance means that the diagnostician fills in the particular management deficits, such as medication or exercise regimen, dietary prescription, follow-up care, or other health-promoting practices. If a client is unable to assume responsibility for any health management practices, total health management deficit would be used. Health, in this category-label, can include inability to manage a disease regimen, as for example: Potential Health Management Deficit (Diabetes) or Health Management Deficit (Diabetes).

Noncompliance is a diagnosis that has received a lot of attention in the literature. Some view this category label as being value-laden, not addressing the real problem, and not reflecting mutual decision making between the client and nurse (Breunig et al., 1986). Definitions of this term vary. If an author views noncompliance as not carrying out doctors' or nurses' orders, it is judged to be a negative label (Stantis and Ryan, 1982). Those that define the term as nonadherence after informed decision and expressed intention (Gordon, 1986) or nonadherence associated with adverse effects (Vincent, 1985) see the term as a point of departure for determining why the client is noncompliant. If the reasons involve *inability rather than choice,* health management deficit (specify) may be a clearer way of expressing the problem. The reasons that the client is not able to handle health or disease management are stated as factors contributing to the problem. *Potential health management deficit* (or *potential noncompliance*) is used when data indicate risk factors are present but the client has had no opportunity to implement the recommendations (e.g., hospitalized person).

Potential for infection, injury, poisoning, and *suffocation* are categories that describe risk factors for specific areas of health management. Only those clients that are at high risk should be diagnosed, as all human beings have some risk for these problems. It should also be noted that clients can be at risk for infection, in a general sense, or for infection in a particular body part or system. It would be more precise and give a clearer base for preventive treatment if this was specified. The same specification adds precision to potential for injury. For example, diagnoses for a particular client may be: Potential for Respiratory Infection, Potential for Wound Infection, Potential for Accidental Injury, or Potential for Falls. Caution should be exercised to ensure that sufficient data are present to support these diagnoses and other professionals should be informed of the high risk state so that their treatment plans take this into consideration.

Developmental health management deficit (specify) may be useful in describing a condition in which a child is not able to assume responsibilities, expected at a particular developmental level, for health promotion, disease prevention, or disease management. This delay may be related to lack of opportunities for learning. Potential for infection, injury, and suffocation is useful for describing conditions encountered in pediatric, as well as adult, health care.

Nutritional-Metabolic Pattern

Diagnoses describing dysfunctional nutritional-metabolic patterns are biopsychosocial conditions related to nutrient intake and supply. Nutrients are necessary for cellular metabolic processes, such as energy production and synthesis of substances used in cellular function, growth, and repair. Nutritional patterns are influenced by (1) maturation, (2) family, social, and cultural patterns, (3) learned psychological associations between food and basic needs, and (4) environmental availability of foods. For example, as growth and maturation proceed, the type of foods ingested, method of ingestion, and the social-psychological milieu of eating changes. Bottles and high chairs are replaced by family silverware and social dining. Biopsychosocial factors (including cultural and spiritual) can lead to dysfunctional patterns, such as exogenous obesity and nutritional deficits.

Sixteen diagnostic categories have been identified in the nutritional-metabolic pattern area. Six describe dysfunctional food and fluid patterns, two describe possible reasons for these patterns, four categories describe local, metabolic problems in nutrient supply to the skin, and four describe metabolic problems in body temperature regulation.

In a review of research this was shown to be a high-ranking area for dysfunctional patterns; as may be seen in Table 5-1, nutritional deficits and problems in skin integrity were high-frequency diagnoses. Consider first the set of categories describing food and fluid patterns. (The terms in brackets in the display lists in this chapter are more concise labels, in the opinion of this author, than the NANDA-approved diagnostic labels.)

Alteration in Nutrition: More Than Body Requirements [or *Exogenous Obesity*]

Alteration in Nutrition: Potential for More Than Body Requirements [or *Potential Obesity*]

Alteration in Nutrition: Less Than Body Requirements [or *Nutritional Deficit (Specify)*]

Fluid Volume Deficit

Potential Fluid Volume Deficit

Alteration in Fluid Volume: [*Excess* or *Excess Fluid Volume*]

Nutritional deficit is followed by the term *specify.* Unless a total nutritional deficiency is present, there should be specification of which nutrients are deficient. For example, less than the daily requirement for protein intake would be labeled: Nutritional Deficit (Protein Intake). *Potential fluid volume deficit* usually responds to nursing treatment. A significant *fluid volume deficit* or *excess fluid volume* may require medical treatment. Two additional categories in this pattern area are:

Impaired Swallowing [or *Uncompensated Swallowing Impairment*]

Alterations in Oral Mucous Membranes

These two categories are useful in describing the possible reasons (etiologies) nutritional deficits occur, such as Nutritional Deficit/Uncompensated Swallowing Impairment. They also may be used as risk factors for a potential nutritional or fluid intake deficit.

Avoid using a medical diagnosis, such as cerebrovascular accident (stroke), as an etiological factor contributing to a swallowing impairment. The brain in fact is not the focus for *nursing* intervention. Also avoid, for example, using alterations in oral mucous membranes (problem) related to stomatitis (etiology) because stomatitis is a type of alteration not a reason for the alteration. It would be clearer to name the specific condition that is amenable to nursing intervention and delete the broad classification category *alterations in.* The conditions that follow pertain to the highly metabolic organ, the skin, or to metabolism:

Potential Impairment of Skin Integrity [or *Potential Skin Breakdown*]

Hyperthermia

Impairment of Skin Integrity

Hypothermia

Impaired Tissue Integrity

Ineffective Thermoregulation

*Decubitus Ulcer (Specify Stage)

Potential Alteration in Body Temperature

The accepted diagnoses *impairment of skin integrity* and *potential impairment of skin integrity* are very general; they include too many conditions to be useful as a focus for definitive nursing intervention. Impairments can range from a surgical incision to blisters. The treatment plan is unclear when a surgical incision is labeled impaired skin integrity; if the concern is preventing infection and if the client is at high risk, use *potential* for wound infection. *Potential skin breakdown* and *decubitus ulcer* (specify stage) describe specific "impairments" and are clearer and more precise. When using *decubitus ulcer* to describe observations, consult a manual (Gordon, 1987) or articles on stages of ulceration to make the diagnosis precise. It should also be noted that certain stages of ulceration require surgical treatment and the problem is temporarily referred to a physician. The diagnosis *impaired tissue integrity* is extremely broad; it is defined as damaged or destroyed tissue such as cornea, mucous membrane, integumentary (skin), or subcutaneous (McLane, 1987). Thus, it includes the diagnoses discussed above and *alteration in oral mucous membranes.* For treatment planning, it is more useful to specify the specific area of damage if the condition can be resolved by nursing actions.

Potential for alteration in body temperature describes risk factors for hypothermia, hyperthermia, or ineffective thermoregulation. When using this diagnostic category, the specific type of alteration needs to be specified before interventions can be determined. Thus, *potential for* hyperthermia, potential for hypothermia, or potential ineffective thermoregulation would be more useful categories. The actual conditions of *hyperthermia, hypothermia,* and *ineffective thermoregulation* may or may not respond to nursing treatment; thus, it is important to determine the etiology of the condition. If nursing can provide only palliative care, or if there is any question about the reason for these conditions, they should be referred for medical diagnosis and treatment.

Altered growth and development is a category in the NANDA taxonomy of nursing diagnoses that could be used to classify specific dysfunctional developmental patterns, such as developmental delays. Development is an inherent characteristic of functional patterns; thus developmental delays may occur in any pattern area. In this pattern, growth delays may result from inadequate nutrition. Diagnoses could be developed to describe those that can be resolved through nursing action. Metabolic (endocrine) problems manifested in delayed growth are referred to a physician.

Elimination Pattern

The ten diagnostic categories within this pattern area describe bowel and urinary elimination patterns. No potential problems have been identified. Let us consider bowel elimination first:

Alteration in Bowel Elimination: Constipation [or *Intermittent Constipation Pattern*]
Alteration in Bowel Elimination: Diarrhea [or *Diarrhea*]
Alteration in Bowel Elimination: Incontinence [or *Bowel Incontinence*]

The NANDA-accepted labels for the above categories have been made more concise [italics]; in this author's opinion it is not necessary to include the broad classification category *alteration in bowel elimination* when the diagnosis is recorded. Each condition is within the scope of nursing practice but the diagnostician should be cautious; constipation, diarrhea, or incontinence can be a symptom of a disease that requires medical treatment. For example, an intermittent constipation pattern usually is due to inadequate roughage and fluids in the diet and poor bowel routines but also can be a symptom of cancer of the bowel. The following dysfunctional urinary elimination patterns have been identified:

Altered Urinary Elimination Pattern
Urinary Retention
Stress Incontinence
Total Incontinence
Functional Incontinence
Reflex Incontinence
Urge Incontinence

In this set we have the broad category *altered urinary elimination pattern* and six specific types of alterations: retention and five types of incontinence, each of which has specific definitions (McLane, 1987). Precise assessment is necessary to differentiate among the types of incontinence and specific interventions are required to assist the client in managing the problem.

Developmental delay can occur in any functional pattern area. In this area the NANDA-approved category *altered growth and development* may provide a focus for clinical identification of specific diagnostic categories to describe, for example, delays in the development of bowel and bladder control. Etiological or related factors that can be resolved by nursing will also need to be identified. In addition, pediatric nurses are concerned with providing anticipatory guidance to prevent dysfunctional developmental patterns; they will need to describe and classify the potential or high risk states encountered in their clinical practice.

Activity-Exercise Pattern

A client's pattern of activity, exercise, and leisure is a result of biopsychosocial factors. The pattern describes the client's *ability* and *desire* to engage in energy-consuming activities, such as play (child), work, exercise, self-care, and leisure. *Ability* is influenced by the development of coordination, strength, skill, endurance, and nutrient supply to tissues (cardiovascular and respiratory reserve). Loss of the ability to engage in activities of daily living is associated with feelings of dependency and lack of control over the immediate environment. The *desire* to do energy-consuming activities and the choice of activities are influenced by psychological and socioenvironmental factors such as motivation, mood state, and personal perception of benefits, risks, skill, and social acceptability.

The 18 diagnostic categories in this pattern area can be grouped into broad and specific dysfunctional patterns and dysfunctional supporting processes. The following set describes broad dysfunctional patterns that influence all energy-consuming activities:

Potential Activity Intolerance
Activity Intolerance (Specify Level)
Impaired Mobility (Specify Level)

Potential activity intolerance is a useful category to describe the presence of risk factors for abnormal response to energy-consuming activities. Clients who have been inactive or on prolonged bed rest frequently have this potential problem. In cardiac rehabilitation this category can be used to describe the risk factors associated with increasing activity after an acute myocardial infarct; it alerts nurses to carefully observe the client's activity response. *Activity intolerance* (specify level) is useful in describing the etiology for problems such as self-care deficit, perceived sexual dysfunction, impaired home maintenance management, or social isolation. Examples would be: Self-Care Deficit (Level III)/Activity Intolerance or Sexual Dysfunction/Activity Intolerance. It would be incorrect to state activity intolerance (Level II)/cancer or activity intolerance (Level II)/peripheral arterial disease. As with some previous diagnoses, avoid stating the medical disease as the etiology for activity intolerance; it is not useful as the basis for planning *nursing* intervention. It is important not to miss signs and symptoms of decreased activity tolerance in hospital care and home care of the frail elderly; this condition can produce a number of problems.

It may be noted that a number of diagnoses in this pattern area require specification of a functional level. Activity intolerance can be specified by levels of *endurance,* such as

Level I: Walks regular pace on level ground but becomes more short of breath than normally when climbing one or more flights of stairs.
Level II: Walks one city block 500 feet on level or climbs one flight of stairs slowly without stopping.
Level III: Walks no more than 50 feet on level without stopping and is unable to climb one flight of stairs without stopping.
Level IV: Dyspnea and fatigue at rest.

Using these levels, the degree of activity tolerance could be specified as Social Isolation/Activity Intolerance (Level III) using the problem/etiological factor format.

Impaired mobility (specify level) is a frequently identified diagnosis (Table 5-1). It can severely restrict a client's control over his or her environment and is frequently due to pain management deficit (as commonly occurs in chronic arthritis) or an uncompensated sensory-motor deficit (as occurs with hemiplegia). Used as an etiology, it describes a factor contributing to problems such as self-toileting deficit or social isolation.

Different levels of impairment require different nursing interventions; thus the level should be included in the diagnostic statement. The client's mobility can be described using levels of *dependency* (McLane, 1987). Level 0 is included below to show the range used in a health status evaluation but would not be used in stating a diagnosis because it indicates that no problem is present:

Level 0:   Is independent in movement.
Level I: Requires use of equipment or device.
Level II: Requires help from another person(s): assistance, supervision, or teaching.
Level III: Requires help from another person and equipment or device.
Level IV: Is dependent and does not participate in movement.

The second set of diagnoses within this area describe more specific dysfunctional activity patterns:

Impaired Home Maintenance Management (Mild, Moderate, Severe, Chronic)
Diversional Activity Deficit
Total Self-Care Deficit (Specify Level)
  Self-Bathing–Hygiene Deficit (Specify Level)
  Self-Dressing–Grooming Deficit (Specify Level)
  Self-Feeding Deficit (Specify Level)
  Self-Toileting Deficit (Specify Level)

Impaired home maintenance management describes the inability to do energy-consuming activities related to shopping, cooking, cleaning, laundering, and general home maintenance. This dysfunctional pattern is often caused by activity intolerance or impaired mobility. Other etiological factors that can contribute to impaired home maintenance management are uncompensated short-term memory deficit or general cognitive impairment, knowledge deficit, reactive situational depression, or family stress. It is important in hospital discharge planning to anticipate this problem, as it may delay discharge. In many cases, inability to manage household activities is diagnosed in a home visit.

Diversional activity deficit may be found in high-risk populations, such as hospitalized clients (adults and children) with "nothing to do," newly retired persons without preretirement plans, or frail elderly confined to their homes. The overstressed "workaholic" may have a deficit because of lack of planning for recreation and leisure time.

Self-care deficit[3] was third in frequency of diagnostic categories in Table 5-1. For precision in the diagnosis of self-care deficits use the previously listed levels of dependency to classify the client's deficit. If assessment data suggest that the client performs all but one self-care activity, then a subcategory is used. In hospital and community nursing, self-care deficit is a common problem that is usually produced by activity intolerance, impaired mobility, uncompensated short-term memory deficits (as in Alzheimer's disease), and uncompensated cognitive or sensorimotor deficits. Hyperactive or withdrawn psychiatric clients or children who have mastered self-care skills also may exhibit this problem.

---

[3]It is important to remember that *self-care deficit* and *self-care agency deficit* are two very different concepts. Self-care deficit refers to the inability to do the daily activities specified above. Self-care agency deficit is an abstract concept within a conceptual model (Chapter 3) and is defined as a discrepancy between self-care agency and self-care demand.

The client's response to self-care deficits may be fear of continued dependency; this could be described in the following diagnostic statement: Fear (Dependency)/Self-Care Deficit (Level IV). Increasing the self-care ability of the client by teaching compensatory methods should begin to resolve his or her fear. This is a more clinically useful way of stating the diagnosis than fear (dependency)/stroke and provides a basis for a *nursing* treatment plan to increase self-care ability.

A third set of diagnostic categories within the activity-exercise pattern describes conditions that may influence energy-consuming activities, such as mobility, self-care, activity intolerance and other problems described above. Some of the following can be prevented or resolved by nursing intervention; others are referred to a physician when signs of the condition are observed and the client is assessed for co-occurring nursing problems:[4]

*Potential Joint Contractures
Alteration in Cardiac Output:
Decreased [or *Decreased Cardiac
Output*]
Alteration in Tissue Perfusion
(Specify Cerebral, Renal, etc.)
Impaired Gas Exchange
Ineffective Airway Clearance
Ineffective Breathing Pattern

Potential joint contractures is a high-risk condition that occurs when movable joints are kept immobile. Tendons at the joints shorten and the joint moves into a flexed position. Independence in walking, feeding, and other body motions require movable joints; thus it is important to recognize the risk factors for contractures, make the diagnosis, and institute preventive nursing interventions.

Decreased cardiac output, alteration in tissue perfusion, and impaired gas exchange are conditions that should be referred to a physician when signs and symptoms are observed. They are within the collaborative, or interdependent, domain of nursing practice. A major nursing role in their treatment is frequent observation. Also, it is important to recognize that clients with these conditions usually have nursing diagnoses.

Ineffective airway clearance refers to a condition in which the client is unable to clear secretions or an obstruction from the respiratory tract. This can produce a state of fear or panic about not being able to breathe. The condition occurs in clients who have reduced awareness of secretions, impaired cough reflex, and debilitation.

The list of approved defining characteristics for *ineffective breathing pattern* (McLane, 1987) suggests that the category describes respiration (and respi-

---

[4]The reason some conditions are approved nursing diagnoses but for which the author recommends referral to a physician will be discussed in the section on collaborative problems in Chapter 9. Briefly, when assessment reveals collaborative problems, they are referred to a physician.

ratory compensations) inadequate to maintain sufficient oxygen supply for cell requirements. This diagnostic category would be more useful for nursing if defined by characteristics describing ineffective patterns of breathing under the voluntary control of the client (rather than the hypoxic results). The client with a chronic respiratory condition could be helped to learn ways to increase vital capacity and air exchange if an ineffective breathing pattern was contributing to self-care deficit or other problems. In other client situations, the following may be useful if treatments within the domain of nursing can lead to their resolution: Ineffective Breathing Pattern/Incisional Pain.

As in other pattern areas, developmental problems can occur in the activity exercise pattern. They include:

*Altered Growth and Development: Self-Care Skills (Specify)
Altered Growth and Development

Altered growth and development: self-care skills (specify) can describe delays in bathing-hygiene, dressing-grooming, feeding, or independent toileting. The term *specify* requires that the diagnostician identify the specific skill that deviates from norms for the age group. Developmental delays in crawling, walking, and other activities should also be described and labeled. Careful consideration needs to be given to the description and labeling of various types of altered growth and development so that a consistent nomenclature results.

Sleep-Rest Pattern

The one approved diagnostic category in this pattern area is *sleep pattern disturbance.* As may be seen in Table 5-1, it is a common condition diagnosed by nurses. All sleep disturbances are not treated in the same manner; therefore, it is more useful to identify the various types of sleep pattern disturbances such as: Delayed Sleep Onset, Interrupted Sleep Pattern, or Sleep Pattern Reversal.

Delayed sleep onset is a dysfunctional pattern that can occur with fear, anxiety, conflict, or with presleep activities that are not conducive to relaxation. *Sleep pattern reversal* describes a condition of remaining awake at night and sleeping or napping in the daytime. This is sometimes seen in elderly clients and produces difficulties for both clients and their families. An *interrupted sleep pattern* can occur in hospital situations where the client is awakened for medications or treatments. It is also common post partum when a parent with a young infant is awakened frequently. Another sleep disturbance, *early awakening pattern,* may be a symptom of depression and should be investigated further. No diagnostic categories have been identified for dysfunctional rest/relaxation patterns.

Cognitive-Perceptual Pattern

Diagnostic categories in this pattern area describe dysfunctional sensory-perceptual and cognitive patterns. All information from the internal and external environment is channeled through sensory receptors and relayed to centers in the brain concerned with perception and cognition. Deprivation or excess of sensory information can affect both perception and cognition. Dysfunction or retarded development of cognitive processes, such as attention, orientation, memory, problem solving, and decision making, can produce dependency on others. Consider first the diagnostic categories describing perceptual problems:

*Uncompensated Sensory Deficit (Specify)
Unilateral Neglect
Sensory-Perceptual Alterations: Input Deficit or [*Sensory Deprivation*]
Sensory-Perceptual Alterations: Input Excess [or *Sensory Overload*]
Alteration in Comfort: Pain
Alteration in Comfort: Chronic Pain
*Pain Self-Management Deficit (Acute, Chronic)

The diagnostic category *uncompensated sensory deficit* requires that the deficit be specified. Examples of problems and etiological factors would be: Impaired Mobility Related to Uncompensated Visual Deficit or Impaired Socialization Related to Uncompensated Hearing Deficit. The modifier *uncompensated* directs the nurse to help the client compensate for the loss. Care may range from full assistance to helping the client obtain simple or complex assistive devices. *Unilateral neglect* describes a condition in which there is lack of attention to the side of the body with a sensorimotor loss and to objects on the affected side; this can occur with a stroke. This deficit can be an etiological factor in self-care deficit and a risk factor for potential for injury. *Sensory deprivation* describes signs and symptoms resulting from a low level of sensory input. This condition may occur in the homebound or hospitalized elderly who already have sensory deficits, intensive care settings, newborns in incubators, and other situations in which the level of sensory input is reduced. The *potential* for this problem to occur should also be recognized. In contrast to deprivation, *sensory overload* describes a condition in which input is greater than the person can handle. Clients with cognitive impairments may experience overload in an environment that has high, sustained sensory stimulation.

Three diagnostic categories describe pain conditions. *Alteration in comfort: pain* was a highly utilized diagnosis in the research reviewed (Table 5-1). It is more useful in clinical situations to drop the classification category *alteration in comfort* and add a modifier such as *chest, joint,* or *incisional pain.* This provides a base for more definitive interventions. It is also likely that acute pain is collaboratively treated and resolved quickly; when the pain experience becomes chronic, clients have to be supported in their management of this condition. More important to the focus of nursing treatment is the category *acute or chronic pain self-management deficit.* Nursing intervention is directed toward helping clients to manage and control their pain through actions such as notification of nurses when experiencing pain, positioning, distraction, and relaxation. Clients with chronic pain self-management deficit have to learn to choose which medication matches the severity of the pain experience.

As may be noted, *discomfort* was second in frequency of reported nursing diagnoses (Table 5-1). This condition is not listed by NANDA and has not been described. Clearly, clinical studies should be done to see if this is separate and distinct from the category *alteration in comfort: pain.*

Dysfunctional cognitive patterns currently described by diagnostic categories are:

*Potential Cognitive Impairment
Impaired Thought Processes
*Uncompensated Memory Deficit
Knowledge Deficit (Specify)
*Decisional Conflict

The first three diagnostic categories provide labels for dysfunctional or potentially dysfunctional cognitive patterns. *Potential for cognitive impairment* describes risk factors for impairment in memory, reasoning ability, judgment, and decision making. Risk factors include low sensory input, hearing and visual deficits, and tranquilizers or sedatives. A combination of these factors, such as sometimes found in the elderly, place the client at high risk for cognitive impairment.

Impaired thought processes and *uncompensated memory deficit* are useful in describing etiological factors for problems in self-care, home maintenance, and other activities of daily living. It is possible in some cases to improve non-reality-based thinking, help the client compensate for memory deficits, and increase attention span when nursing intervention is focused on these etiological factors.

It was interesting to note that *knowledge deficit (specify)* was not among the highly utilized categories in a 1973–1985 review of clinical studies (Table 5-1). Health education and counseling has been a professional activity highly valued by nurses and repeatedly documented as a nursing responsibility. This category describes inability to state or explain information or inability to demonstrate a required skill necessary for health (or disease) management. The term *specify* requires that the particular area of knowledge deficit be included when using this category. Specification could include medication, diet, activity, or health practices such as exercise or relaxation.

Decisional conflict (specify) describes a state of uncertainty about a course of action to be taken when choice involves risk, loss, or challenge to personal life values. Clients may experience this condition when faced with surgery, certain therapies, divorce, or other life events. This category can be used to describe a problem or as an etiological or related factor for other problems.

Developmental delays may occur in the cognitive-perceptual pattern. These can be described and classified within the currently approved taxonomic category *altered growth and development.* Nurses in pediatric settings frequently encounter conditions in which development of cognitive abilities is not consistent with norms for the age group. Delays in a child's cognitive development can occur in a low-stimulus environment or with parental overprotection. Potential developmental problems and the risk factors they describe also need to be described and classified.

Self-Perception–Self-Concept Pattern

This pattern includes nine dysfunctional patterns of perception, mood, and ideas or attitudes about the self and self-competency (cognitive, affective, or physical). Two diagnostic categories, *anxiety* and *self-concept disturbance* (and its sub-components), were highly utilized by nurses in the studies reviewed (Table 5-1). All of the categories describe subjective feelings of clients and thus, require verbal reports for diagnosis. The currently identified dysfunctional patterns of self-perception–self-concept are:

Fear (Specify Focus)
Anxiety (Mild, Moderate, Severe)
Anticipatory Anxiety (Mild, Moder-
ate, Severe)
*Reactive Situational Depression
Hopelessness
Powerlessness (Severe, Moderate,
Low)
Self-Esteem Disturbance
Body Image Disturbance
Personal Identity Confusion

Fear and anxiety are two conditions encountered in all nursing settings. Be aware in using these diagnostic categories that a discrimination has to be made between these two conditions that share many of the same defining characteristics. (This type of discrimination is referred to as *differential diagnosis*.) *Fear* is a focused feeling of dread, threat, or danger to the self and the focus of the fear is to be specified, as may be seen above. Intervention is directed toward helping the client deal with the specific fear. In contrast, *anxiety* is nonspecific in focus. The client may express feelings of dread, threat, or danger but cannot identify a specific reason for these feelings. One of the first steps in treatment is helping the client to identify the focus. *Anticipatory anxiety* describes an increased level of arousal associated with perception of a future threat (unfocused) to the self or significant relationships. Both fear and anxiety may be seen at various levels of severity. Designating the level of severity is helpful in making treatment decisions. If a client is in a panic state it may be necessary to obtain a medication order before nursing treatment of the condition can begin.

Reactive situational depression describes feelings of sadness, despair, or dejection regarding a particular situation. Usually the condition is transitory and responds to nursing intervention. A discrimination has to be made between this condition and *hopelessness* in which the problem is an all-pervading sense of no hope, choices, or alternatives. *Powerlessness* describes a subjective feeling of lack of control over a situation and that one's actions will not significantly affect the outcome. This condition is frequently seen as a factor contributing to the client's reactive situational depression. *Hopelessness* describes a subjective state in which an individual sees either very limited or no alternatives or personal choices. When in a state of hopelessness, clients are passive and cannot mobilize resources in their own behalf. Discrimination is required between this condition and reactive situational depression, as hopelessness may be symptomatic of depression.

Self-esteem disturbance is a category used to describe negative feelings or conceptions of the self. Norris and Kunes-Connell (1985) point out that a defensive self-esteem may mask a self-esteem disturbance. Self-report of high self-esteem may be a defensive reaction to negative feelings about the self. This category is useful in describing adolescents and adults with such a problem; in pediatric settings it may be useful to use *developmental self-esteem disturbance. Body image disturbance* is closely related to disturbances in self-esteem. This category describes negative feelings or perceptions about characteristics, functions, or limits of the body or body parts. It may occur with loss of a body part or function, with underdevelopment, or after large weight losses. Some clients who are dependent on machines for long periods of time will suffer body image distortions. *Personal identity confusion* describes the inability to distinguish between self and others and feelings of "not knowing who I am." Oldaker (1985) has studied this condition in adolescents; it is also seen in psychiatric settings.

Delays can occur in the development of a functional pattern of self-perception–self-concept. Diagnostic categories are needed to describe these delays and dysfunctional developmental patterns of self-concept, personal identity and competency, body image, and the perception and control of mood states. Delays should be suspected when behavior does not meet norms for the age group.

Role-Relationship Pattern

People establish relationships to meet the human need for contact and interaction with others. Roles and relationships serve as a structure for family units, friendships, work and play, community groups, and a society. Dysfunctional patterns of role performance, interactions, and relationships can be the source of developmental problems or role stress in persons, families, or communities. Consider first the diagnostic categories that describe dysfunctional patterns influencing any type of interaction:

Impaired Verbal Communication
Impaired Social Interaction
*Unresolved Independence-Dependence Conflict
Potential for Violence

Language permits the communication of ideas, needs, purposes, feelings, and intentions. *Impaired verbal communication* describes the reduced or absent ability to use language in these human interactions. The category is broad; currently it is used to describe clients who are unable to speak, have speech impairments, or do not speak the dominant language.

There is an affective component to human communication that includes nonverbal sensitivity to others, facial expression and body posture, and tone and

inflection of speech, as well as culturally appropriate behavior in social interactions (the so-called social graces). These components of social interaction
can be influenced by lack of knowledge and skill, as well as neurological conditions, such as cerebrovascular accident (stroke), or mental illness. *Impaired
social interaction* is a diagnostic category that may be used to describe an
ineffective quality of social exchange that leads to discomfort in social situations
and an insufficient or excessive quantity of exchange. The problem that most
commonly occurs because of impaired social interaction is social isolation or
rejection; thus the diagnosis may be expressed in the problem/etiology format
as: Social Isolation/Impaired Social Interaction.

Unresolved independence-dependence conflict describes the need or desire to be independent (activities of daily living or decision making) in a situation
that requires some dependence. This conflict may be present in therapeutic,
maturational, or social situations. For example, the need for complete rest may
be required but produces conflict because the desire for self-care and ambulation is equally strong. The client may have the inability to move but this conflicts
with the desire for mobility and an adolescent may be in conflict over the wish
to be independent but also realize (or be reminded) that full maturational competency has not been attained. Accepting help from others when needed may
generate conflict for a person who has a history of independence and a strong
desire to be independent. *Unresolved dependence-independence conflict* is
also a useful category. It describes the situation where a person or family
experiences conflict between the insecurity of more independence and the
present security in being dependent. In both diagnostic categories the term
unresolved helps to direct nursing intervention; the goal is to help the client
resolve the conflict.

Potential for violence describes a set of risk factors for self-directed harm or
trauma to others during anger, rage, agitation, or depression. This condition is
usually associated with psychiatric settings where the aim of treatment is to
reduce person-environmental risk factors. Yet, the category is equally useful
when delivering care to communities, families, or individuals. A further specification may be inserted to increase applicability: *potential for self-violence,
potential for family violence,* or *potential for community violence.*

Now let us consider a set of diagnostic categories that describe patterns that
involve loss of relationships or reduced human interaction relative to the client's
need:

Anticipatory Grieving
Dysfunctional Grieving
*Translocation Syndrome
*Social Isolation
Social Isolation [or *Social Rejection*]

Grieving is a subjective state that follows loss or change in a pattern of
relationships. The loss can involve a person, possessions, job, status, home,
ideals, and parts or processes of the body. *Anticipatory grieving* describes the

expectation of a disruption in a familiar pattern or in a significant relationship; sadness and sorrow are expressed in anticipation of the loss. The normal grieving process should not be confused with *dysfunctional grieving* which describes an extended length or severity of grief and mourning. When risk factors are present for delayed grieving or for severe reactions to loss, the need for preventive intervention may be based on the diagnosis of *potential for dysfunctional grieving.* In using any of these three diagnostic categories, it is important to keep in mind that grief and mourning are culturally influenced and that observations of the person, family, or community should be evaluated in the context of their culture. Some have also suggested that the term *specify* would make the category more useful, as for example: Dysfunctional Grieving (Loss of Spouse). It may also be noted that *loss of spouse* is the focus of grieving and not an etiological factor. As discussed previously, etiological factors are the focus for intervention. Then to be useful the primary factor should be something that responds to nursing intervention. An example would be: Dysfunctional Grieving (Loss of Spouse)/Unavailable Support Systems. This etiological factor would suggest interventions, such as helping the person to talk about feelings, reactions, hopes, and plans and to make contact with bereavement groups in the community.

Translocation syndrome describes a set of biopsychosocial problems that occur particularly in circumstances of dependency and environmental change. Common examples of environmental change are transfer from a critical care unit to a convalescent unit, transfer from home to a nursing home, and change of room and location within a long-term care facility. For a person who is dependent or whose adaptive capacity is limited, the change from familiar surroundings, routines, people, and relationships can produce dysfunction in a number of patterns.

Social isolation describes interpersonal interactions below a level desired or required for personal integrity. The category is useful in describing the condition that results from voluntary or therapeutic isolation from others. It can occur with therapeutic isolation in hospitals, impaired mobility, fear, or body image disturbances. In contrast, the NANDA-accepted diagnosis *social isolation* has a different orientation; the author has relabeled it as *social rejection.* This category describes a condition of aloneness perceived as imposed by others and as a negative or threatening state. Other diagnoses have to be developed. One example is *support system deficit.* This would describe a condition in which there is insufficient access to, or utilization of, help from others during a crisis period. The help needed by a client may be instrumental, such as assistance with child care, obtaining a job, or locating a community service. In other instances the need for support may be expressive, such as caring, trust, intimacy, and empathy during a crisis period. Interventions differ for the two types of support system deficit (instrumental and expressive); thus, it is more clinically useful to specify the type of support systems that the client needs when developing this category.

A third set of diagnostic categories within the role-relationship pattern describes dysfunctional primary relationships:

Alteration in Family Process
Potential Alteration in Parenting
Alteration in Parenting
*Weak Mother-Infant (Parent-Infant) Attachment

Alteration in family process is currently defined as the inability of the family (or household members) to (1) meet the needs of members, (2) carry out family functions, or (3) maintain communications for mutual growth and maturation. This category is very broad and inclusive; the specific alterations need to be identified. The previously given caution against using a classification category as the problem ("alterations in . . .") and the specific diagnosis as the etiological or contributing factor pertains here also. Using "alteration in family process related to dysfunctional family communication patterns" would be similar to expressing a medical condition as "respiratory disease related to viral pneumonia."

Alterations in parenting and *potential alterations in parenting* are also broad and inclusive categories that do not focus thinking on a particular alteration. Specific diagnostic categories need to be identified to increase clinical usefulness. One alteration in parenting designation that is in an early stage of development by clinicians is *weak mother-infant attachment* or *weak parent-infant attachment.* This category describes an unreciprocal bonding relationship between the parent or primary caretaker and the infant. The term *unreciprocal* refers to behaviors on the part of the parent(s) *and* the infant. Thus, assessment has to be concerned with (1) the parent(s), (2) the infant, (3) the interaction that exists between them, and (4) the environment that can facilitate or inhibit attachment. If risk factors for weak attachment are observed during the prenatal period, *potential for weak mother-infant attachment* would be appropriate as a focus for preventive intervention. As in some of the previously considered diagnostic categories, conditions involving family or parent-child relationships have to be evaluated in the cultural context of the client. Otherwise, diagnostic errors may result.

The common developmental problems that may occur in this functional pattern area include:

*Altered Growth and Development: Speech-Communication Skills
*Altered Growth and Development: Social Skills

Altered growth and development: speech-communication skills describes a condition in which speech and language patterns do not meet norms for the age group. When a child's social skills, such as those discussed above in regard to impaired social interaction, do not develop according to developmental norms for the age group the condition can be described by the diagnostic category *altered growth and development: social skills.* As with previous diagnoses, the taxonomic category *altered growth and development* may be dropped from clinical recordings when developmental delays are clearly described in diagnostic terms.

Sexuality-Reproductive Pattern

Diagnostic categories within this pattern area describe client's perceived disturbances in sexuality or reproduction. Although closely tied to the role-relationships pattern, the sexuality-reproductive pattern is seen as a distinct functional health pattern for assessment. Five diagnostic categories have been identified:

Sexual Dysfunction
Altered Sexuality Patterns
Rape Trauma Syndrome
Rape Trauma Syndrome: Compound Reaction
Rape Trauma Syndrome: Silent Reaction

Sexual dysfunction describes perceived problems in achieving desired sexual satisfaction. The term *perceived problems* is used to indicate that it is the client's perception of problems, not the care provider's personal values regarding what constitutes sexual dysfunction, that is the focus of diagnosis. The category is very broad and inclusive and specific dysfunctions amenable to nursing intervention need to be identified. Clients with limitations on sexual expression imposed by disease or therapy may come to the nurse's attention. In other instances sexual dysfunction may be a symptom of a relationship problem. The diagnosis *altered sexuality patterns,* accepted in 1986, appears similar to *sexual dysfunction.* The criteria for diagnosis are less well defined. There is one defining characteristic: reported difficulties, limitations, or changes in sexual behaviors or activities (McLane, 1987).

Further work is needed to identify dysfunctional developmental patterns, such as those that do not meet expected developmental, cultural, or social norms for an age group. When developed, diagnostic categories can be classified under the NANDA-approved category *altered growth and development.*

Rape trauma syndrome and the two types of reactions are diagnostic categories describing the biopsychosocial problems following rape. A compound reaction includes the reactivation of physical or psychiatric illness or the reliance on alcohol, drugs, or both. *Rape trauma syndrome: silent reaction* is associated with no verbalization of the occurrence of rape in the presence of abrupt changes in relationships and sexual behavior, sudden onset of phobic reactions, and increased anxiety (McLane, 1987).

Coping-Stress Tolerance Pattern

Coping is defined as the cognitive and emotional processes used by a person, family, or community group to manage stress. When an event or relationship is perceived by the client to tax or exceed personal resources and to present a threat to well-being, stress exists (Lazarus and Folkman, 1984). (Many view the terms *stress* and *anxiety* as overlapping.) Stress tolerance is essentially a measure of vulnerability; persons with low stress tolerance are susceptible to ineffective coping. Currently there are seven diagnostic categories that describe dysfunctional patterns of coping-stress tolerance:

Ineffective Coping (Individual)
*Avoidance Coping
Ineffective Family Coping: Compromised
Ineffective Family Coping: Disabling
Family Coping: Potential for Growth
Post-Trauma Response
Impaired Adjustment

As currently defined by NANDA, *ineffective coping* describes the impairment of adaptive behaviors and problem solving abilities used to meet life's demands and roles. Essentially, the category describes ineffective or nonproductive management of stress or anxiety. Avoid using this diagnosis to describe excess food or alcohol intake, noncompliance, or uncooperative behavior unless anxiety, perception of life stress, and inability to problem solve are also present (Vincent, 1986).

Avoidance coping is a type of ineffective coping. It is used to describe minimization or denial of information (facts, meanings, consequences) when a situation requires active coping. Avoidance can be problematic if the reality of chest pain is distorted or denial of diabetes results in health management deficits. In using this category it is important that avoidance coping is not confused with hope or adaptive denial. For example, avoiding the facts or implications of a situation may be adaptive in the early stages of a crisis and would not be labeled as a diagnosis requiring resolution.

Two of the above diagnostic categories describe ineffective family coping. The term *compromised* refers to the situation where ineffective family coping results in insufficient or ineffective family support to members. *Ineffective coping: disabling* describes neglect, rejection, abandonment, and other coping behaviors that are detrimental to family members.

The diagnostic category *family coping: potential for growth* describes a situation where coping is effective and family members have the potential to grow through the experience of coping with stress. Nursing is directed toward helping the client use the experience of coping with stress to attain higher levels of personal or family development.

Post-trauma response describes a sustained crisis-reaction to an overwhelming traumatic event. It can interfere with cognitive, affective, and sensory-motor activities and is characterized by repetitive dreams or nightmares, guilt, and flashbacks. This condition may follow war experiences, disasters, epidemics, rape, assault, torture, or other events that are viewed as crises by the person. *Impaired adjustment* describes a state of inability to modify life style or behavior in a manner consistent with a change in health status (McLane,

1987). As defined, this diagnostic category would be used to describe behaviors consistent with impaired adjustment to illness.

Diagnostic categories have not been identified to describe dysfunctional development of coping strategies and the ability to tolerate stress. In addition current diagnostic categories may describe conditions encountered in the care of children but the defining characteristics (behaviors) sometimes pertain only to the adult.

Value-Belief Pattern

Values, beliefs, goals and life commitments guide the choices made by a person, family, or community; they can influence the evaluation of situations in terms of personal meaning. Thus, values, beliefs, goals and commitments can explain why a situation may be stressful for one client and not another and why one person is highly motivated in a situation and another is not. Currently, one diagnostic category has been identified by NANDA in this pattern area:

Spiritual Distress (Distress of the Human Spirit)

As currently defined by NANDA, *spiritual distress* describes "disruption in the life principle which pervades a person's entire being and which integrates and transcends one's biological and psychosocial nature" (McLane, 1987). It is used when clients express concern with the meaning of life, death, suffering, or their personal belief system. No diagnostic categories have been developed to describe dysfunctional development of this pattern area. A number of theories exist to describe and explain children's spiritual and moral development and the evolution of ethics and values in adulthood. These theories plus clinical observation of conditions encountered in caring for children may help to identify diagnostic categories in this area.

SUMMARY

Early in this chapter a distinction was made between functional, dysfunctional, and potentially dysfunctional patterns. When data indicate a pattern is *functional* in the context of the whole person's (family, community) functioning, this indicates a strength that may be mobilized to deal with health problems. *Dysfunctional patterns* (actual problems) and *potentially dysfunctional patterns* (potential problems) are described by diagnostic categories. Various types of patterns were discussed, including unhealthful changes from baseline and developmental delay or dysfunctional development.

When an actual problem is diagnosed the search begins for etiological or related factors which are the focus for intervention. In contrast, when diagnosing potential problems, one must delineate the risk factors which contribute to the high-risk state—intervention focuses on risk factor reduction.

Currently identified categories that provide labels for nursing diagnoses were discussed. These are terms used to describe actual or potential problems. It was noted that the categories are in an early stage of development. Yet most have been demonstrated as useful for describing problems encountered in clinical practice and as a focus for treatment planning. The overview of current diagnostic language in this chapter should be followed by intensive study of the conceptual basis, definition, and critical defining characteristics for each diagnostic category. This brief introduction to diagnostic categories will prepare the reader for considering the diagnostic process which employs information collection, interpretation, clustering, and naming the condition judged to be present.

BIBLIOGRAPHY

Bruenig, K., Brickwitzki, G., Schute, J., Crane, L., Schroder, P. M., & Lutze, J. (1986). Noncompliance as a nursing diagnosis: Current use in clinical practice. In Hurley, M. (ed.), *Classification of nursing diagnoses: Proceedings of the sixth conference.* New York: Mosby.

Gettrust, K., Ryan, S., & Engleman, D. (1985). *Applied nursing diagnosis: Guides for comprehensive care planning.* New York: Wiley.

Gordon, M. (1987). *Manual of nursing diagnosis.* New York: McGraw-Hill.

Gordon, M. (1985). Practice-based data set for a nursing information system. *Journal of Medical Systems.* 9:43–55.

Hurley, M. (1986). *Classification of nursing diagnoses: Proceedings of the sixth conference.* St. Louis, MO: Mosby.

Institute of Medicine. (1979). *Report of a study: Sleeping pills, insomnia, and medical practice.* Washington, DC: U.S. National Academy of Sciences.

Lazaruus, R., & Folkman, S. (1984). *Stress, appraisal, and coping.* New York: Springer.

Lin, N., Woelfel, M., & Light, S. (1985). Buffering effect of social support subsequent to an important life event. *Journal of Health and Social Behavior,* 26:247–263.

McLane, A. (ed.)(1987). *Classification of nursing diagnoses: Proceedings of the seventh congress.* St. Louis, MO: Mosby.

Oldaker, S. (1985). Identity confusion: Nursing diagnoses for adolescents. *Nursing Clinics of North America,* 20:763–774.

Stanitis, M. A., & Ryan, J. (1982). Noncompliance: An unacceptable diagnosis. *American Journal of Nursing,* 82:941–942.

Taylor, F. K. (1971). A logical analysis of the medico-psychologic concept of disease (Part 1). *Psychological Medicine,* 1:356–364.

U.S. Department of Health, Education, and Welfare. (1979). *Healthy people: The Surgeon General's report on health promotion and disease prevention.* Washington, DC: Government Printing Office, DHEW (PHS) #79-55071.

Vincent, K. (1986). Validation of a nursing diagnosis: Nurse-consensus survey. In Hurley, M. (ed.), *Classification of nursing diagnosis: Proceedings of the sixth conference.* St. Louis, MO: Mosby.

Vincent, P. (1985). Letters to the editor. *American Journal of Nursing,* 33:266–267.

Voith, A., & Smith, D. (1985). Validation of the nursing diagnosis of urinary retention. *Nursing Clinics of North America,* 20:723–730.

CHAPTER 6

CLINICAL INFORMATION COLLECTION

The diagnostic process was defined previously as including four activities: *information collection, information interpretation, information clustering,* and *naming the cluster.* Chapters 3 and 4 began the discussion of information collection. The focus was on *what* information is to be collected. This chapter continues the discussion, but the focus is on *how* information is collected during assessment.

Assessment,[1] a term used frequently in nursing, *is a health status evaluation which requires the collection and interpretation of clinical data.* It continues during all professional, nurse-client interactions. Assessment never stops but at points in time a diagnosis may be made, revised, or discarded as a basis for directing nursing treatment. Can assessment occur without diagnosis? Yes. When the information reveals no health problems the clinical data are summarized and recorded as the health status evaluation.

Professional responsibility to the client requires that diagnoses be based on assessments that are *deliberate* and *systematic.* These characteristics of data collection increase the likelihood of obtaining accurate information and, thus, making accurate diagnoses. Deliberate assessment has purpose and direction. It is based on many of the ideas already discussed, such as:

1 Awareness of the professional domain and scope of practice responsibilities (Chapters 2 and 3)
2 Clear concept of the clinical data needed to fulfill responsibilities to clients (Chapter 4)

[1]Variation exists in use of the word, assessment (Bloch, 1974). Some use the term to refer to four activities of the diagnostic process; in this book it will mean the collection and interpretation of clinical data.

3 Use of focal questions and observations that conserve clients' and nurses' time and energy (Chapter 4)

A systematic approach implies organized information collection and logical sequencing of questions and observations. Three main factors can influence organization during assessment; they will serve to structure the content in this chapter. The first is the *the situational context* which includes the physical and interpersonal characteristics of the situation and how the assessment is structured. The second is the *nature of the information* which influences both how it is collected and how it is used. The *diagnostician's cognitive and perceptual capabilities,* which are important tools for collecting health-related information, is the third factor. All three factors operate simultaneously in every clinical situation where information is being collected. For example in a hospital room (situational context), a nurse (diagnostician) anticipating that a client may be having pain looks closely for facial grimacing related to pain (nonverbal nature of information). How is information collected for health evaluation and diagnostic judgment? By knowing the nature of the desired information, setting up the ideal situation for its collection, and finely tuning the senses required for perceptual recognition.

SITUATIONAL CONTEXT FOR ASSESSMENT

The *context* of assessment situations refers to the circumstances in which information collection occurs. Although information collection is the objective in all assessment situations, contexts differ in terms of the immediate purpose and scope of data to be gathered, probability of health problems, and structure of the physical and interpersonal environment. These contextual factors will be examined in relation to common types of assessment occurring in clinical practice:

1 Initial assessment which occurs when a nurse adds a client to his or her caseload

2 Problem-focused assessment which is done daily (or more frequently if needed)

3 Time-lapse reassessment that occurs in clinics, health maintenance organizations, or occupational, school, and residential settings

4 Emergency assessment which is required when initial impressions indicate a life-threatening situation

Take particular note of differences in the *probability of a health problem.* These differences directly influence the diagnostician's approach to information collection and the inherent difficulty of the task. Clearly, if one knows what one is looking for (problem-focused assessment), the search is easier than if one does not (universe of possibilities). As will be seen in a later chapter, nurses have strategies for quickly narrowing the universe of possibilities during initial assessments.

Admission Assessment

Whenever a client is added to a nurse's caseload, an admission assessment of the 11 previously described functional health patterns is completed. This establishes the *nursing data base.* Initial assessments are referred to as a data base because (1) basic historical and current information about all health patterns is collected and (2) the information is used as baseline criteria against which any further changes are evaluated.

Purpose and Scope   The purpose of initial assessment is to evaluate a client's health status, identify any problematic functional patterns, and to establish a therapeutic, helping relationship. As described below, the *components of the admission assessment are a nursing history of functional patterns and an examination of pattern indicators.* The former is done by interviewing the client, significant others, or both. The latter requires observation and other examination techniques. Generally, a comprehensive assessment is necessary. If a client's condition is critical (physiological or psychological instability exists), only screening assessment of patterns may be warranted (see Chapter 4).

Collection of data can be influenced by the psychological set of the clinician and by clients' view of a nursing history and examination. How each of these influence the purpose and scope of data collection will be described in the next sections.

Psychological Set: The Nurse   A psychological set is an inclination to take certain actions or hold certain attitudes. A disposition or set influences what is attended to and overall motivation. Thus, it *directly influences the clinician's purpose and scope of data collection, as well as expectations of the probability of health problems. During history and examination the set, or motivation, is to describe and evaluate functional health patterns and subsequently to offer the client help or guidance as necessary.* This fact should be kept in mind, because it is not the common, everyday social set. Most interpersonal interactions are not descriptive-evaluative, nor are they purposefully diagnostic. Neither are they necessarily or deliberately therapeutic.

The nurse's motivation in the interaction complements the client's role set. Although sometimes disguised, the client's objective generally is to obtain help in health evaluation, problem solving, or physical activities. The first step in providing help is to describe and explain current health patterns. Then professional decisions can be made regarding the need for help and the goals of helping.

The most productive motivation of a professional health care provider doing assessment is to *explain* the data. It has been suggested that *a diagnostician approaches clinical observations with a descriptive-explanatory set related to the question, Why?* This set should predominate over a concern (1) about personal self-maintenance (What is the client in relation to me? or Can the client help me meet my needs?), (2) about personal role (Who is the client in relation to me? or What role shall I play?), or (3) about acceptable and unacceptable behavior of the client (How well does the client meet my expectations of a client?). Sets to perceive and interpret greatly influence the way client behaviors are categorized (Sarbin, Taft, and Bailey, 1960, pp. 144–159).

Imagine what would ensue if one's primary set in a psychiatric setting was self-maintenance. Clients' behavior might be instantly interpreted as potential violence. Or a nurse with a set to evaluate how a client "stayed in line" with the patient role might be quick to see too much independence and "taking over" during assessment. Far too often care providers slip into nonproductive sets during interactions with clients.

Part of socialization into professional nursing is to learn role behavior, for example, that the motivation predominating in assessment is the descriptive-explanatory, or *why*, set. This is not to say that the other sets are never used. An experienced nurse may reflect on how sensitive the client is to another's (the nurse's) needs. Are social cues to roles (the nurse's role) received? How well does the client assume various role expectations? The nurse-client interaction is used as the object of observation. The nurse pays attention to her or his own affective reactions and impressions generated by the client's behavior. These personal reactions are used as hypotheses about how others react to the client and may provide data about health problems in the role-relationship pattern area. These techniques are particularly useful in specialty areas such as psychiatric nursing assessment.

Psychological Set: The Client   Assessment is accomplished more successfully when one is aware of one's own perspective and takes account of the motivation and perspective of the client. According to one school of social psychology, behavior is greatly influenced by the way a person "defines the situation" (Cardwell, 1971).

Extending this idea to assessment would suggest a number of things. Initially, both client and nurse bring past experience, expectations, and values to the situation. Individually, both synthesize these predefinitions with current perceptions. Unspoken questions, may arise: What is happening? What role shall I play? How shall I behave? *Personal definition of the assessment situation is one factor that influences behavior in interpersonal interaction.* This idea provides food for thought. How does the nurse help the client to define and understand the "situation" of assessment and health care? Before discussing approaches, let us extend this idea further.

Diagnosis is also a "definition of situation"; it is a way of defining the health situation. A client usually has some idea of the health problems when assessment begins. This idea includes notions, expectations, and feelings, and they may be realistic or unrealistic. By telling his or her health history and thinking about the questions asked, a client may even be disposed to define the situation in a new way. Simultaneously, the nurse gains information to define the situation diagnostically.

Prior to assessment, the individual, family, friends, or society must define the situation as requiring health consultation or care. Otherwise, no action is taken. The client's predefinition of the problem, the data collection process, and the health care system need to be taken into account.

Herzlich and Graham (1973) identified the meanings people attributed to the terms *health* and *illness*. Of interest to our discussion are the findings about when and why people consult health care providers. In these researchers' middle class, urban sample and in other studies (Koss, 1960; Mechanic and Volkart, 1961; Zola, 1979) it was found that perception of symptoms was not sufficient to initiate health consultation. Passage from a perceived state of health to perceived sickness occurred when symptoms interfered with work or social activity. People then defined themselves as needing to know "what is the matter."

Symptoms were viewed as ambiguous; they could either mean nothing or be important. This produced uncertainty. Most importantly, symptoms interfered with activity. These were the reasons consultation was sought. The expectation was that the health care provider would define the situation and give it meaning. Routine health examinations were sought even in the absence of symptoms, for the same reasons; the care provider would reassure that absence of symptoms meant health (Herzlich and Graham, 1973, pp. 78–87). *Interference with functional activities involved in daily living was the main concern that initiated health consultation.* Therefore, diagnosing disease is an insufficient response to the client. Diagnosis should also focus on management of functional activities and on the associated capabilities required. This is the province of nursing diagnosis, although it is not a diagnostic area that has been offered to the consumer in a systematic, organized way by nurses.

Most clients will view consultation or entrance into the health care delivery system as focusing on medical diagnosis, medical treatment, and the prognosis of physical or mental disease. This is how they have been socialized. The details of health management are usually left for them to work out as best they can. As the literature reveals, one result is a high incidence of noncompliance with therapeutic recommendations (Haynes, Taylor, and Sackett, 1979).

Two reactions from clients are common when nurses begin to assess things other than the physical aspects of a disease. One is amazement that the nurse would be concerned. The second is the "something else is the matter with me" reaction. (The latter also occurs when three or four doctors plus a medical student see a patient.)

Consumers have to become accustomed to defining the health care system as offering both nursing and medical consultation and as oriented to both health and disease. Purposeful communication to inform people about this distinction and about nursing's role in health care is needed. The communication can be incorporated into nursing assessment of the functional health patterns described in Chapter 4.

Consider some examples of initiating an assessment so as to help the client define the situation. The nurse could say, being purposefully vague, "Ms. Klein, I'd like to see if I can help you. Let's talk about some things regarding your care. . . ." The more direct approach is, "Ms. Klein, I'd like to do a nursing assessment. There may be things you would like help with, so we'll talk about the way you plan your diet and . . ." (mentions a few relevant things). The latter clearly implies a strategy for educating the consumer about nursing. It familiarizes the client with vocabulary (*nursing assessment*), definitions, and what benefits may be derived. When the situation is perceived clearly, the client is in a better position to respond to assessment questions. Over and over again this has been demonstrated in psychological studies of cognition (Bruner, Goodnow, and Austin, 1956). *Responses are more appropriate when a person knows what is expected, and involvement increases when the benefits are clear.* These are points sometimes neglected in clinical practice.

Probability of Health Problems   The initial assessment cannot be problem-focused at the start; no current data are available. *The hypothesis of no dysfunctional pattern is as probable as the hypothesis that dysfunctional patterns exist.* The question directing assessment is: *Does a health problem exist?* The universe of possibilities is open. On the basis of initial cues (age, medical problem, initial observations or impressions), likely possibilities are generated.

Structure for Information Collection   The interpersonal situation in which initial diagnoses are established is important. Generally, the person, family or community group does not know the nurse. Therefore, consideration has to be given to establishing trust and rapport during assessment. *Interpersonal factors* are critical for obtaining valid information and for a future helping relationship. The *environmental setting* is also critical to the initial assessment. When people are asked to share information about personal "ways of living," privacy must be ensured. The clinician and client, trying to structure a therapeutic relationship characterized by confidence and rapport, need a *comfortable setting free from interruption and distraction.*

Structure is provided for information collection during an initial assessment by the nursing history and examination. The history contains the client's subjective reports of functional health patterns, whereas the examination consists of nursing observations. A format for history taking and examination was discussed in Chapter 4; how to do this type of assessment will be discussed in some detail in this chapter, as it is a complex and important nursing activity that initiates the professional relationship.

Nursing History and Examination   The nursing history can be done by interview, by questionnaire, or by a combination of both. Important differences exist. If the client fills out an assessment form, the responses have to be taken at face value. No interpersonal interaction occurs as the questions are answered. During an interview further clarification can be derived by branching questions. Some health care settings combine both approaches; this occurs most commonly when entering clients are not acutely ill or cognitively impaired, as for example in ambulatory or day surgery settings, when prior scheduling of admission permits sending an assessment form to the home for preentry completion, or when the admission office distrubutes forms. Follow-up questions are asked during an admission interview. The advantages of this procedure are that a portion of the nurse's time is saved and the opportunity still exists to follow through on problematic or potentially problematic patterns. In addition, the client can relax and fill out the information at his own pace. The interpersonal contact in either situation is designed to clarify the issues, permit elaboration by both parties, and thus allow the nurse to arrive at an understanding of the client's responses. Currently, history taking by interview is most common. A successful interview is guided, not dominated, by the nurse. Actually, the client should be talking about 80 percent of the time and the nurse, 20 percent. The nurse guides the interview by opening a topic (pattern area), assisting with the narrative, focusing, and closing a topic (Froelich and Bishop, 1977, p. 89). The first decision is how to begin; the last involves termination.

Beginning an Assessment   An initial assessment begins with the nursing history. Introductions are important because people consider names personal. Address the client by name, introduce yourself, and state your title, for example, student nurse, registered nurse, or clinical specialist. Explain your purpose. All of the following introductions have been observed in clinical settings; which one begins to establish a professional relationship?

1 Mr. Jones? I'm Ms. Arnold, a student nurse at the university. I'd like to talk to you about your health and how you're managing.

2 Hi, Mr. Jones. I'm Ms. Arnold, a student. I have to do a nursing assessment on you.

3 Mr. Jones? I'm Joan, but most of my friends call me Jo. I'd like to see if you have any problems.

4 Bill Jones? I'm Ms. Arnold; before I go off duty I have to do your nursing care plan.

The over-friendly approach of numbers 2, 3, and 4 is not appropriate in initiating an admission assessment. Examples 2 and 4, with the "have to do" phrase, may communicate that other activities would be preferred. In number 4, especially, the client is made to feel that he is delaying the nurse from going off duty; this situation generates the expectation of a rushed job. Rather than focus on a task to be done, focus on the client's needs as in number 1, which is the preferred introduction. The idea of how to begin health pattern assessment will be expanded further in later chapters on diagnostic strategies.

Helping the Client to Describe Health Patterns   Both the knowledge of what to assess and the interpersonal skills that facilitate history taking are important in helping clients describe their health patterns. Much has been written about communication and interviewing techniques; in this section a few major points will be considered: topic transitions in health pattern assessment, creating questions, and the use of selected techniques to facilitate communications.

TOPIC TRANSITIONS As each pattern is assessed, try to relate the next pattern area to a previous statement. Use an appropriate transitional comment; then follow with a question. Otherwise, the nursing history appears to be an interrogation. Note the difference in use of transitional comments in the following two assessments of the sleep-rest pattern of a hospitalized adult:

ASSESSMENT 1

Nurse: You mentioned before that you felt tired during the day; when you get up most mornings do you feel rested and ready for work?

Client: No, not lately; I guess I'm not getting enough sleep.

Nurse: That certainly can contribute to being tired during the day. Has this been a few days, weeks, or longer?

Client: It's been about a month now.

Nurse: About how many hours do you sleep, on the average?

Client: About 4; I try to go to sleep about 11:00 and I'm still awake between 3:00 and 4:00; then I have to get up at 7:00.

Nurse: That can be irritating, to lie awake in the dark. I'm sure you've thought about what might be causing this and what would help you get to sleep (*questioning tone*).

Client: I start thinking about all the problems and I worry that my husband will have another heart attack at night. I guess I finally fall asleep around 3:00 from exhaustion. I don't take any pills.

Nurse: He's been home 4 weeks when you had to come into the hospital, right? How has he been doing?

Client: Well he seems to be doing good; his doctor is very pleased with his recovery. I guess I'm silly to worry but . . . (*voice trails off*).

Nurse: Well, sometimes thinking can help work out things but maybe we need to talk further about your concerns. I could come back this afternoon after you have your x rays. Are you concerned right now about him being alone?

Client: No, my daughter is staying over; but you'll come back later?

Nurse: Yes, let's talk this afternoon; I notice you have glasses; are they for reading or . . . (*nurse uses this to introduce the cognitive-perceptual pattern assessment*).

ASSESSMENT 2

Nurse: I'd like to ask you about your sleep pattern now. When you get up in the morning, do you feel well rested?

Client: No, not lately.

Nurse: How many hours do you sleep at night?

Client: Not more than 4; I have to get up at 7:00 to go to work.

Nurse: When do you go to bed?

Client: Eleven.

Nurse: So you don't get to sleep until 3:00?

Client: Yes . . . (*nurse asks the next question as client hesitates.*)

Nurse: How long have you had this problem?

Client: About 4 weeks; I just can't seem to get to sleep before 3:00 most every night. It's terrible lying awake.

Nurse: Do you take anything to sleep?

Client: No, but the doctor ordered some sleeping pills here.

Nurse: Well, that should help. Do you know why you have the trouble sleeping at home?

Client: No . . . not really.

Nurse: Any nightmares or bad dreams?

Client: No.

Nurse: Well maybe you'll sleep better with the pill and after you have your tests and go home things will be better. How's your vision? (*Nurse introduces the cognitive-perceptual pattern.*)

In the first assessment the transition from pattern to pattern and from question to question is smoothly made. The interview is personalized and the nurse exhibits interest and concern. In the second assessment one gets the impression that there are a set of questions to be asked and the history taking is an *interrogation.* Generally, both nurses asked the same questions and obtained data to support a sleep onset disturbance. Which one was most effective in establishing a supportive relationship? Which obtained better data for diagnosing the probable cause of the sleep onset problem?

Short abrupt questions or reading questions one by one from a paper is not effective in establishing an interpersonal relationship that communicates caring. In fact, the nurse in the second assessment did not obtain any information about the probable cause of the sleep pattern disturbance. At the point where the second nurse asked about nightmares, the client may have been ready to share her concerns about her husband but the nurse continued the questioning. Instead, when the client hesitantly said "No, not really," the nurse could have responded with a supportive tone of voice: "Sometimes worries can keep us awake at night; do you have any concerns?" Even without knowledge of the client's concern about her husband having a heart attack, fear and anxiety should have been considered. These are two of the most common causes of sleep onset disturbance.

Some further examples of smooth transitions may be helpful. A number of problems may be verbalized while the client reports data about his or her health-perception–health-management pattern. The transition to nutritional pattern can be made by saying, "Let's jot down those problems; we will want to talk further about them. I seem to need more specific information about some things. You mentioned that planning meals was difficult. What kinds of foods have you been eating at breakfast, lunch, dinner, and for snacks? Let's begin with breakfast." This leads into the nutritional pattern.

Attempt to construct a comfortable transition, especially in areas usually considered personal. For example, after inquiring about family structure and relationships, move on to sexuality patterns: "You mentioned that you've been married nearly 10 years; do you both find sexual relationships satisfactory?" or less direct, "Do any marital problems arise now and then?" or "Has this illness been associated with any problems in sexual relationships?" Creating transitional statements will take practice. *The main idea to keep in mind is to personalize the interview.* Pick up on something that has been said and relate it to the next topic for discussion.

CREATING QUESTIONS In Chapter 4 the content of questions for individual, family, and community assessment are listed. These need to be formulated in the context of the ongoing assessment. In addition, branching questions will need to be constructed to clarify, elaborate, or validate information.

There are various types of questions and remarks that facilitate history taking. One is the *open-ended question; the topic for discussion is specified in a general question and usually elicits descriptions and current concerns.* An example would be "What's it like for you when all the children are at home for the day?" This is in contrast to the *direct question, which requires a specific yes or no answer.* An example is, "Do you get upset when all the children are home for the day?" After a client has responded to an open-ended question, direct questions may provide particular cues. When a specific diagnostic possibility is being considered, the critical characteristics (diagnostic criteria) of the category guide the formulation of questions.

Probing questions are frequently needed to obtain clarification. These are questions that permit the client to elaborate. They are commonly used when a client employs abstract terms or offers judgments such as *nervous, depressed,* or *ulcer.* Beware of accepting such words at face value: the client may define them totally differently than you do. Probe with a follow-up inquiry such as, "What feelings do you notice when you're nervous?" Sometimes it will be discovered that cardiac rhythm irregularities are occurring. Similarly, *ulcer* may mean a skin abrasion.

It is also not uncommon for clients to circumvent an area that is emotionally charged, such as death. They may not be sure the nurse can accept their beliefs or feelings. The nurse who suspects this must probe with care and at the same time be accepting and supporting.

FACILITATING COMMUNICATION Support, reassurance, empathy, and silence are communications that assist the client in describing health patterns. *Support demonstrates interest, concern, and understanding.* It can enhance description or close it off, depending on when understanding is communicated. *Reassurance communicates that the client has worth and self-reliance. Empathy accepts or clarifies feelings or behavior. Supportive silence permits the client to continue a response when description is difficult.* Examples of these communications follow:

Support

Client: I have a terrible time trying to get to sleep at night.
Nurse: That must be difficult. What seems to be . . . ?

Reassurance

Client: I have a terrible time trying to get to sleep at night.
Nurse: I think we can come up with some things you can do. What seems to be . . . ?

Empathy

Client: I have a terrible time trying to get to sleep at night.
Nurse: That can cause you a lot of worry and concern. What seems to be . . . ?

Silence can communicate interest or withdrawal. For example, when the client uses the words *terrible time,* the nurse could shift forward very slightly, holding eye contact. This movement indicates interest and concern. Shifting away from the client and from eye contact indicates withdrawal from the problem, irrespective of what the nurse says or the silence that intervenes. The client may be sensitive to this body language and may not elaborate, thinking the nurse is uncomfortable or not interested.

Questions and remarks can be *reflective* or *confronting. A reflection echoes a portion of what the client just said.* For example, a child may say, "I get upset in school"; the nurse then says, with a gentle, supportive, questioning tone of a voice, "Upset?"

Confrontation focuses attention on feelings or behavior. It is used to probe more deeply. A client may describe some change. Three or four sentences later it is evident that this change began 2 months after a divorce. The nurse, feeling attention should be focused on the time sequence, may say, "Do you think that was related to your feelings after your divorce?" Confrontations can be based on the need to validate an inference or an observation during the diagnostic process; confrontation during an intervention may have other objectives, such as insight development.

During the assessment of emotionally charged areas, a client may begin to cry. Accept this demonstration of feeling without feeling guilty. Feelings of guilt are a sign to the nurse that his or her focus has turned inward toward self rather than outward toward the client. Crying is a cue to depth of feelings, such as frustration or sadness. Empathy, reassurance, or silence combined with touch usually is helpful. After the client gains some composure the nurse can ask whether he or she can help in any way. This is better than suggesting that the interview stop; the only recourse then would be to leave, since presence indicates waiting to continue.

Early indications of fatigue or increasing anxiety need to be observed. Try to validate these impressions with the client. Both fatigue and anxiety during the interview should be treated as data. Fatigue is a cue to activity tolerance. It should be noted and a decision made about shifting from a detailed assessment to a few screening questions. Judgment has to be used regarding the signs of increasing anxiety. Either the topic or the discussion of the topic with a not-yet-trusted nurse may be producing a personal threat to the client. The client can be asked whether he or she wishes to talk further about the topic or to continue later. There are many good books about interviewing and assessment that deal with situations such as these and prepare the beginner for handling this type of situation if it arises.

Examination Following the nursing history an examination is done. Observations are made of physical characteristics such as gait and mobility, skin integrity, heart rate, and range of joint movement. Cues obtained during history taking provide impressions of speech (tone, rate, and quality) and possibly interactions if another person is present (parent-child or client-other relationships).[2] Assessment occurring in the home provides opportunities to observe living conditions, safety hazards, and the client's neighborhood.

Five sensory modalities (vision, hearing, cutaneous touch, smell, and kinesthesia) provide a means for obtaining clinical data during examination. (Taste, the other sensory modality, is rarely used.) The nurse is a sensitive measuring device for listening, interpersonal interaction, observation, inspection, and examination (auscultation, palpation, and percussion). An amazing amount of information can be collected through the use of the five sensory modalities and these four methods of data collection. As educational programs incorporate additional physical examination skills into clinical courses, the areas listed under examination in Chapter 4 can be expanded. (Many excellent books about the methods of clinical data collection are available; some are listed in the bibliography at the end of this chapter.)

All of the above observational and examination methods provide information about functional health patterns. For example, a pattern of exercise-activity described in the history can be understood in the context of an observed gait impairment. A school child's poor hygiene may be understood after examination of living facilities.

Deeper understanding of functional patterns is acquired *only* if physical assessment findings *are collected for this purpose.* Seems obvious? Apparently it is not, because sometimes physical examination data are separated from nursing history data by using a biomedical systems format (gastrointestinal, cardiovascular, and similar categories). If functional health patterns are a reasonable focus for nursing assessment and diagnosis, think about *all* clinical data as indicators of these patterns. What is observed during examination may be the outcome of existing or emerging functional patterns the client described during the history. Or the observational data may explain why certain patterns exist, have changed, or are emerging developmentally.

Examination of the client and situation verifies or expands understanding gained during history taking. Generally, dysfunctional patterns are elicited during the history; examination provides further data, not surprises.

---

[2]Interaction in the full sense of the word cannot be accomplished when a patient is unconscious, extremely hyperactive, or markedly out of contact with reality. In these instances information is acquired from a knowledgeable person or by examination.

Terminating the Admission Assessment After information is collected through history taking and examination, termination of the initial assessment begins. There are three objectives at this time:

1 Offer the opportunity to the client to add further information or express additional health concerns.
2 Summarize the assessment.
3 Make plans for treatment of problems.

As one's experience in diagnosis increases, it becomes possible in most cases to structure diagnostic hypotheses simultaneously with history taking and examination. After asking whether the client has further information or concerns, the nurse summarizes and makes plans in the context of ongoing events. The table on p. 176 is an example of terminating an initial assessment of a 60-year-old female client admitted one day before gallbladder surgery; the diagnoses are moderate anticipatory anxiety related to perceived postoperative dependency, exogenous obesity related to caloric intake-energy expenditure imbalance, high risk for atelectasis, and social isolation related to stress incontinence.

Summarization and planning with the client at the time the assessment ends may not always be possible, especially when the nurse is in the early stages of learning diagnosis. Secondly, even the experienced diagnostician may not be able to formulate diagnoses "on the spot" because of complexity of the health problem or because of missing data. The nurse should not feel pressured to diagnose, summarize, and plan at the end of the assessment; it is better to discuss concerns at the symptom level than to share early judgments that may be incorrect. For example, a nurse could say, "We've talked about a number of things; while you're thinking about anything we've missed, I'll just look over what we talked about. . . ." Or, when data are missing or time is needed to formulate a problem, an expression of interest and concern may be sufficient. This could be stated as, "You've mentioned a number of things; I think you can work out some solutions if we talk about these some more" or "Let's both think about what could be causing your family to react this way."

The idea to be gained from the above examples is that *after assessment clients should* (1) *perceive that something will be done with the information that has been shared* and (2) *have a feeling of future competency for handling any identified problems with (or without) assistance from the nurse.* Basically, what is being described is a sharing of interest, concern, and understanding— the caring response even before the actual care plan has been designed.

This section began the examination of *how* information is collected in the admission assessment. Various terms are used to refer to this activity, including *assessment, data collection,* or the *admission nursing history and examination.* A history is obtained by interview; examination requires observation and other techniques. These techniques were described briefly and will be further discussed in other chapters.

Both clients and nurses have expectations for assessment. The nurse seeks

Interaction	Purpose
Nurse: You've mentioned a few things that we can help you with while you're in the hospital. Is there anything we haven't talked about that is of concern to you?	Give cues that summarization is forthcoming.
Client: No, I can't think of anything; the worst thing is not being able to control my urine when I can't find a bathroom quickly.	
Nurse: That can be troublesome; there are ways to manage that and we'll also have to see what ideas the doctor may have. Is that something that will be troublesome now?	Summarization and plans for the concerns that have been expressed. (Notice that in summarization the actual diagnostic labels need not be used.)
Client: Oh, no, the bathroom is right here and I have a bedpan in my table.	
Nurse: You mentioned wanting to lose weight; that's another thing we can work on after your surgery. It seems that your diet and fluid intake have been good. Also, you mentioned bowels have been regular the past week. All these things are important for healing after surgery. Your concern about the surgery is something we'll want to talk about after lunch. I've got some ideas that might help you control what happens. This afternoon we'll go over how you can manage things like discomfort and prevent other problems with particular exercises. Read the little booklet; if your daughter comes in this afternoon, should we include her?	Summarization and plans for expressed concerns. (Notice that for some diagnoses the nursing care will not be started until after surgery.) Leave client with feeling of ability to cope with problems or concerns identified.
Client: Oh, yes, she would like to know all about it, too.	Preoperative preparation plans and plans to further discuss anxiety response.
Nurse: Good. See you around 2:30. Enjoy your lunch.	

information to describe and explain functional health patterns. Clients expect to learn the meaning of symptoms or to be reassured about their health and health practices. In addition to the care provider's interpretations of physiological symptoms, clients wish to know the meaning of symptoms relative to the human functions they engage in day by day. These functions are the focus of nursing, and assessment begins the process of nursing. The client may need to be told why nurses wish information so that interview purposes are clear.

Problem-Focused Assessment

One might assume that diagnoses are made, care is planned and carried out, problems are resolved, and outcomes of care are evaluated. This sequence, proceeding so neatly through time, is the "textbook picture" of clinical practice. In reality, people change, events occur, and diagnoses get added, deleted, or revised. When a treatment plan is implemented, the expectation is that the client's health problems will begin to resolve. To know whether or not the treatment is effective, periodic assessment of the status of the problem is done; thus the assessment is problem focused.

Purpose and Scope   The *purpose* of doing a problem-focused assessment is to evaluate the *presence or absence of a particular diagnosis.* The scope of data collection is narrower than in an initial assessment of a new client and, naturally, time required for assessment is less. As will be seen below, guidelines for information collection are based on the previously made diagnosis. The anticipation of new problems and alertness to discover missed problems or misdiagnoses accompanies this type of assessment.

Probability of Health Problems   As the name implies, in problem-focused assessment a problematic health pattern is assumed to exist when information collection begins. The *hypothesis of a dysfunctional health pattern is more likely than the hypothesis that no dysfunctional pattern exists.* The question pursued is, *Does the problem exist now and, if so, what is the status of the problem?* The assessment task is relatively structured.

Structure for Information Collection   The structural context in problem-focused assessment differs from that of an initial assessment. Change has occurred in the interpersonal dimension; now the nurse and client are not strangers to each other. Whereas in the first encounter trust, confidence, and rapport had to be built, successive encounters focus on extending and maintaining these. In addition, in the admission assessment, the setting was structured to promote sharing of information in a relaxed manner. In problem-focused assessment, the nurse most likely interweaves assessment and care activities such as teaching, bathing, or treatments. Yet, judgment has to be exercised regarding privacy and whether activities are a source of distraction.

Information collection can be structured by using the assessment parameters of the problem. These are derived from the defining characteristics in manuals (Gordon, 1987). For example, consider the diagnosis *self-bathing/hygiene deficit* related to activity intolerance (level III) which means the person's tolerance is quite low. Transforming the major characteristics of this diagnosis into assessment parameters is easy. During problem-focused assessment, information is collected on the following assessment parameters that are applicable to the situation:

1 Ability to get to water source
2 Ability to regulate water source
3 Ability to wash upper and lower body
4 Verbal report of ease of breathing pre- and post-bathing/hygiene
5 Heart rate and rhythm pre- and post-bathing/hygiene

Parameters 3, 4, and 5 would be assessed in every client with this diagnosis. If the client is known to walk to the bathroom without activity intolerance and has sufficient strength and coordination to turn on the faucets in a shower, then items 1 and 2 are deleted. If problem-focused assessment reveals *no change* in the bathing/hygiene deficit, assessment of another parameter is necessary:

6 Use of energy conservation measures in bathing/hygiene

Interventions are directed toward teaching general energy conservation techniques and those particularly related to bathing and hygiene. Therefore, this assessment parameter provides a check on the effectiveness of the nursing intervention and a possible explanation of no change in items 3–5.

How often is a problem assessed after treatment has begun? This depends on the diagnosis and the predicted time for a treatment response. For example, the status of self-esteem disturbance may be checked daily. This would be too infrequent for a diagnosis of severe anxiety; cues to potential for violence may be checked every 15 minutes. Problem-focused assessment is multipurpose; it can reveal:

1 Validation or lack of validation of the original diagnosis and etiological factors (recheck)
2 Changing levels of acuity, severity, or function that necessitate revision of the diagnosis
3 The progress of a problem toward resolution (outcome attainment)
4 The effectiveness of the treatment plan

Emergency Assessment

When a client is admitted to a critical care unit, enters the emergency room, or has a life-threatening episode in any setting, emergency assessment is indicated. This has to occur within seconds in order to institute immediate treatment.

Purpose and Scope   A life-threatening emergency is always expressed, however subtly, in *all* functional patterns. Yet to determine that an emergency exists, a few pattern indicators need to be assessed. The purpose of assessment is (1) to identify the situation as either an emergency or a nonemergency, (2) to determine the *nature* of the emergency quickly, and (3) to intervene quickly.

Although probably without much conscious recognition, a nurse scans for certain overt, perceptible cues *every time* a nurse-client interaction occurs. This takes approximately 2 to 7 seconds and is done in a particular order. For example, a primary scan of three indicators of change in metabolic and activity patterns (skin color, posture, and facial expression) provides a wealth of information on the heart-lung-brain complex in less than a second. Additional information, if indicated, includes the radial or apical pulse and feeling for passage of air at the mouth. This information dictates whether further emergency assessment is done.

The preliminary scan of skin, posture, and face is usually done simultaneously with a question addressed to the person. Verbal or even nonverbal response would indicate changes in the cognitive-perceptual pattern. Environmental factors are often the major importance to the assessment. For example, if a person in a restaurant develops inability to breathe, panic, and bluish cast to the skin, a "cafe coronary" may be suspected (acute strangulation occurring from aspiration of incompletely chewed food).

Certain crises occurring in the life of a person, group, or community also require emergency assessment. For example, psychotic breakdown and potential for suicide or violence are crises requiring immediate assessment, diagnosis, and intervention. Indicators of critical changes in self-concept (which may lead to suicide) or relationship patterns (which can result in violence) are cues to whether or not a crisis exists. In community health practice, emergency assessment may be required on the rare occasion of impending mob violence, riot, epidemics, or natural disasters.

Probability of Health Problems   Obviously, in an emergency admission *the hypothesis of an acute dysfunctional change in a pattern is more likely than the hypothesis that no acute change has occurred.* The question is, What is the nature of the dysfunction?

Structure for Information Collection   Emergency assessment differs from other assessments (Corrigan, 1986). Time between observation and action, and the purpose of intervention, are different. In emergency assessment the life-threatening "diagnosis" is usually identified as a cluster of signs and symptoms. Immediate action and thoughts about cause are simultaneous. The purpose is to preserve life. Consequently, emergency assessment may not impose as high a *cognitive* demand as other types of assessment. Yet emotional and situational demands can be high. Also, time and risk factors contribute to the nurse's overall cognitive-affective state. Human life is valued. This value contributes to the heightened emotional state of care providers when a life-threatening emergency occurs.

Time-Lapse Reassessment

In this type of assessment the time lapse since a previous assessment may be considerable. Three, six, twelve, or more months may have elapsed since the last clinic visit or since the last health status review in a residential center. Functional patterns and the client's situation may have changed. Natural growth, health management practices, or long-term care can have demonstrable effects over time. Equally possible, nonproductive patterns may have emerged because of health practices or situational factors.

Purpose and Scope   The basic purpose of a time-lapse reassessment is to evaluate changes in functional patterns. It is similar to the problem-focused assessment as a review of the current status of previous problems is done. Depending on the time lapse, new patterns may have emerged and require assessment; accordingly, a total screening of all patterns is done in somewhat less depth than the initial assessment previously discussed. If problems are perceived it may be necessary to elicit an in-depth history since the last evaluation.

Probability of Health Problems   When a client has not been seen for a few months, it is difficult to predict problems with any certainty before information has been collected. *The preencounter hypothesis, either that a dysfunctional change has occurred or that none has occurred, is influenced by previous knowledge of the client.* The question is, Has change occurred over time, and, if so, what is its direction?

Structure for Information Collection   Time-lapse reassessment is common in the follow-up of clients in ambulatory care settings and in periodic assessment in residential facilities, long-term care facilities, long-term home care, and school and industrial nursing. Situational factors play a similar role in this type of assessment, as in the other types of assessment discussed above. The information load and cognitive strain vary with the complexity of changes in the client's health status over time.

Summary of Situational Context for Assessment

As is evident in this discussion, the structure of the assessment situation differs in accordance with the possibility that problems are present and the questions used in assessment. The differences among the four types of assessment are shown in Table 6-1. This summary table suggests that it is important to know the purpose of assessment so that assessment procedures can be structured

TABLE 6-1
COMPARISON OF THE FOUR ASSESSMENT SITUATIONS AND THEIR STRUCTURAL INFLUENCES

Assessment situation	Preencounter probabilities	Questions directing the assessment	Structure of the environment
Initial (admission) assessment	The hypothesis of no dysfunctional pattern is as probable as the hypothesis that dysfunctional patterns exist	Does a problem (dysfunctional pattern) exist?	Establish a setting for obtaining accurate data (lighting, quiet, etc.)
			Establish an interpersonal atmosphere conducive to sharing thoughts, feelings, beliefs
Problem-focused assessment	The hypothesis of a dysfunctional pattern is more likely than the hypothesis that no dysfunctional pattern exists	Does the problem exist today? If so, what is the status of the problem?	Extend and maintain an interpersonal atmosphere conducive to sharing thoughts, feelings, beliefs
Emergency assessment (client classified by instantaneous perception of life-threatening cues)	The hypothesis of an acute, dysfunctional change in a pattern is more likely than the hypothesis that no acute change has occurred	What is the nature of the dysfunction?	Establish a setting for obtaining data quickly and for immediate life-sustaining action
Time-lapse reassessment	The hypothesis that no dysfunctional change has occurred or that dysfunctional change has occurred is influenced by previous knowledge of the client	Has change occurred over time? If so, what is its direction?	Establish a setting for obtaining accurate data (lighting, quiet, etc.)
			Reestablish interpersonal atmosphere conducive to sharing thoughts, feelings, beliefs

to obtain valid and reliable data. The next section should further expand the notion of just how valid and reliable data can be. Additionally, it will become evident that the nature of the information influences *how* it is collected.

NATURE OF CLINICAL INFORMATION

In this section, discussion will focus on the specific nature of clinical information and how its characteristics can influence the accuracy of health assessments and diagnostic judgments. During an admission assessment a large number of cues to the health status of a client are collected. *A cue is defined as a piece of information which influences decisions (to collect more information, diagnose a dysfunctional pattern, or judge that a pattern is functional).* They are the "building blocks" (Cutler, 1979) or "raw data" used to understand health patterns. Many difficulties can be avoided if one understands the nature of clinical cues and how to use them.

Psychologists classify judgment tasks on the basis of the number and complexity of the cues involved. Clinical judgment ranks high in both the amount of information that has to be processed and the complexity of the information. Cues can have multiple values, only some of which are significant and take on different meaning when occurring alone or in combination with other cues. Generally, clinical cues are probabilistic, which means they are not perfectly dependable indicators of a person's *actual health state.* In addition, cues can be labelled in different ways:

Valid-invalid	Subjective-objective
Reliable-unreliable	Historical-current
Relevant-irrelevant	State-contextual
Diagnostic-supporting	

Each of these characteristics influence how data is used in making accurate diagnoses; they will be the subject of discussion in this section.

If the listing of characteristics seems overwhelming, be assured that most human beings already have an intuitive grasp of each of the above. For example, early in life we learn to make a *judgment* about when it is safe to cross a busy street. The judgment is *probabilistic.* A probability exists that one or more drivers will not stop for the red light. The light itself is a cue that can take on *multiple values* (red, green, yellow), each of which has meaning. We have learned that the speed of the car approaching a traffic light is *relevant data,* although it is a *subjective* rather than an *objective* cue.\ Sometimes information is available about how many accidents have occurred at a particular crosswalk (*historical data*) but the most *valid diagnostic cue* to safety is that all cars have stopped. (Yet there is still the chance that a car will start up because of an irrational driver.) *Supporting data* helps if this possibility occurs to us; looking at the drivers as we cross provides some *contextual data,* such as a "behavior reading." No cue is a perfectly dependable cue (*reliable*) but in combination they do increase the probability of making an accurate judgment about when it is safe to cross.

Valid and Reliable Cues

Two of the most important characteristics of data used in diagnosis are validity and reliability. These terms help to specify the degree to which a cue, or cluster of cues, lead to accurate diagnosis.

Valid Cues   Good diagnostic judgments are based on good data and valid cues are valued as "good" data. *A cue is valid if it represents the properties of what is being judged.* A description of food and fluid intake represents one property of a nutritional-metabolic pattern; thus it is one piece of information that is valid for making a judgment about this pattern. Is the client's description of what her husband prepares for each meal valid information about her dietary pattern? No, information on the type of meals prepared does not provide direct information about intake and leads to risky judgments based on assumptions.

There are degrees of validity. *Highly valid data represent critical properties of a functional health pattern. Information of lower validity requires assumptions that may or may not be true.* The clearer the definition of functional health patterns, the easier it is to seek valid data with which to make judgments about patterns. Thus definitions of the critical properties of a pattern have to be continually improved as new knowledge accumulates. In addition, during assessment keep in mind the definition and components of each health pattern so that the data collected is relevant. This leads to a valid, functional assessment.

Let us now apply this information on validity to diagnostic categories. Accurate diagnoses are associated with the use of highly valid cues. *A cue to a health problem is highly valid if it contains information on the critical properties of a diagnostic category (critical defining characteristics or diagnostic criteria).* In the example above if observation suggested a possible nutritional problem, the actual food ingested would be a more valid indicator of nutritional deficit than the husband's cooking practices. (The cooking practices may be further explored when the search for etiological factors begins.) Validity in assessment and diagnosis may be summarized in the maxim: "If you came to count trees, don't spend your time looking at the acorns on the ground."

Reliable Cues   Reliable information is also valued as "good." *Information is reliable if it is (1) a dependable indicator of a functional pattern or of a diagnosis and (2) obtained through accurate measurement.* For example, which measure of food and fluid intake is most dependable, and therefore most reliable, as data for assessing the nutritional-metabolic pattern?

1 A client's description of food and fluid intake
2 A nurse's daily observation of fluid and fluid intake
3 The husband's description of the meals served to the client

To make a judgment about food and fluid intake, most would prefer to use the second option, the nurse's observations. This preference is based on the idea that an outside observer (and a professional) is free of bias and more accurate. It may be that the client is just as accurate as the nurse but we do not know this. The husband's description of meals served to the client has the lowest reliability; we do not know if the client eats all of her meals.

The above example has further implications. The *cost of obtaining information* through observation is high. If there is no reason to suspect that the client is unreliable, her verbal report may be accepted. In some situations observation is impossible; client reports are then accepted as the most reliable information obtainable. In other situations judgments are so important that, irrespective of time and costs, direct measurements are performed. Situations have to be judged individually.

Reliable cues to a diagnosis occur always, or nearly always, when the condition is present. Reliability, in addition to validity, is a dimension of critical defining characteristics (diagnostic criteria). As work on nursing diagnoses progresses, these cues will be contained in manuals and will be the most dependable information for accurate diagnosis. To return to the maxim above and apply it to reliability, the acorns are not a dependable measure, even if all the trees are oak.

The second aspect of reliability, accuracy of measurement, contributes to "good" information in both health evaluation and in diagnosis. This is why the following points always have to be considered during information collection:

1 Observational and interviewing skills
2 Accurate measuring devices (e.g., equipment)
3 Good lighting for observation
4 Well-formulated questions
5 Careful listening to verbal cues
6 Constructing a situation of acceptance, interest, and caring

In summary, valid and reliable cues obtained by accurate measures provide a data base for judgments about functional health patterns of a client and about diagnoses.

Cue Values

Cues can take on different values. For example the characteristic *marital status* has six values: married, divorced, separated, widowed, single, and the recent addition, never married. Some cues, for example, blood pressure or heart rate, can be represented by numerical values. Quantification (numerical values) allows more precise measurement. Yet many cues to a client's health status are subjective impressions of quality or quantity, such as estimates of respiratory depth, moistness of the skin, or severity of discomfort. As Norris (1982) has pointed out many of the very common conditions encountered in practice have not been adequately described and precise measures developed; fatigue, restlessness, and nausea are examples. As much as possible, data should be scaled (and scales carefully defined) or quantified numerically. Quantification increases reliability of measures, and subsequently the reliability of judgments and communications.

Probabilistic Cues

The word probability means the same as chance. The diagnostic task is a probabilistic one. This means that nursing diagnoses are made at some level of probability, not absolute certainty. In contrast, there are other types of categorizations in which information permits one to infer with certainty. These situations are not too common in the everyday world or in clinical practice.

In the previous discussion of validity and reliability of data, the impression may have been given that reliability and validity can be totally controlled. In this section it will be seen that (because of the nature of cues about people) the degree of control over validity and reliability of data and of clinical judgments varies. Much information is probabilistic. Nurses have to learn to deal with uncertainty when it cannot be totally eliminated by assessment methods.

From the time one first notices things in the surrounding world, one learns about probabilities. They involve whether or not trains are apt to come on time, the possibility of a good grade or pay raise, and the chance that a driver will stop at a stop sign. From childhood on, each person works on learning the *likelihood of events* and *what predicts what.* For example, if an object looks like a book, it probably has printed pages.

In nursing, interest centers on the probability, or likelihood, that a problem exists, given a set of cues, or signs and symptoms. *Even the critical, defining cues for a diagnosis may not allow certainty in diagnostic judgments.* The probabilistic nature of nursing practice has been described by Hammond. He argues that client conditions produce different cues, and the same cue can be produced by different conditions (1966, p. 34). In other words, the cues available for diagnosing a health problem are not always completely reliable.

Consider an example: *A smile is a cue to friendliness.* Let us say that 80 percent of the time when people are friendly, they smile. On the other hand, smiling may be present 20 percent of the time when people are really hostile and angry. Smiling does not predict friendliness with 100 percent certainty. It is a *probabilistic cue.* If these figures are correct, this cue is associated with only 80 percent predictive validity. That is, inferring friendliness when a person smiles will be a valid inference in 80 out of 100 cases. An error will result in 20 cases.

The ideal situation would be to find cues that are *certain.* Then clinicians could be "sure" of their diagnoses. Yet human behavior is variable and the ideal probably can never be reached. At least at this point in scientific development one cannot actually "stand in the shoes" of another person and know what the other knows, feels, or believes.

Anxiety is a good example for further demonstration. Consider first of all two people. In reality, they both feel anxious. Yet they manifest different signs or cues; that is, they express anxiety differently. Now consider one person who is anxious. This person will not necessarily demonstrate the same signs of anxiety in two different social environments or at two different times. Thus a set of cues may be unreliable in terms of various *individuals* and also in terms of one individual in different *situations* and through *time.*

Hammond (1966) describes clinicians as hard pressed to point to one set of cues that *always* indicates a diagnosis. Most textbooks reflect this lack of predictability. Look at the way authors describe the signs and symptoms of nursing or medical diagnoses. They use words such as "*usually* presents the symptoms of . . . ," "*nearly always* associated with these signs . . . ," or "*frequently* demonstrates an elevated . . . ." This "hedging" reminds one of the kind of language used in another probabilistic, uncertain situation—weather forecasting; it has the same built-in uncertainty.

Clinicians generally consider *physical cues* to be more reliable and valid indicators of a diagnosis than *social cues.* For example, redness and blanching over bony prominences of the back are highly reliable and valid signs of potential skin breakdown in white- or yellow-skinned persons. Signs of altered body image are more variable from one individual to another; thus they are less reliable predictors of the diagnosis. This difference in the reliability of signs results in a greater feeling of uncertainty in making the latter diagnosis than in making the former.

To identify subjective states (feeling states) or self-perceptions of clients, it is critical to obtain verbal reports of the person. Subjective data increase the clinician's confidence in the diagnosis, as well as validity and reliability of the diagnosis. In the case of objective phenomena, such as potential skin breakdown, it is not critical that the client confirm the clinician's observation (that the skin is red or blanching).

The cues gleaned from interview and examination have a wide range of predictive accuracy. Additionally, many times judgments have to be made with limited information and time.

Handling Uncertainty   There is a way of dealing with uncertain information in situations where errors have to be controlled. The method of approach is to use the cues with the highest validity. Every time a cue that is a valid indicator of a diagnosis (critical defining characteristic) is present, there is a high probability that the health problem is present. Such a cue is, in addition, a reliable indicator across clients.[3]

Highly reliable, highly valid cues are referred to as the *critical defining characteristics* of a diagnostic category. They increase confidence in diagnostic judgments. If one or more cues point to the possibility of a health problem, the remaining critical defining cues should be assessed before the diagnosis is

---

[3]By definition a valid indicator of a health problem is also a reliable indicator. This statement is based on the assumption that assessment of the cue has been accurate.

made. (As discussed previously, not all currently identified diagnostic categories have critical signs and symptoms specified.)

Clinical inferences about subjective states, such as pain, body image, or conflict, are plagued with uncertainty unless a combination of observations and verbal reports is used. Subjective feeling states are not observable; only the client's response to the feelings can be assessed. For example, consider the signs of restlessness and facial grimacing, combined with a history of abdominal surgery 24 hours previously. A possibility is that the client is having incisional pain. How confident would you be about making this inductive inference from that data?

The more knowledge you have about postsurgical care, the *less* confident you will be! These cues are highly uncertain predictors of pain; they do not discriminate among three or four other conditions that are manifested by restlessness and facial grimacing. Suppose the postoperative client says, "I've tried turning and taking the medicine; nothing helps the pain." Does this cue increase confidence in the diagnosis of pain management deficit? Yes; now the other cues become supporting cues. When the cluster is put together, confidence is sufficient to make the diagnostic judgment.

Can doubt always be erased by more information? No, not unless the cue is a more valid and reliable indicator than the information already secured. A verbal report of pain increases validity in the above example because pain, by definition, is a subjective state really known only by the client. It also must be noted that a verbal report *alone* is not always sufficient data. An adequate level of confidence to infer pain and give a narcotic usually requires both verbal report and observational data; this is because, although feeling pain is a valid indicator, our methods of *measuring* feelings (assessing the client's subjective report) are not always reliable. Verbal reports are used to measure feelings and may be biased by conscious or unconscious motives of the person reporting.

The above considerations are important. Good diagnostic judgments are made on the basis of the most valid and reliable cues that can be acquired in a particular situation. *The more valid and reliable the cues, the less uncertainty and the higher confidence the nurse will have in his or her judgments.* Of course, the better the diagnostic judgments are, the higher is the probability that the care plan devised for the client will be effective.

It may be an interesting exercise to determine which of the following cues and inferences from data are highly valid and reliable. Evaluate each independently. The task is to select information that is absolutely necessary for accurate diagnosis of an intermittent constipation pattern. For the moment, disregard the etiological factors. These are the cues:

1 Decreased activity level
2 Hard, formed stool today
3 Palpable mass in abdomen
4 Reports feeling of pressure or fullness in rectum
5 Reports history of frequent straining at stool

6 Appetite impairment

7 Headache

8 Reports two or three episodes per month (history) of hard, formed stool following period of no bowel movement

What needs to be determined are the necessary and sufficient criteria for diagnosing an intermittent constipation pattern. The first inference, number 1, decreased activity level, is obviously insufficient for making the diagnosis; it may be either a factor contributing to severity or an etiological (causative) factor in this diagnosis. Hard, formed stool today, item number 2, indicates the possibility of the presence of constipation. It does not provide data about an intermittent pattern. A cue such as this should be investigated in terms of the frequency and precipitating factors.

The third cue, palpable mass in the abdomen, is not definitive. It does not differentiate between stool and a tumor. The fourth cue is similar; a rectal tumor could cause the same sensation but usually would also be associated with other symptoms. Number 5 is history of frequent straining at stool; this indeed does provide a valid cue. Is it sufficient information? No, but it is a key piece of information which we will hold for the moment.

The sixth cue, appetite impairment, is interesting; it may be secondary to constipation but deserves investigation to ensure that it is not a cue to another condition. It could be a predisposing or causative factor of constipation if sufficient fluids and bulky foods are not being ingested. Headache, cue number 7, is not unusual with constipation but is not diagnostic. It does deserve explanation even in isolation. Thus far we have one cue; the rest of the information could be signs or symptoms of other conditions. Therefore the cues represent unreliable and nondifferentiating evidence for the diagnosis under consideration. They could be supporting cues for the presence of a *current* state of constipation, but not an intermittent pattern.

The eighth cue, a history of hard, formed stool two or three times per month following a period of no bowel movement, is a highly valid predictor of the diagnosis being entertained. It is a verbal report; unless the reliability of the client is questionable, it does provide sufficient confidence for the diagnosis. Is this one cue sufficient to identify the health problem? Is it a necessary or critical cue, without which the validity of the diagnosis would be questionable? Is it a conclusive sign? The answer to these questions is yes. Cue number 5, frequent straining, is redundant; it really does not provide any further information but only supports that the stool, as described in cue number 8, is probably hard to evacuate.

Redundant cues serve a function. They provide a check or support for a diagnostic judgment and can increase confidence level when information is uncertain. Up to a point, redundant cues are probably psychologically necessary. In excess, they provide quantity, not quality, in a data base.

The etiology of this health problem still has to be identified. A number of options are open. If the eight pieces of data were actually collected in a real situation, questions would arise. Should etiological factors be investigated immediately? Or should the problem be referred to a physician for differential medical diagnosis?

The cues *appetite impairment* and *palpable mass,* in conjunction with the problem of intermittent constipation, suggest the need for differential medical diagnosis. Could a tumor be present? It is highly advisable to refer the problem to a physician if the nurse is not competent to discriminate among the etiological factors of intermittent constipation, especially a tumor. A second option is to discuss with a physician the findings and the possibility of administering an enema. The palpable mass may be stool accumulated in the colon; if so, it would disappear when the enema was expelled. In the absence of abdominal tumor, the client's constipation problem may be amenable to nursing therapy. Etiological factors to be investigated by the nurse include dietary patterns, abdominal muscle tone, bowel habits, anxiety, and decreased activity.

This example illustrates the need to examine the data collected, predict alternative explanations, and test possibilities. It also demonstrates the uncertain nature of clinical data. Essentially, two main factors should influence judgment. These are the validity and reliability of information available *and* theoretical knowledge one can bring to bear in interpretation.

In the next section relevant and irrelevant cues will be discussed; again it will be seen that highly valid and reliable cues are the relevant data for assessment and diagnosis. Sometimes in practice one hears the comment: "There isn't much relevant information in that note [on the client's chart]." Consider now what that comment could mean.

Relevant Cues

The key to efficiency (save time) and effectiveness (accuracy) in both functional health pattern assessment and diagnosis is to focus on relevant information. The terms *relevant* and *irrelevant* are used frequently to pertain to validity. The relevance of a cue depends on the purpose for collecting information. Overall evaluation of functional health patterns is one purpose of an initial assessment. Specific information about the essential properties of each pattern is considered *relevant* data. This information is what makes the data base informative.

For example, if the health-perception–health-management pattern is being assessed, relevant cues will be found in:

1 The client's perception of his/her general health
2 General level of resistance (e.g., colds, infections)
3 Health practices (things done to keep healthy, including any prescribed drugs, treatments, etc.)
4 Health beliefs (perception of whether health practices make a difference)
5 Use of tobacco, alcohol, drugs
6 Compliance

7 If illness present: perceived cause; actions taken; results of action; if no illness present: management of everyday health problems[4]

In contrast, irrelevant information for health-perception–health-management would include repeating the physician's history of the illness; in most settings this can be found on the client's record. The nurse is interested in how the client perceives and manages health and illness.

The second purpose of assessment is to identify dysfunctional patterns (nursing diagnoses) if they are present. Early data may suggest a tentative diagnosis. The cue search then becomes focused on the critical characteristics (signs and symptoms) that define the diagnostic categories under consideration; that is, the characteristics that are relevant to the diagnoses. *Relevant cues correspond to the highly valid and reliable characteristics of a category. Even when using relevant cues, studies have shown that adding a lot of irrelevant information increases errors, takes more time, and increases difficulty* (Ciafrani, 1984; Gordon, 1980).

These findings may be explained by the difficulty human beings have in holding large amounts of information in working memory. When searching for cues to support or reject a possible diagnosis, zero-in on the critical defining characteristics and, one by one, assess for their presence or absence. As frequently stated: "Go where the money is." Yet, caution must be exercised in discounting what appears irrelevant in regard to a particular diagnosis. When investigated it may prove to be an indicator of another problem.

Irrelevant information can produce interference. Large amounts cause cognitive processes to become overloaded with noncontributory or redundant information, the "chaff" as opposed to the "wheat." For example, before completing the assessment of a client's nutritional pattern, one should have sufficient data to determine whether any type of nutritional deficit or excess is present and how the client manages this functional pattern. This necessary information is the wheat. It may be interesting to know also that the client's father was a good cook, but this information in isolation is probably irrelevant.

The advantage of focusing on relevant data is that less time is needed for the assessment. For example, one could ask five questions about a client's sleep pattern. Suppose instead the client is asked, "Most mornings when you get up, do you feel rested and ready for the day?" If the response to this question is yes, is it relevant in a screening assessment to know the hours of sleep and other particulars? These details would be relevant only if a problem was present. *Each piece of clinical data collected should provide additional information relevant to judgment about a functional health pattern.*

On occasion a client may provide a great deal of unsolicited irrelevant information, such as stories about life successes of each of his or her children. Be aware this may signal (1) a need for attention, (2) need to impress (pay attention to self-perception-self-concept data), (3) unclear orientation of the

---

[4]These are components of a screening assessment; components for other patterns may be found in Chapter 4 and Appendix E.

client at the beginning of an admission assessment, or (4) hesitancy of the nurse in conducting the admission interview. In handling this type of situation consider that increased amounts of irrelevant data can interfere with information processing and cause errors in judgment. To interrupt tactfully, one might say: "Your children's success must give you a lot of pleasure (*supportive, interested comment*), tell me when you . . . (*go on to a related question in the history*)."

Diagnostic and Supporting Cues

As previously mentioned, diagnostic cues, or criteria, are the critical characteristics of a diagnostic category. They are the cues that must be present if the diagnostic label is used because they coincide with the formal definition of the category. *When diagnostic cues or criteria are fully identified, it is expected that they will be highly valid and reliable, few in number, and relevant to only one diagnostic category.* For example, when a client repeatedly verbalizes negative feelings about an actual or perceived change in structure or function of the body or body part, this is a *diagnostic cue* to body image disturbance. Other cues may be present in the situation, such as anxiety, fear, or hiding, overexposing, or ignoring a body part. These are *supporting cues* that increase the diagnostician's confidence and serve to validate a client's verbal expression of feelings. Supporting cues may be useful, but are not highly reliable indicators of a diagnosis. There are two reasons for low reliability. One is that supporting cues usually describe behaviors which may or may not be present with the condition. Secondly, supporting cues can be indicators of other conditions and, therefore, do not permit discrimination among conditions. This idea is illustrated in Figure 6.1, where diagnostic cues and overlapping, supporting cues are diagrammed. The situation in diagnosis is similar to everyday tasks of discrimination, such as telling "this from that"; we learn which cues to rely upon and which are variable in situations.

In general, cues or clusters of cues that require attention and are important in diagnosis are of three types:

1 Cues to change in a client's functional patterns
2 Deviation from pattern norms (population, cultural-ethnic, baseline)
3 Cues to delays or to dysfunctional pattern development (developmental assessment)

The first type is the cue that signifies change in a client's usual patterns that is unexplained by expected norms for growth and development. Change can be positive and health-supporting or it may be negative and potentially dysfunctional. An example of the latter would be change in the role-relationship pattern so that the client becomes socially isolated.

The second type of cue that requires attention is deviation from an appropriate population norm. For example, a person may have *no change* in frequency of elimination but depend on laxatives and enemas to maintain regularity. This represents a deviation from "normality."

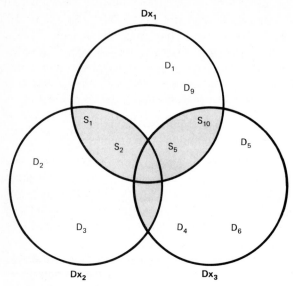

FIGURE 6-1
Example of 3 diagnoses (Dx) with overlapping supporting cues (S) and distinctive diagnostic cues (D).

In another situation a client may be within the norms of his or her ethnic group but deviant in terms of the general or dominant social norms. This situation can produce problems for the person within one or many functional pattern areas, a possibility that would need to be validated with the client.

A person may have no change in nutritional pattern. This does not mean that the pattern is productive for the person. It may be causing an elimination problem, or a nutritional deficit may be present if requirements have increased. These problems are detected only by evaluating information relative to the whole.

The third type of cue or cue cluster important for nursing diagnosis is that which indicates pattern development. Each of the functional health patterns is continually evolving as the person grows older. For example, it is expected that a young child's activity-exercise pattern will evolve as neurological development permits more coordinated movement. Similarly, value-belief patterns change with life experiences, including experience with dying. Cues to development of functional health patterns are important. They may signify developmental lags or evolving patterns that are dysfunctional for the client.

Describing signs and symptoms only from the viewpoint of the nurse can lead to errors of omission. The way a client "defines the situation" must be taken into account. For example, it may be "apparent" that a particular mother and father are very concerned, caring, and capable. But if their child says, "Mommy doesn't love me," this statement is a cue. It should not be brushed aside with some superficial reassurance. If that is how the child defines the situation, that is how it is for her. Similarly, if a person says there is no other recourse than suicide, in reality as that person perceives it there may not be another way. When a person newly diagnosed as diabetic says, "I can't manage," the response "Of course you can" may cut off critically important cues.

Dismissing cues with superficial reassurance may decrease the nurse's anxiety and the time spent in assessment. Yet the underlying problem will not go away. It will probably come back to haunt the staff in a different guise because the original communication was not attended to. "Uncooperative" behavior (from the nurse's or doctor's perspective), frequent calls, and repeated visits to an emergency room are common ways clients express unresolved problems.

Any discussion of important cues must consider the cues that define currently accepted nursing diagnoses. These are health problems within the scope of nursing practice, and cues to their presence must not be missed. For example, if dietary pattern, body weight, and other characteristics are not assessed, a nutritional deficit may be missed.

A dilemma exists. Most diagnoses are not well defined. Therefore, what are the "important" cues? At this stage of development the list of accepted diagnoses (Appendix A) and their defining criteria (with their deficiencies) are the best available in the nursing literature (McLane, 1987; Gordon, 1987). A discussion about what needs to be done to ensure that critical criteria for using diagnostic labels are available is contained in Chapter 11.

Subjective and Objective Cues

Frequently in practice a subjective-objective classification of cues is used. This is probably a false distinction. All observations have some subjectivity because the stimulus has been processed through the observer's mind.

Common usage defines *objective data* as characteristics perceived by some outside observer, whereas *subjective data* refers to characteristics perceived by the client and not the observer. The latter includes subjective perceptions and feelings, such as self-concept or pain. In contrast are the so-called objective data the nurse observes, such as skin color, heart rate, or parent-child interaction. Clinical data are commonly categorized as subjective or objective within the format of the problem-oriented recording system in many health care agencies.[5]

The objective-subjective designation has relevance to the processing of information. The trained observer credits himself or herself with more objectivity than the client. Thus objective data are considered to be free from personal biases, emotions, and the like that can influence information processing. This supposition, of course, is not always true; many times people, nurses included, see what they are ready to see. Yet the clinician *tries* to put aside biases or

---

[5]The problem-oriented recording system is a charting format that requires the separation of objective observations and subjective reports. Its use with nursing diagnoses will be discussed in a later chapter.

predispositions and to be objective when analyzing clinical data. Some nurses are more successful than others.

It is well to recognize that there are two primary value systems that relate to subjective and objective data. In the diagnosis of disease or disease complications, objective data are valued for their diagnostic significance. Thus when a nurse transmits data to a physician, the emphasis is usually on objective data. Objective and subjective data are of *equal* diagnostic significance to nurses. Some examples will clarify these two sets of values.

In the process of diagnosing disease, the physician considers subjective reports to be tentative until verification can be obtained by objective measures. In the extreme case, physical symptoms may be categorized as hypochondria if objective measurement does not support subjective reports. A somewhat paradoxical situation exists: if a lesion is observed on x-ray, the situation is reversed; support for the presence of the lesion is sought in subjective data from the client. For example, if lung pathology is found by objective x-ray examination, the patient is asked whether pain, dyspnea, or other subjective symptoms have been experienced. A conflict between the two types of data is resolved either by greater reliance on objective measurements or, in some cases, a "wait and see" attitude.

In psychiatric diagnosis subjective data are essential but are complemented by objective examination to rule out organ pathology. For example, signs of a behavioral disorder would not be given a psychiatric label without ruling out organic problems, such as a brain tumor.

Nurses are concerned equally with both objective and subjective data. They shuttle back and forth between their own observations (the so-called objective data) and the subjective reports of the client. Many manage to arrive at a synthesis. For example, a nurse may objectively measure a pressure sore. Yet there is *equal* diagnostic concern about the individual's coping response to this condition and personal and environmental factors that brought it about.

Subjective client reports have diagnostic value because they help the nurse understand the client's perspective. These subjective data are valued because nurses' *primary* emphasis is on people and their total situation, including, but not limited to, the disease. Medical care providers of course do not totally ignore the person's ideas, actions, feelings, values, or beliefs, but these are not diagnostic of disease.

When a nurse acts within a nursing framework, the concerns, the data, and the diagnoses are different from those of physicians. When a nurse operates within a biomedical framework and transmits data to a physician, objective data are valued more than subjective reports. Both frameworks are used in nursing practice.

A related typology of clinical cues is the *sign and symptom classification. The term symptom designates an experience related by a client.* Information about symptoms is subjective. It includes the client's perceptions of body temperature, skin sensations, palpitations, feelings of competency or esteem, beliefs, attitudes, and values.

In contrast, *a sign is an objective indicator of a health problem.* A symptom can be a sign, and a client can perceive a sign but may not interpret it. If this is thoroughly confusing, the reader will appreciate why the terms *sign* and *symptom* are frequently used interchangeably. For the reader who wishes to pursue the distinction further, King's (1968) treatise on the subject will be of interest.

Historical and Current Cues

Another useful way of thinking about the clinical data collected for purposes of nursing diagnosis is from a *time perspective.* An understanding of a client's functional patterns is constructed from historical and current cues. This way of classifying clinical data permits one to examine the cues used in nursing diagnoses. Are they based on historical information, current information, or both? Secondly, are diagnoses based only on cues to the client's state or also on cues about the situational or environmental context?

To appreciate the distinction between historical and current information, keep in mind that current data come from the "the here and now." Historical data may pertain to last night, 2 days ago, or 10 years ago.

Historical measures of client characteristics provide historical state cues. These are previous values of characteristics, such as blood pressure, appetite, family roles, and body perception. In community assessment, traffic fatalities or cardiovascular death rates in previous years may be historical cues.

The data described above provide an individualized base line. One common example is blood pressure. What does a current value of 95/78 mean? If the value for the past 2 years has been 150/190, the interpretation is different than if blood pressure has been consistently in the 90–100/70–80 range. As another example, knowing the past number of hours of sleep helps the nurse interpret and evaluate the present value of this characteristic. *Historical state data provide baseline cues for interpreting the current state of a client within the context of the client's own functional pattern.*

A nursing diagnosis should never be made exclusively from historical cues. Can you think why this is so and how it could ever occur? Inferences about a particular client's behavior can be derived deductively by combining some information (in this case, historical data) and generalizations from memory. For example, a nurse may infer that because a patient was "angry and complaining about the staff" on the day of admission, this is the current emotional state. In a sense the client is never allowed to escape the history. *Using only historical cues predisposes to diagnostic error.* Clearly, the current state of the client must be assessed. Also, it must be recognized that an inference is created in the mind of the clinician and may or may not stand up to the test of reality. This paragraph contains ideas so important in avoiding diagnostic errors that it may be worthwhile to reread it.

Current data about attributes of the client are current state cues. These are the current values for blood pressure, comfort level, activity level, caloric intake, age, laboratory test values, emotional state, and other client characteristics. This type of information, in combination with historical base lines, is used to identify health patterns and detect changes.

Current state cues should always be sought before making diagnoses. The etiology of a self-care deficit, or any other problem, is determined by current or historical cues. To determine whether a change in pattern has been abrupt or gradual, historical data are used.

In addition to collecting information about the state of the person, the nurse measures characteristics of the client's situation. These describe the context within which functional patterns arise. Attention is focused on both historical and current situational cues.

Previous values of unchangeable characteristics of the person (birthdate, for example) or situation are historical contextual cues. Events that have already occurred are part of one's life history. Not only are they history, but they are the context (not the state) out of which current functional patterns may have evolved. It is worthwhile to consider a few examples, since this type of cue is very useful in diagnosis.

First consider a rather obvious relationship. During assessment, the nurse elicits the information that the client avoids high-roughage foods. For example, no bran, leafy vegetables, nuts, or other foods with bulk are reported in the diet. This has been the pattern for a decade or more. (Note the historical and current *state* information.) The nurse thinks that the client is missing a good source of vitamins and is susceptible to constipation because of the lack of bulk in the diet.

There are two options: one is to plunge ahead and try to correct this behavior; the other is to wonder why the client avoids roughage. Choosing the latter option, the nurse can ask questions to determine whether there is any explanation in past history. The nurse learns that about 15 years ago the client was diagnosed as having diverticulosis[6] and was told to avoid high-roughage foods. This contextual event (being diagnosed and instructed) happened in the past but is the reported reason for the current dietary pattern.

Historical contextual cues (situational cues) not only are helpful in understanding functional patterns but also play an important role in prediction. There is an indication from research (Gordon, 1972, 1980) that nurses use situational cues to predict the most likely health problems. In an admission assessment, prediction is necessary because the universe of possibilities is open. To fully investigate every conceivable functional health problem is impossible. Therefore predictions (inferences, or hypotheses) are made about the likelihood of various problems. Problems estimated to be of high likelihood are investigated.

Predictions are made on the basis of historical contextual cues and knowledge of relationships stored in the nurse's memory. For example, a recent historical event in the life of a person, such as a first heart attack, is information

---

[6]Diverticulosis is a condition in which there are small outpouches and weak points in the wall of the colon. Older methods of treatment included the avoidance of high-roughage foods.

that can be used to predict the likelihood of certain dysfunctional problems the nurse knows are often associated with heart attack.

Historical information about the environmental context also helps one understand the background from which functional health patterns arise and develop. This information includes prior living environments, economic conditions, the health and welfare resource systems and the interpersonal and sociocultural environment. In addition to contributing to the nurse's understanding of health patterns, this information may be useful in the prediction of problems. The reader may be wondering, Why bother to think about possibilities? Why not just collect the assessment data?

The perceptually sensitive observer anticipates. An inference is made from relationships stored in the observer's memory. This inference then forms the basis for a set of probing questions and the search for further cues. *Predictive inference is anticipation, and it largely depends on contextual cues.*

Assumptions or inferences drawn on the basis of the person's history are useful but must be used with caution if incorporated, without validation, into diagnosis. Although the historical event (two days ago) of having an amputation or breast removal may be associated with an alteration in body image, amputation is an insufficient rationale for diagnosis of body image disturbance. A tentative diagnostic hypothesis (body image disturbance) should be generated to guide cue search. Diagnosis based on only historical cues about the situation can result in an error of *historical stereotyping.*

A final type of clinical cue is the *current contextual cue.* This is derived from assessment of the current situation. For example, assessment usually includes the structure of the interpersonal environment. Is the person a hermit or part of a large, closely structured family network? What are the neighborhood and community like? What health services are available? What are the current events in a client's life, such as an episode of physical illness, a divorce in process, or a husband dying at home? *The current context of the client's life, when combined with the historical context, permits the nurse to construct the client's situational or environmental pattern.*

This discussion has separated out for definition, analysis, and attention types of client and environmental cues. In actual practice these cues are not collected in separate packages but are obtained within the assessment sequence. What usually happens is that a piece of information is collected and attended to, and then a question arises: What kind of information is necessary to derive meaning from this cue? One may branch to *historical* information about the client and past environment. This information is usually obtained by questions posed to the client or others possessing the historical data. Branching may also point toward the need for more *current* data. This is obtained by questions to elicit subjective reports about the client's state. The nurse may also need to examine the current situational context, such as home environment. *Obviously, if one knows what type of information is needed (historical or current), assessment proceeds more rapidly.*

Why bother with a clinical cue classification? Mainly because cognitive operations need some checks and balances. Habits can arise that affect efficiency and accuracy. Feedback is not always available after student days are over. One can fall into a pattern of *diagnosing only on the basis of here and now, which is probably cognitively inefficient,* as will be seen in the discussion of diagnostic strategies. Another habit pattern is *diagnosing only on the basis of historical information; this is close to stereotyping and is very risky. Examining the cues one habitually uses provides checks and balances on the needed mixture of historical and current information.*

Summary of Nature of Clinical Information

This discussion of clinical cues has provided an introduction to the nature of clinical information used in assessment and diagnosis. Four important types of clinical cues to the health status of the client were identified. These were cues indicating change in a functional pattern, deviation from pattern norms, dysfunctional patterns, or pattern development.

The uncertain, or probabilistic, nature of clinical data was described. Because of the human capacity for variability in behavioral expression, signs and symptoms predict with less than perfect certainty. Nurses have to learn to deal with this uncertain environment. It was suggested that highly valid and reliable information has to be used. Additionally, the nurse must recognize that judgments based on uncertain data are subject to error. A continual openness to new contradictory or supporting information has to be maintained.

Clinical data can be relevant or irrelevant to the purpose of assessment or to a particular diagnostic hypothesis. Knowing what data are needed prevents cognitive processes from being overwhelmed with irrelevant information. Information that does not increase the reliability or validity of judgment is irrelevant. The focus in data collection has to be on the cues that "pay off" in terms of health status evaluation.

The distinction between subjective and objective data was discussed. It was suggested that when a nursing framework is being used, both types of data provide important cues. Nurses are equally concerned with so-called objective observation of the client and the client's situation and with the person's subjective perceptions, responses, beliefs, and attitudes. The client's perspective on his or her situation is considered as important in assessment as the nurse's perspective on it. Rather than discount clients' subjective, personal biases and feelings, nurses use these data in diagnosis.

Historical and current client and contextual data were related to functional health pattern assessment. For understanding a pattern, both types of data are necessary; this is why assessment consists of both history-taking and examination. The errors and decreased efficiency resulting from an overemphasis on either historical or current data were pointed out. The section may be summarized by saying *important cues* are relevant; they may be historical or current, subjective or objective, and related to the client's state or situational context.

Lastly, important cues are those that represent the most reliable and valid data available.

DIAGNOSTICIANS' BASIC TOOLS

This section will focus on the diagnostician, who can be thought of as both a measuring device and an information processor. Thinking of oneself as a sensitive measuring device permits some objectivity. It is possible to stand aside and examine the way cognitive and perceptual processes can influence information collection.

Cognitive and perceptual abilities are the basic "tools" used in information collection. Nurses have been developing these capabilities since birth. They include *perception, memory,* and the use of *categories.* In fact, a complex skill used in nursing diagnosis began to develop during infancy. Learning that a toy ball did not cease to exist after rolling behind the chair ushered in the development of inference. Diagnosis requires sharpening cognitive and perceptual abilities and one important additional ingredient, clinical knowledge. The discussion will begin with this factor because, as will be clear later, people perceive on the basis of previously acquired knowledge.

Clinical Knowledge

Knowledge is a necessary, but not a sufficient, condition for expertise in nursing diagnosis. What is an adequate knowledge base? It is difficult to say. Minimally, knowledge of the functional pattern areas described in Chapter 3 is needed for health status evaluation and diagnosis. Specifically, the following are necessary areas of knowledge for nursing diagnosis (other areas would be required for nursing intervention):

1 Range of norms for the 11 functional health patterns (age norms)
2 Natural development of functional patterns during the life-span
3 Variations in patterns related to culture, environment, disease, and other influences
4 Common dysfunctional patterns (nursing diagnoses)
5 Indicators of dysfunctional patterns

The practical approach is to gain a working knowledge of the functional patterns and of high-incidence nursing diagnoses. It is most important to use the patterns consistently in assessment. From this practice and from further study one learns *what patterns clients exhibit, what factors are associated with the patterns, what nursing treatment is successful,* and *what outcomes result.* Knowledge develops with experience, but the clinician has a responsibility *to see that experience contributes to knowledge.* Fulfilling that responsibility takes analysis and reflection; it does not happen automatically. The cognitive and perceptual abilities discussed in the following sections are the means used to learn about clients; they are also the means used to continually increase clinical knowledge.

Perceptual Recognition of Cues

Attaching a name to the sensory event is an act of *perceptual recognition and categorization.* The process of recognition and categorization is evident in statements such as "the new patient is a *male*" or "his skin is *warm.*" *Male* and *warm* are examples of concrete perceptual inferences and concrete identity categorizations. In a particular situation these kinds of perceptions may be cues to a diagnosis if the nurse uses them to go beyond mere recognition. Vast amounts of information impinge on the nurse's sense organs at any given moment. This information enters what is called sensory memory. Information decays quickly in sensory memory unless it is *recognized* and *transferred* to short-term memory. Recognition involves an inference about identity. Coding a sensory experience makes it possible to categorize it—to say, for example, *this* is a textbook and *that* is a novel.

There are three major requirements for becoming a sensitive observer. One is to *have knowledge categories available for coding relevant sensory data* so that the identity and meaning of what one observes can be determined. A second factor in becoming a sensitive observer of health-related cues is to *anticipate, or look for, cues* on the basis of knowledge that certain client behaviors are likely in particular situations. Third, observers have to *focus attention* so that sensory data are not missed. These three factors influence *perceptual sensitivity to cues* and subsequently influence diagnostic judgments.

Coding Perceptual Data Categories may be detailed discriminations (mottled skin) or global representations ("poor" skin color). This is determined by the interests and needs of the person and, basically, by past interactions with the environment. For example, English teachers pay close attention to grammar and sentence structure. They have categories available for coding auditory or visual data about grammatical errors, such as dangling participles. Compared to nurses, English teachers may fare poorly in perceiving and categorizing heart rhythms or nonverbal messages. They lack discriminating categories and category systems in these areas. Many sophisticated discriminations are required in nursing. For example, nurses learn to discriminate among at least nine changes in skin color: jaundice, mottling, flushing, bronzing, sallowness, ashenness, glossiness, pallor, and cyanosis.

Categorization helps one learn to respond to things judged as equivalent (things in the same category). When skin is categorized as *mottled,* nurses derive certain meanings from this perception. A different meaning is derived when sensory data are put into another category, *sallow* skin.

Ways of representing the perceptual world of nursing practice are learned primarily from others. Descriptions, names for things, and meanings are provided in nursing's "cultural heritage." During learning, images are constructed and stored in memory. Think for a minute; conjure up an image of a thermometer. Describe it. Presumably the reader does not have one handy; thus some mental image from past learning has to be scanned. Images are also referred to as categories.[7] They are representations in memory from past interactions with the world. In fact, categories and their interrelations are each individual's own personal descriptions of the world. If, when verbalized, they are not reasonably congruent with others' descriptions, the discrepancy is called madness or creativity!

Much of nursing education involves learning to use categories. The nurse learns (1) to isolate important details from the environment and categorize observations, (2) to work with the descriptive labels used in health care, (3) to recognize relationships among categories, and (4) to plan treatment for categorized situations. Most importantly, learning to categorize permits the nurse to order and relate one thing to another, such as one cue to another, clusters of cues to a diagnosis, and then diagnosis to treatment. It also permits anticipation of things not immediately observable (Rosch and Lloyd, 1978, p. 1).

Anticipation *Sensitivity* is a term used frequently in nursing. Clients use it in the context "such a sensitive nurse." Supervisors, clinical specialists, and nursing instructors may use the term similarly *or* in the negative: "She's just not sensitive to clients." One can surmise that sensitivity is highly valued in a nurse because people rarely confront each other directly with accusations of insensitivity to people. Sensitive observers see not only the very obvious and apparent things but also the not-so-apparent. They anticipate and predict.

Perceptual sensitivity to client behavior depends in part on anticipation of behavior. If something is anticipated, or expected, less information is needed for recognizing and coding sensory input. This is because categories for recognizing the input are more accessible in memory. To become aware of relationships among cues and to know the meaning of cues, one must learn the appropriate categories for coding clinical data and must know the relationships among categories.[8] Knowing the likelihood of events permits anticipation and perceptual readiness. Perception is accurate as long as what is expected corresponds with the events that actually take place.

An example may further clarify how anticipation increases perceptual sensitivity. Suppose a nurse knows that 3 days of bed rest can produce muscle weakness. When a client begins to get out of bed after confinement, a slight buckling of one knee may be sufficient to identify the possibility of muscle weakness. Lacking background knowledge of the expected likelihood of muscle weakness, another nurse might miss the relatively subtle cue of knee buckling

---

[7]Earlier in the book, nursing diagnoses were described as *conceptual categories.* In this section the focus is on *perceptual categories* that are the cues, or building blocks, used in attaining a diagnosis.

[8]Categories and relationships could be constructed, but the disposition, curiosity, and time to do this are not constantly present. *Thus a tendency exists to ignore information that cannot be coded.*

and the client might not be supervised as ambulation begins. An impressive cue, such as falling, might be necessary before recognition could occur.

Focused Attention   In addition to having categories for coding sensory inputs and knowing the likelihood of events, sensitive observers focus their attention. People have the capacity to direct their attention selectively to particular aspects of their environment. The functional advantage of focused attention is that one is more apt to "see" what is important relative to the goal of the moment; distraction by extraneous stimuli is reduced. This selectivity can be lifesaving when one is crossing a busy street and advantageous when looking for a friend in a crowd.

During client health assessment, focusing of attention increases sensitivity to relevant information. For example, the functional health patterns previously discussed focus one's attention on 11 areas of health-related behavior relevant to nursing. This focus increases readiness to perceive cues to these patterns.

In summary, unless appropriate categories and category systems are available for coding sensory events, perception can be delayed or inaccurate. Inability to place sensory input into an appropriate category, when one is motivated to do so, results in a "long, close look." This prolonged observation is common in the child or adult who pauses to stare at something of interest that cannot be immediately categorized. Learning, asking questions, and curiosity increase availability of categories. In contrast, ignoring observations or events that one cannot classify or understand inhibits learning and may lead to diagnostic error.

Various causes of failure to recognize cues have been identified (Holt, 1961, p. 378); these causes and recommendations for prevention are contained in the following listing:

1 Lack of categories in memory (for example, lack of clinical knowledge). Study and memorize the words used to describe client behaviors and health problems named in textbooks.

2 Lack of training in discrimination (for example, discrimination of skin color changes or between fear and anxiety). Seek opportunities in clinical practice for discriminating among levels of a cue and differentiating one diagnosis from another.

3 Blocks to retrieval of categories when needed because of fatigue or emotional upset. Avoid these.

4 Demanding too exact a degree of fit between sensory data (cues) and categories in memory or accepting too gross a fit (insufficient data). Discuss observations and diagnoses with instructors or clinical specialists to get feedback. Obtain a grasp of the subtle differences in cues across clients with the same diagnosis; seek out repeated experiences (same diagnosis, different clients).

5 Lack of precise criteria for recognition (category in memory has not been, or cannot be, precisely defined by observable data). Learn the criteria for recognizing cues and diagnoses; help to further specify these.

Everyone has experienced failure to recognize something because of the above reasons. In clinical practice, steps have to be taken to reduce the causes of failure to a minimum. If perception depends on stored representations of the world and retrieval from memory when sensory input occurs, a question arises: How does one store the clinical information required for thinking and perception?

Memory: Chunking, Note-taking, Organization

Humans retain information for long and short intervals. For example, nurses observe and retain information about a pulse rhythm for a minute (the usual observation period); they remember a telephone number until dialing is complete; and they recall the type of surgery a person had last year. The concepts of short- and long-term memory storage are used to explain remembering and forgetting. They are important ideas in assessment, because lost information can lead to error.

Images, thoughts, and information of which one is currently aware are the contents of *short-term memory stores.* Information can be held for seconds or a minute or more. According to a current theory of memory, features (for example, the features of a blister) are held for scanning until *long-term memory store* (knowledge) can be retrieved, placed in the short-term store, and scanned (Atkinson and Shiffrin, 1971). This is the way identification occurs. The person finds the best fit and labels the perceived features. In this example, features of the lesion under observation would conform to *blister* features stored in memory, and the label stored in memory (*blister*) would be applied.

Chunking Information   Short-term storage is "working memory" and consciousness. It is within this short-term memory that perceptual inference, conceptual thinking, problem solving, and decision making go on. Miller (1956, pp. 81–97) suggests that the human mind can hold only about five to nine separate pieces of information in the short-term store. To overcome limited memory capacity, "chunking" is used. Pieces of information are put into broader categories, or "chunks," by abstraction. For example, in listening to a client relate a typical dietary pattern, one could use the four basic food groups to "hold" information as the person recites all the foods eaten in a typical day. Diagnostic concepts are also a form of chunking clusters of signs and symptoms into broad categories.

Chunking prevents overload. Without chunking, loss of pertinent pieces of information can occur. In clinical situations the nurse must hold information in short-term memory storage until it can be recorded, processed in decision making, or understood by retrieval of other past experiences from long-term memory.

If short-term memory images are lost within a number of seconds, how does a nurse remember a pulse rate or rhythm? Indeed, how does one remember the last numbers of a 7- to10-digit telephone number after dialing the first few?

Rehearsal of information, such as repetition of a telephone number, decreases the rate of loss of the digits and sequence. Yet if similar information, such as other numbers, enters the short-term store, forgetting occurs (Atkinson and Shiffrin, 1971, p. 88). This is a common event everyone has experienced.

Transfer of information to long-term memory storage explains humans' ability to remember after long time lapses. Long-term recall is partially dependent on intentional rehearsal of information to be remembered. (What is thought to occur in rehearsal is that neurons maintain reverberating circuits or undergo some type of structural or functional change.) In addition to intentional rehearsal, constant thinking or rumination about an event can firmly establish memory. Note taking can also assist memory.

Note Taking New information can cause loss of information if rehearsal is interrupted. It is well to remember this when collecting all the nursing history and examination data. Inventions to compensate for the limited capacity to hold information in consciousness include the pencil and paper!

Some nurses do not take notes during a history and examination. This could give the client the impression that the information provided is not important enough to write down. In addition, research findings suggest that it is highly unlikely that continuous information over a period of even 20 minutes can be retained (Atkinson and Shiffrin, 1971). Five to ten minutes are necessary for minimal consolidation in long-term memory and an hour or more for maximum consolidation (Guyton, 1976, p. 752).

Organization Another important point relevant to assessment is that remembering and forgetting seem to be influenced by information coding. Experiments have demonstrated that ability to remember (to recall memories from long-term storage) depends on (1) the way in which information was rehearsed and stored and (2) the retrieval probe that is used (Atkinson and Shiffrin, 1971, p. 89).

Have you noticed that some nurses have to retrieve nursing knowledge by using a disease category probe? This is because their clinical knowledge was originally learned and stored in this way. This cognitive organization around disease categories facilitates practice if nursing is only disease-related. Person-focused nursing requires that knowledge be organized within categories that describe any human being, with or without disease. The 11 functional pattern areas are an example. In long-term memory these areas are then "cross-referenced" with the likelihood of alterations in patterns associated with disease. This method of categorization enables the nurse to organize nursing knowledge *and* medical knowledge and to integrate the two classes of information. A retrieval probe can retrieve all three bodies of knowledge (nursing, medical, and integrated) if the situation warrants. If the client is seen only for health promotion, a disease-oriented probe is not necessary to retrieve clinical knowledge of functional patterns.

The idea of memory probes and long-term memory retrieval can also be applied to assessment. Suppose one wished to get rid of those pages and pages of an assessment tool that defy memorization. Assessment items could be coded in memory under the 11 functional pattern areas. For example, a nurse would learn, that is, place in long-term storage, the items to be assessed in the nutritional-metabolic area (Appendix E). The specific items of data in each area could be retrieved and used to guide questions and observations during history taking and examination. A small sheet with items listed could be devised until learning was complete.

A set of categories, such as the functional health patterns, serve as advanced organizers for storing specifics. *Advanced organizers are "ideational scaffolding" for the retention of details* (Ausabel, 1968, pp. 148–152). The payoff in this type of cognitive organization lies in ease of retrieval; the succinct list of patterns can be used as quick probes for the data to be collected in each area. The key to any retrieval is an appropriate "search set." The key to learning is to organize and categorize details in meaningful ways—meaningful for clinical practice.

SUMMARY

In this chapter the most critical component of the diagnostic process—information collection—has been explored. Unless valid and reliable information is used as a base, health problems may be ideas constructed by the diagnostician rather than descriptions of the client's real signs or symptoms. To avoid having imagination take over, diagnoses must be firmly based in clinical data.

In the first section of this chapter, assessment was defined as health evaluation based on collection of information (data). It was emphasized that this component of the diagnostic process is continuous during all nurse-client interactions. Four types of assessment situations were identified. These included the *initial assessment* at admission, which includes both history and examination. The purpose of the initial assessment is to establish diagnoses (if health problems are present) that can direct care planning. The *problem-focused assessment* has as its purpose the daily or periodic evaluation of the status of a diagnosis. In some situations, such as residential or long-term care, the time lapse between health status assessments (*time-lapse reassessment*) may be long. A complete history and examination are recommended; yet problem-focused assessment and time-lapse reassessment are designed as follow-ups to previous assessment data. An *emergency assessment* differs from the three other types of assessment in the level of problem formulation and the immediacy of intervention. The differences in scope of data, context, and purpose of these four types of assessment were discussed.

The admission assessment was examined rather closely. Both the client and the nurse have a psychological set toward the interaction; their sets are complementary in most instances. The client wishes to resolve ambiguities and seek help; the nurse has a descriptive-evaluative set and wishes to offer help. Ideas were explored in regard to beginning the assessment, assisting the client to describe his or her health patterns, and terminating the assessment. Assessment was considered in the context of establishing a therapeutic relationship.

After this overview of information collection, discussion turned to other factors that influence a nursing data base. The situational context that permits a client to share information was discussed.

Two other influential factors were examined. One factor is the *nature* of clinical information and its influence on data collection. The probabilistic, or uncertain, nature of clinical data influences subjective confidence in diagnoses. In an uncertain situation, collecting more and more data is not the answer; rather, the most valid and reliable predictors have to be sought. Important cues were described as those that contribute to evaluative judgments. These cues may be of various types: subjective, objective, historical, and current. Important cues are relevant to health status evaluation and permit reliable and valid judgments.

The last section of this chapter focused on the diagnostician's influence on what data are collected. The diagnostician was viewed as a sensitive measuring device. An examination of perceptual recognition and perceptual sensitivity to cues emphasized the importance of clinical knowledge. It is on the basis of knowing what to expect that sensory input is coded, cues are anticipated, and attention is directed. Examination of short- and long-term memory storage resulted in suggestions for collecting information and for organizing clinical knowledge necessary for assessment.

At this point the reader should have a beginning grasp of nursing diagnosis. The process of arriving at a diagnosis has been outlined in a broad sense. This chapter and the one preceding it have emphasized one component of the process, information collection. Information is continually collected throughout all nurse-client interactions. At certain points, when the data indicate, diagnoses are formulated. If diagnoses are present they are used as a focus for the initial nursing care plan.

Information collection is not a random process. Professionals know why information is needed—the long-range goal for which it is collected. Stated differently, they have a conceptual framework from which they view the client, their goal, and the ways that may be used to reach the goal. A framework for professional practice focuses attention on *what* information is important.

It has been suggested that people of all ages, at all levels of health, and with any type of disease have certain functional patterns. Behavior within these pattern areas may be viewed as adaptations, as self-care, or from other perspectives. Irrespective of the conceptual framework applied, the behavior exists and constitutes the basic data of concern to nurses.

After preceding chapters established that a framework is necessary for determining *what* data to collect, the present chapter focused on factors influencing *how* data are collected. Yet nurses do not just collect data; they also make evaluative judgments. If health problems are present these judgments are referred to as diagnostic judgments, or nursing diagnoses.

The reader is being led through the diagnostic process. The question at this point is what to do when a cue or cluster of cues seems to indicate a dysfunctional health pattern. The answer is to generate the likely possibilities and collect data to test each one. Chapter 7 will expand on this answer.

BIBLIOGRAPHY

Atkinson, R. C., & Schiffrin, R. M. (1971). The control of short-term memory. *Scientific American,* 225: 82–90.

Ausabel, D. (1968). *Educational psychology: A cognitive view:* New York: Holt, Rinehart and Winston.

Block, D. (1974). Some crucial terms in nursing: What do they really mean? *Nursing Outlook,* 22: 689–694.

Bruner, J. S., Goodnow, J. J., & Austin, G. A. (1956). *A study of thinking.* New York: Wiley.

Cardwell, J. D. (1971). *Social psychology.* Philadelphia: Davis.

Ciafrani, K. L. (1984). The influence of amounts and relevance of data on identifying health problems. In M. J. Kim, G. McFarland, & A. McLane (eds.), *Classification of nursing diagnoses: Proceedings of the fifth national conference.* St. Louis: Mosby.

Corrigan, J. (1986). Functional health pattern assessment in the emergency room. *Journal of Emergency Nursing,* 12:163–167.

Cutler, P. (1979). *Problem solving in clinical medicine: From data to diagnosis.* Baltimore: Williams & Wilkins.

Froelich, R. E., & Bishop, V. M. (1977). *Clinical interviewing skills.* (3d. ed.). St. Louis: Mosby.

Gordon, M. (1987). *Manual of nursing diagnosis,* 1986–1987. New York: McGraw-Hill.

Gordon, M. (1980). Predictive strategies in diagnostic tasks. *Nursing Research,* 29: 39–45.

Gordon, M. (1972). *Probabilistic concept attainment: A study of nursing diagnosis.* Unpublished doctoral dissertation. Boston College.

Guyton, A. (1976). *Textbook of medical physiology.* (5th ed.). Philadelphia: Saunders, p. 752.

Hammond, K. (1966). Clinical inference in nursing: A psychologist's viewpoint. *Nursing Research,* 57: 27–38.

Haynes, R. B., Taylor, D. W., & Sackett, D. L. (1979). *Compliance in health care.* Baltimore: Johns Hopkins University Press.

Herzlich, C., & Graham, D. (1973). *Health and illness: A social psychological analysis.* New York: Academic Press.

Holt, R. (1961). Clinical judgment as a disciplined inquiry. *Journal of Nervous and Mental Disease,* 133: 369–382.

McLane, A. (ed.) (1987). *Classification of nursing diagnoses: Proceedings of the seventh conference.* St. Louis, MO: Mosby.

King, L. S. (1968). Signs and symptoms. *Journal of the American Medical Association,* 206: 1063–1065.

Koos, E. L. (1960). Illness in regionville. In D. Apple (Ed.). *Sociological studies of health and sickness.* New York: McGraw-Hill.

Mechanic, D., & Volkart, E. H. (1961). Stress, illness behavior and the sick role. *American Sociological Review,* 26: 51–58.

Miller, G. A. (1956). The magical number seven, plus or minus two: Some comments on our capacity for processing information. *Psychological Review,* 63: 81–97.

Neisser, U. (1978). Perceiving, anticipating, imagining. In C. W. Savage (Ed.), *Perception and cognition: Issues in the foundations of psychology,* Minnesota Studies in the Philosophy of Science. Minneapolis: University of Minnesota Press, vol. 9.

Nisbett, R., Krantz, D., Jepson, C., & Kunda, Z. (1983). Use of statistical heuristics in everyday inductive reasoning. *Psychological Review,* 90: 339–363.

Norris, C. M. (1982). *Concept clarification in nursing.* Rockville, MD: Aspen Systems.

Rosch, E., & Lloyd, B. (1978). *Cognition and categorization.* Hillsdale NJ: L. Erlbaum (Distributed by Halsted Press Division. New York: Holt, Rinehart and Winston.)

Sarbin, T. R., Taft, R., & Bailey, D. E. (1960). *Clinical inference and cognitive theory.* New York: Holt, Rinehart and Winston.

Zola, I. K. (1979). Culture and symptoms: An analysis of patients' presenting complaints, In R. E. Spector (Ed.). *Cultural diversity in health and illness.* New York: Appleton-Century-Crofts.

INFORMATION INTERPRETATION AND CLUSTERING

INFORMATION INTERPRETATION AND CLUSTERING

In previous discussions information collection has been treated independently of the overall diagnostic process. This separation permitted an emphasis on important topics but neglected the fact that information is interpreted and clustered while it is being collected. It may be recalled from Chapter 1 that the following four activities occur not as steps but as continuous actions during the diagnostic process:

1 Collecting information (continuous)
2 Interpreting information (continuous)
3 Clustering information (continuous)
4 Naming a cluster or problem formulation (occurs at certain confidence points)

The focus of this chapter is on how to use information obtained during assessment.[1] Using information for health status evaluation requires interpretation and clustering of cues on the basis of their meaning. (Naming the cluster of cues in the full sense of the recorded problem and etiological statement is discussed in Chapter 8.) There are various levels at which these aspects of the diagnostic process can be described. At the observable level nurses are seen to ask questions and examine a client; then they verbalize and record a diagnosis. How do we explain this behavior, especially when their diagnoses are valid and reliable?

At a deeper level of explanation it is said nurses use diagnostic strategies.

---

[1]Various types of assessments are discussed in Chapter 6. Emphasis in this chapter will be on the initial assessment, which is the most complex.

The selection of information to be collected, the sequence of collection, and the way information is used are a sequence of decisions, which by definition is a *strategy* (Bruner, Goodnow, and Austin, 1956, p. 51). Learning how to make a diagnosis requires probing to a deeper level. Exactly what is going on when a diagnostic strategy is employed? Rather, what do we think is going on? From studies of diagnosticians and others, it appears that decisions are based on *diagnostic hypotheses* generated from the clinician's *interpretations* of the information collected. In fact, over and above routine assessment questions and examination guidelines (Chapter 4), information collection is directed by hypotheses.

Hypotheses (possibilities) are *alternative interpretations* of the data. They are investigated by collecting more information. Some hypotheses may be discarded, some held, and others revised; also, new diagnostic hypotheses may be generated as assessment continues. In other words, diagnosticians structure and organize the initial data by their hypotheses. They focus the search for further information on a likely set of possibilities. If the information collected "fits the picture" of a particular diagnostic category, then their thinking is made "public." A nursing diagnosis is stated and a treatment plan is recorded. The reader is probably thinking:

How do you know when the cues "fit the picture"?

How do nurses know what questions to ask and what to observe if these things are not specified by the routine assessment tool?

Where do hypotheses come from?

Answers to these questions are at a deeper level of explanation where the diagnostic process is explained in terms of clinical reasoning, inference, and judgment. These cognitive processes were introduced in Chapter 6 as the diagnostician's basic tools for interpreting and clustering information. They are extremely important in professional nursing because decisions that result from these processes can have an impact on the client's comfort or life.

In the discussion that follows, interpretation of assessment information will be emphasized in the first section and clustering of information in the second. It should be noted that these usually occur together. In most instances the meaning of a cue depends on the cluster of interrelated cues in which it is embedded. Figure 7-1 illustrates the process to be discussed in this section.

INTERPRETATION OF INFORMATION

To be useful information collected during an assessment has to be interpreted. *To interpret means to assign meaning to a cue or determine what it signifies.* There are different levels of meaning that can be derived from information. Higher, complex levels require more cognitive skill and ability. For example, it will be seen that interpreting whether a cue indicates a functional or dysfunctional pattern requires less skill than interpreting whether a set of cues mean that a particular diagnosis is present or absent.

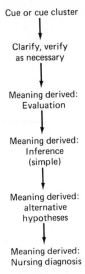

Cue or cue cluster

Clarify, verify
as necessary

Meaning derived:
Evaluation

Meaning derived:
Inference
(simple)

Meaning derived:
alternative
hypotheses

Meaning derived:
Nursing diagnosis

FIGURE 7-1
Interpreting the meaning of clinical clues.

Recognizing a Diagnostic Cue

The recognition of a diagnostic cue from among client responses and observations collected in assessment of a pattern is extremely important. *If attention is not paid to a diagnostic cue, the shift from routine assessment to the diagnostic process does not occur.* The decision point is depicted in Figure 7-2.

Information collected during assessment may contain client responses or nurse-observations that *point directly* to one or more diagnoses. When this occurs the diagnostic interpretation is simple. The cue or cluster of cues corresponds to the characteristics stored in memory of one or more diagnoses. These diagnoses are used as hypotheses for structuring further data collection. The question "What is the problem in this functional pattern?" has been quickly narrowed down to a few dysfunctional patterns (possible diagnoses). As the reader may have anticipated, diagnostic interpretations of the meaning contained in assessment data are not always this simple.

Before the *diagnostic meaning* emerges it may be necessary to clarify, verify, or determine the basic meaning of cues. Consider an example of pieces of information in the self-perception–self-concept pattern from two clients scheduled to begin chemotherapy for cancer:

Client A: I'm so afraid of what will happen to me.
Client B: Someone I knew very well had this same treatment.

Client A's statement provides a diagnostic cue ("I'm so afraid") that *directly* suggests the diagnostic hypotheses of fear and anxiety. Neither clarification nor verification of "afraid" is necessary; it is viewed as meaning "feelings of concern about a threatening event," which is a defining characteristic listed in diagnostic

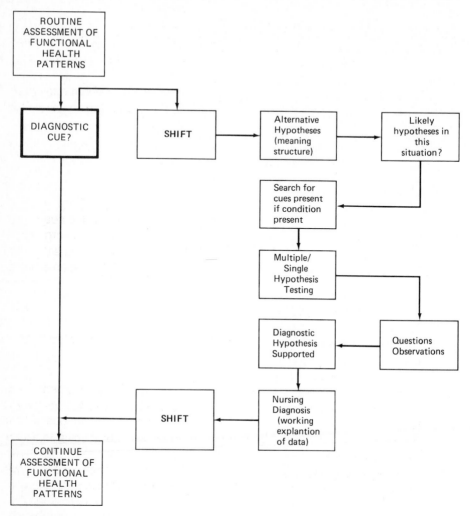

FIGURE 7-2
Representation of shifts from routine assessment to the diagnostic process.

manuals for both fear and anxiety. The next step is to determine if the feeling is focused on something specific (fear) or is diffuse (anxiety).[2] In contrast, Client B's statement raises the possibility that "someone's" experience may be used by the client to predict his own experience. Is this positive or negative? He "knew" this person—interestingly, he uses the past tense. He could be referring to many years ago or that the person is deceased. It may or may not be that

[2] Are you thinking it is fear of the chemotherapy? That is a good example of an inference. You have put together *afraid* and *chemotherapy* and inferred that they are related. Next you must validate this "creation."

the person's death is viewed as related to treatment and it may or may not be that Client B identifies with this person. Before jumping to any diagnostic interpretations (for example, fear or anxiety), clarification and verification are necessary.

Information collected during assessment will not always match the textbook listing of diagnostic signs and symptoms. Thus, the diagnostician has to be prepared to

1 Clarify and verify cues when necessary before interpreting their meaning.
2 Recognize the meaning of direct dues (Client A).
3 Derive meaning from concealed cues (Client B).
4 Put initial cues together so that their basic meaning emerges.

Let us consider each of the above elementary processes as "the search for meaning" when it is not immediately apparent. The discussion will be organized by a series of questions that diagnosticians ask themselves (consciously at first and then unconsciously) while interpreting and structuring information early in the diagnostic process:

Is there a need for clarification?
Is there a need for verification?
Is the meaning clearly interpreted relative to norms, and in the context of other cues?

Need For Clarification   Before attempting to interpret assessment data, clarification may be necessary. *Clarification refers to the search for clearer understanding.* Whenever clients use vague, abstract, or ambiguous terms, data has to be clarified; otherwise misperceptions may occur leading to errors in diagnosis. For example, what does the client mean by a "poor" marriage? What are the feelings the client is classifying as "anxious"? What does "I eat good" mean? Do *specific* fears underlie a statement such as "I'm afraid of dying"? What does the client mean by "I feel weak." *Without clarification, clinicians tend to place their own meanings on these ambiguous words and statements.* They may *assume* they know what the client means and later be shocked to find their assumptions totally wrong. For reliable information collection put aside personal meanings, especially for important cues; clarify what the client means by further questions.

Need for Verification   *Verification of data means double checking.* This is necessary when (1) the diagnostician has doubts about his or her perception, (2) there is a conflict, or contradiction among cues, or (3) an inference or assumption has been made and is being used as an important piece of data to influence nursing actions. This may be as simple as making sure the blood pressure really was 180/80 or as complex as saying to a client after a visitor leaves: "You seem very angry." Verification is also used to validate diagnostic impressions with the client. For example in the case of noncompliance, the client may be asked: "You seem to be having trouble managing *all* those medications; I think it might be due to trouble remembering what-to-take-when; do you think that might be the reason?" Lastly, when cues appear to be conflicting or contradictory, double checking can reveal if the nurse's perception was inaccurate.

Deriving Meaning: Evaluation of Cues   After clarifying perceptions and understandings (as necessary) and verifying ambiguous information, the diagnostician begins to interpret the meaning of a client's response. The *first level* of interpretation requires evaluation. The purpose is to determine if the verbal report or the observation is "normal" or "abnormal," that is, a cue to a functional pattern (healthy behavior) or a cue to a dysfunctional pattern (diagnostic cue). Cue evaluation is an important step because it determines whether the routine assessment is to continue or a shift to the diagnostic process is necessary (see Figure 7–2). In evaluating a cue or cluster of cues, *the diagnostician compares the information obtained from the client with knowledge of norms and criteria retrieved from memory.*

Example A

A measure of heart rate reveals 126 beats per minute. To evaluate whether this finding means normal functioning or dysfunction, the nurse considers other information: that the measure is from an infant; this particular infant's baseline heart rate pattern is 120–130; that infants have a normal heart rate of 120–160. Therefore, 126 is evaluated as normal.

The heart rate now *begins to take on meaning;* it is normal. Evaluation is based on a comparison of a cue to a norm or criterion for health. A problem may be missed if a verbal report or observation is judged as indicating a functional pattern, when in fact the health pattern is dysfunctional. The reverse error, an incorrect judgment of dysfunctional pattern (when functional), leads to overdiagnosis.

The level of meaning derived from the data above is limited because the information has not been interpreted in the context of the whole person-situation. To decrease the risk of errors, *a second level of interpretation* is necessary in most instances. *Each cue has to be interpreted in the context of other cues that are present.* Example B will illustrate this:

Example B

The nurse inquires about protein intake of a 25-year-old woman. Her intake is sufficient when evaluated against norms for adult women. Yet, when interpreted in the context of other data from assessment of her reproductive pattern (the woman is two months pregnant), the cue takes on a different meaning. In fact, the woman has a potential for protein deficit.

Determining whether an isolated cue is a functional or dysfunctional indicator of a pattern takes the nurse to one level of meaning (Example A). *Interpretation of cues in the context of other data reveals the level of meaning necessary for accurate nursing diagnoses (Example B).*

The above examples illustrate how a reliable estimate of the meaning (functional or dysfunctional) of cues depends on (1) the use of norms or criteria and (2) other cues that are present. Both single cues and clusters of cues need to be compared to some norms or criteria. At this point it will be useful to stop and consider the knowledge stored in memory that is used as norms, or criteria, in first-level interpretation of data.

Comparison to Norms   Evaluating health pattern data involves comparing the *observed value* with the *expected value.* Population values (norms) from research, individual baselines, or (in some instances) the clinician's past clinical experiences provide the expected values. These are the criteria with which clinical data are compared. The importance of this evaluation must not be underestimated. It is the basis for subsequent diagnostic judgments.

Caution must be exercised in selecting the expected values to be used for evaluating clinical data. *Population norms* specify a range of normal limits for particular groups, frequently age groups. These norms are used as guidelines when evaluating physical attributes such as visual acuity, blood pressure, or protein intake. For evaluating data such as values, beliefs, self-perceptions, or role relationships, general population norms may be inadequate. Cultural, ethnic, racial, national, and religious patterns, as well as personal ones, need to be considered. For example, evaluation of data on toilet-training practices may be in error if specific cultural norms are ignored.

Secondly, when a social norm is in flux, it may not be useful as a criterion for evaluation. Sexuality patterns are an example; evaluation may have to be based partly or entirely on the client's perception of whether a problem exists.

Individual baselines, if available, are important in evaluating data. *Baseline data* provide individualized criteria that permit evaluation on the basis of the client's own functional health patterns. The difficulty arises in obtaining baseline measures. A human characteristic can be influenced by the context of the assessment situation, *including the nurse doing the baseline assessment.* Previous records may be helpful and should be consulted. If true baselines are not available, data obtained in the admission history and examination are used as baseline criteria for evaluating change in subsequent assessments.

The critical need for baseline data is the reason many hospitals require a nursing assessment within 6 to 8 hours of admission. Ideally, the assessment should be made as soon as a client enters a hospital, clinic, nursing home, or other health care service and has an opportunity to relax and obtain orienting information. The importance of this assessment in establishing baselines is the rationale for (1) having the history and examination done by a professional nurse; (2) doing the assessment in an environment conducive to relaxation; (3) establishing an interpersonal situation that facilitates development of rapport, trust, and confidence; and (4) ensuring privacy, quiet, and adequate lighting to facilitate conversation and examination.

Deriving Meaning: Simple Inference More complex meaning can be derived from assessment information than merely "that's not normal," "wouldn't expect that in this patient," or "that's not usual" as in the levels of interpretation already discussed. When data obtained during assessment do not meet expected health norms, the diagnostician tries to understand the meaning of the cues and whether or not they indicate a dysfunctional health pattern. Interpretation of clinical information at this level requires *inferential reasoning.* That is, an inference, or judgment, is made about what a client's verbal report or an observation means. *Inferential reasoning is the process by which the unknown meaning is tentatively inferred or predicted from known clinical data.*

As was discussed in Chapter 6 inferences range from simple, immediate judgments, such as "limping gait," to complex chains of reasoning that are deliberate and within conscious awareness. Whether simple or complex, an inference represents *going beyond the information collected* to make a judgment. This probably raises the following questions:

Why are inferential judgments necessary?
Aren't they dangerous?
When do you infer rather than use observations?

Inferences further elaborate the meaning of information collected. Consider an example of a relatively low level of inference that requires going beyond observations made at 7:00 in the morning. Note that cues had to be combined in order for an inference to be made and that the inference became a diagnostic "cue":

> The patient's bed linen is pulled out from the bottom of the bed and is lying twisted in a wrinkled lump, the blanket is half on the floor, the undersheet is wrinkled with the mattress cover exposed, and the pillow case is sliding off the pillow. *Inference: bed is in disarray.* The patient, a 50-year-old man, sighs and turns to one side of the bed and then to the other. When he notices the nurse he states he had a "quite a night." *Inference: Most nurses would infer that the patient has been, and currently is, restless.*

As can be seen in this example, an interpretation of the meaning of a set of observations both summarizes the data and provides a selective focus for attention. The expert immediately recognizes restlessness (it acts as a diagnostic cue). The novice may have to analyze the nine cues above before inferring that the data indicate restlessness and then go on to infer what diagnostic interpretations are suggested by restlessness.

Inferences can be "dangerous" as the previous question implied. This is because inferences or assumptions are *created* in the mind of the diagnostician. In contrast, observations are open for others to see and validate. On the other hand as the above example illustrated, isolated observations do not have diagnostic meaning unless interpretations are made. To *prevent errors, always remain open to new information and new interpretations of data.*

As we have seen, interpretation occurs at various levels of complexity; therefore, one or more of these levels of interpretation may be required before further meaning (diagnostic significance) of client responses and nurse observations can be inferred:

1 *Initial interpretation of meaning and evaluation relative to norms.* First the diagnostician determines whether the information points to a functional or dysfunctional pattern through a comparison with expected health norms. This is a superficial level of data interpretation.

2 *Interpreting the meaning of a cue or cue cluster in the context of data available.* The meaning of a cue may be very different when considered in the context of the whole person-situation.

3 *Interpreting meaning of cues to arrive at a simple level of inference,* such as restlessness, anger, or withdrawal. This level of interpretation involves placing some structure on the data and arriving at an inference.

There are two reasons why assessment data need interpretation. One is because the human mind cannot manage the large number of isolated bits of information in either one pattern area or the total assessment. (Recall the discussion of "chunking" in Chapter 6.) The other is that interpretations (hypotheses) guide the search for information beyond the routine screening assessment. (Hypotheses are complex inferences about data.)

Selective Attention to Diagnostic Cues

Selective attention is focused attention. It involves "pulling out" a cue(s) from the stream of ongoing assessment and focusing attention (and thinking) on the cue(s). This is not to suggest that attention is not continuous during assessment. Rather, certain cues alert thinking processes more than others. Levine (1973) refers to these cues or cue clusters as *provocative facts;* they "provoke" thinking. Others use the term *forceful feature* to refer to data that "force" a response (Gale and Marsden, 1983; Thyne, 1966). Irrespective of the terms used, there are cues that nurses select, attend to, and think about during assessment. They are the *diagnostic cues* that serve to generate hypotheses. The reader may ask:

What is it about information that causes attention to be focused?
How do you learn to recognize these cues?

During learning, *key* features of health problems and the meaning of these features are stored in memory. These include the critical cues of diagnoses that nurses are taught to pay attention to and those they have learned, through practice, to value as important. They include, but are not limited to, diagnostic cues. When these cues are encountered during an assessment or when other information suggests their presence, attention is aroused. This is because the data are seen as having either *diagnostic* or *therapeutic significance.* This motivates the clinician to think about the possible meanings of the data and subsequently to gather more information.

Why don't some nurses recognize and pay attention to important data? First, they may not have learned to recognize a cue and its significance. Second, the way they have organized their knowledge in memory may not permit easy retrieval of possible interpretations. Third, there may be only subtle manifestations of the behavior and, thus, it is missed by a novice. Last, as a number of researchers report, clinicians can become distracted by other cues that capture their attention and thinking processes.

Focusing attention on cues that have diagnostic significance is one of the major ways of reducing errors in nursing diagnosis. To enhance attention to diagnostic cues, learn the critical cues for each diagnosis and use these in practice. Distraction by other data can be partially overcome if all assessment information is reviewed before a final judgment is made about the diagnosis. Of equal importance is "putting things together" during assessment. Previous data can take on significant meaning when combined with other information elicited from the client. Thus, a cue may not receive selective attention at the time, but may gain significance and "provoke" thinking after other pattern areas are assessed. *To prevent errors, always remain open to new information and new interpretations of the data during assessment.*

Generation of Diagnostic Hypotheses

During the diagnostic process, attention and thinking are focused on information that has diagnostic and therapeutic significance. As will be seen in this section, this leads to the generation of hypotheses. Diagnostic hypotheses provide *further* interpretations of the possible meaning of data and serve to structure the diagnostic task.

Clinicians go beyond the information contained in inferences, cues, or cue clusters to generate a set of *possible* diagnostic meanings. For instance in the previous example, restlessness can mean pain, anxiety, fear, anoxia, and a number of other problems because it can be present in all these conditions. The diagnostic meaning of restlessness can be interpreted in a variety of ways depending on how the available data are clustered. These possible meanings are called *diagnostic hypotheses.* Usually one of these diagnostic hypotheses turns out to be the actual diagnosis.

Studies have demonstrated that diagnosticians structure an ill-defined task, such as "Does this client have a health problem?" by (1) selectively attending to early diagnostic cue(s), (2) thinking of likely hypotheses that will explain the meaning of cues, and then (3) testing (or "checking out") their hypotheses by collecting further information (Elstein, Schulman, and Sprafka, 1978; Gale and Marsden, 1983). There are a number of reasons why this is a useful strategy for managing large amounts of information. First, the initial cues and those derived from hypothesis testing can be clustered (grouped into "chunks" of information) under the related hypotheses. It is easier to think (in working memory) about three or four diagnostic hypotheses than possibly 10 to 20 isolated bits of information. Second, hypotheses provide some structure for thinking about "what to do next." For example, if cues suggest three possible diagnoses, the task is to check major, critical defining characteristics of the three diagnoses. Third, diagnostic hypotheses narrow the universe of possibilities. For example, rather than having to hold all the diagnoses describing dysfunctional activity-exercise patterns, the universe is narrowed to the likely diagnoses suggested by the initial data. In simple terms, hypothesis generation "brings to mind" alternative meanings or explanations for a diagnostic cue or cluster of cues.

Before considering how to generate diagnostic hypotheses, be assured that this is not a new behavior for most children and adults (Levine, 1975). We are all familiar with "cues" from the comic strip:

Distant speck in the sky,
Moving toward us.

Three "hypotheses" are generated to explain these "cues":

IT'S A BIRD!
IT'S A PLANE!
IT'S SUPERMAN!

This provides a commonplace example of *hypothesis retrieval* from memory. Interestingly, this children's expression is consistent with *likelihood estimates.* In real-life experience birds are the most frequently seen things in the sky. Thus, *bird* is a good tentative hypothesis to raise first. Planes are the second most frequent possibility to explain the distant speck in the sky. Estimates of the likelihood of events suggest that the least likely hypothesis (outside the world of fantasy) is Superman.

Hypothesis generation is critical to the accuracy of the diagnostic process. If the pool of hypotheses generated to explain diagnostic cues does not contain the actual diagnosis, errors can result and we hear the comment: "I never thought of that." The following example of data and the pool of hypotheses will help to grasp the idea of hypothesis generation:

A 50-year-old male client with high blood pressure and heart failure is being seen in the clinic. He looks exhausted (dark circles under the eyes, expressionless, slow gait) and during assessment of his sleep-rest pattern he reports that he is tired and having trouble sleeping.

This cluster of cues which contain the diagnostic cue, "trouble sleeping," suggests a sleep pattern disturbance. Having interpreted the cluster of cues in this way, the next thought is: what kind of disturbance? What pool of alternative possibilities could explain his appearance and verbal report? The following hypotheses provide alternative structures for this diagnostic problem and some direction for further cue search:

Sleep onset disturbance
Interrupted sleep pattern
Sleep pattern reversal
Early awakening pattern

Further information may reveal that one of these diagnostic hypotheses accounts for "trouble sleeping." If so, the diagnostician would then generate etiological hypotheses to explain the problem. Although the data is sketchy at this point, nocturnal dyspnea and fear, anxiety, or depression over deteriorating health should be considered.

The discussion of thinking processes that cannot be seen, heard, or touched is sometimes hard to understand. An idea that may be useful for imagining hypothesis generation is *branching*. Aspinall's study (1979) suggested that performance in the diagnostic process improved with conscious awareness of the idea of branching. Carnevali and her colleagues (1984) also discussed the concept in regard to cue interpretation.

Branching from a diagnostic cue to generate multiple hypotheses is like the branches on a tree that reach out in various directions. The small twigs coming off the branches represent the questions and observations that are made in testing hypotheses through a search for further cues. Generation and subsequent testing of hypotheses can be thought of as a decision tree similar to that shown in Figure 7-3. Consider the following data:

Ms. J. is a 45-year-old, white, married woman with cancer of the liver and jaundice.[3] She is going home in 2 days and is physically able to resume all activities. She states she doesn't know how friends will react to her color.

Figure 7-3 depicts three hypotheses, or branches, generated from considering the cues and patterns areas (role-relationships, self-perception–self-concept, and health-perception–health-management). All three branches represent viable hypotheses, given the clinical data available. Underlying the branching are propositions, deductions, and inferences, all of which are probabilistic statements. The reasoning in two of the areas of branching is as follows:

1 If jaundice, then abnormality in skin color
2 If abnormality in skin color, then change in outward appearance
3 If change in outward appearance, then feelings of being different
4 If feelings of being different, then negative perception of body or self
5 If feelings of being different, then decreased family and social contacts
6 Check client's perception of self
7 Check for social isolation

The experienced clinician rarely needs to go through this reasoning process. Having cared for many patients with jaundice, he or she probably thinks:

Jaundice → altered body image perception
Jaundice → social isolation

Information is then collected to support or reject the hypotheses. If one were pressed to explain the above reasoning, Goffman's (1965) conceptual model of stigma and social identity could be cited.

---

[3]Jaundice is a yellow coloring of the skin and whites of the eyes associated with bile pigment in the blood, in this case due to changes in liver cells and obstruction.

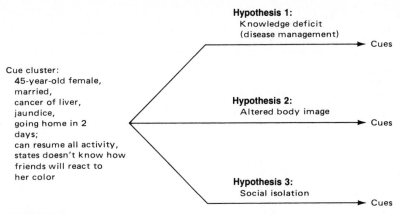

FIGURE 7-3
Branching hypotheses that guide cue search.

Consider another example of branching. In an emergency room a nurse has done a screening for problems in the 11 pattern areas of human function. When the role-relationship pattern (work role and relationships) was being assessed, the client said he was a plumber. While dressing the severe laceration of his right hand, the nurse asked him how he will manage at work. This branching question was based on a reasonable inference that the laceration would interfere with use of the right hand. The inference was being checked in a nondirective manner to elicit the client's ideas or plans. The basis for the question was the proposition that plumbers work with their hands, lifting and twisting things. The nurse could also question whether or not this man lives alone. How is he going to manage self-care, such as dressing, bathing, and cooking? These questions represent branching from a set of cues, background knowledge, and a sensitivity to human needs for self-care.

Imagine the branching that would direct the search for cues if a plumber's work activities became impossible or contraindicated because of neuromuscular, cardiac, respiratory, or psychiatric problems. To anticipate or predict functional problems from a set of situational or contextual cues is an ability that in many instances makes care effective or ineffective. The ability to branch from a set of cues requires cognitive sensitivity to the likelihood of events. Clinical knowledge and logical deduction are employed in branching. Conclusions are inferences, or hypotheses; when turned into questions, they direct further cue search.

How is this done? Some clinicians say certain cues are "automatically" associated with certain diagnostic hypotheses. Others say the possibilities for branching "just pop up" or "come to mind." These explanations do not help the beginner. When just starting to acquire clinical knowledge for interpreting assessment data, the novice needs to learn how to activate hypotheses stored in memory. This process is depicted in Figure 7-4. The following discussion will suggest some useful ways to "zero in" quickly on likely possibilities by finding the right problem area.

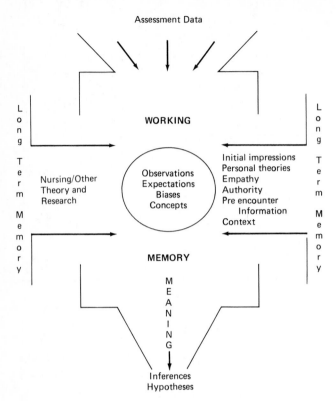

FIGURE 7-4
Transformation of information: from data to hypotheses.

Finding the Problem Area The initial information in a pattern area may be so specific and diagnostic that it suggests only one problem area. This was the case in the earlier example of sleep pattern disturbance. Cues (appearance and verbal report) were clearly diagnostic for a sleep problem and specific hypotheses were immediately apparent. They could be generated by the knowledgeable clinician without much cognitive strain. In many instances this is not the case. The actual problem area is not clear or, as with potential problems, likely possibilities have to be anticipated. Cognitive "work" has to be done to find *the most likely area in which the problem lies* before a pool of diagnostic hypotheses can be generated.

Some hints about using the assessment format and knowledge stored in memory for hypothesis retrieval and generation may be useful. These include use of the functional health patterns, pattern sequence, and expectancies with points of reference.

Use of Pattern Areas Initial hypotheses are usually formulated as broad problems, such as sleep pattern disturbance. These first hypotheses would be inadequate as diagnoses but they serve to structure thinking. Newell and Simon

(1972) are two cognitive theorists who propose that the universe of possibilities is narrowed to a limited "problem space" by early information. A problem space can be thought of as an area of clinical knowledge as, for example, thinking that it "seems like a nutritional problem." Generally, when assessment is being done in a pattern area, the *name of the health pattern* may be used as a broad prediagnostic hypothesis for the initial data. Each of the 11 pattern areas can narrow the universe of possibilities and focus thinking. As data accumulate, broad hypotheses become more specific. For the beginner it may also be useful to structure the assessment using the following questions:

1 Does this client have a health-perception–health-management problem?
2 A nutritional-metabolic problem?
3 An elimination problem?
4 An activity-exercise problem?
5 A sleep-rest problem?
6 A cognitive-perceptual problem?
7 A self-perception–self-concept problem?
8 A role-relationship problem?
9 A sexuality-reproductive problem?
10 A coping–stress-tolerance problem?
11 A value-belief problem?

As assessment of a pattern proceeds, the list of diagnoses grouped within each pattern area[4] provide a pool of hypotheses to explain the data. The following list would encompass currently identified nutritional problems:

Alteration in nutrition: potential for more than body requirements *or* potential obesity
Alteration in nutrition: more than body requirements *or* exogenous obesity
Alteration in nutrition: less than body requirements *or* nutritional deficit (specify)
Potential nutritional deficit
Uncompensated swallowing impairment
Alterations in oral mucous membranes
Potential fluid volume deficit
Fluid volume deficit
Alteration in fluid volume: excess *or* excess fluid volume
Potential impairment of skin integrity *or* potential skin breakdown
Decubitus ulcer (specify stage)
Impaired skin integrity

Let us examine some data. The following small collection of clinical data provides an example of hypothesis generation and sequential decisions about information collection. Try to determine the hypotheses that arose and how

---

[4]This type of grouping of nursing diagnoses can be found in the Manual of Nursing Diagnosis (Gordon, 1987) and Appendix C.

these may have controlled the cue search. Breaks in the nurse's recordings will be made for comments.

Mr. D is a healthy-appearing, single, 60-year-old salesman with well-controlled high blood pressure.

Health-perception–health-management pattern Views self as healthy and enjoying life. Takes medications as prescribed.

Nutritional-metabolic pattern In reviewing dietary pattern he states that he avoids meats except hamburger, doesn't like eggs or fish, and rarely eats raw vegetables or fruits. He comments that everything has to be cooked well.

The initial impression, "healthy appearing," indicates that body weight, facial expression, speech, skin, and mobility do not *globally* appear problematic. This tentative impression provides a background for the rest of the assessment.

When the nutritional-metabolic pattern was assessed, the nurse began by raising the question (broad hypothesis), Does this client have a nutritional problem? The first component reviewed (consistent with the broad hypothesis) was dietary intake pattern. Note the client's response. It supports the broad hypothesis and indicates the possibility of problems. He is eating only soft foods. This kind of diet can be associated with an inadequate nutritional pattern. The report of a soft diet initiated a search for cues guided by less broad hypotheses: Does the client have a nutrient, caloric, fluid, vitamin, or mineral deficit? Inferences from the medical diagnosis, essential hypertension, and initial impression suggested a 50 : 50 chance that any dysfunctional pattern existed. This is typical in the admission assessment, in which there is an equal probability that a problem does or does not exist. Now data are collected to test the hypotheses generated.

Detailed review of typical daily intake reveals less than minimum requirements for protein and vitamin intake. Other nutrient intake is sufficient. When asked if this dietary pattern represents a change, Mr. D replied, "Well . . . yes, I guess in the last year or so."

The nurse's hypothesis, nutritional problem, led to a search for details of the daily intake, comparison to standard requirements, and an evaluative judgment of the data. Note how some of the original hypotheses are discarded and the problem narrows to protein and vitamin deficit. The next question to the client established that there has been a pattern change that evidently occurred over a year. At this point the decision should be to raise the question of *why change occurred* and pursue some causal hypotheses. A broad question about the reason for change did not elicit useful information; questions became more specific.

No indigestion or "stomach trouble" was reported. A question in regard to chewing difficulty produced the report that Mr. D had had a lot of back teeth pulled as a teenager. Examination revealed many missing back teeth, multiple dental caries, and broken teeth.

Three cue-search decisions are evident. One was to elicit cues in the area of gastrointestinal tolerance for food. The second decision was to seek cues to chewing difficulties. This cue-search led to a third decision, to examine the client's teeth as a possible reason for the soft diet. Two questions were asked, one in the area of gastrointestinal tolerance for food and the other in regard to chewing. The hypothesis of chewing difficulty directed the search for cues by examination.

The nurse's inquiry about indigestion was probably based on the proposition that *if* symptoms or concerns exist about a gastrointestinal problem, *then* soft foods are eaten. Based on this proposition, the hypothesis that the problem was *gastrointestinal* was tested. The client reported no indigestion or "stomach trouble." This, plus the absence of any pathology noted on medical examination, was sufficient information for discarding this causal hypothesis.

A second causal hypothesis, chewing difficulty and dental problems, was raised. It probably rested on the proposition that discomfort in chewing could produce a change to soft foods. The age of the client and his verbal report were supporting data. A decision was made to examine the client's teeth, and the data provided support for the hypothesis of dental problems.

The example illustrates hypothesis generation and hypothesis-directed decisions. More information is needed before stating a diagnosis. This would include the client's perception of the dental problem, actions he has taken to deal with the problem, and factors in other pattern areas that may be interacting to produce this problem. The possibility that Mr. D. has a knowledge deficit about minimum daily dietary requirements would also need to be investigated.

In this example multiple hypotheses were tested simultaneously by asking about dietary pattern. Notice how this narrowed the possibilities quickly. Causal hypotheses about digestive disturbances and dental problems were pursued later, one by one. Different hypothesis-testing procedures yield different costs and benefits. For example, one procedure may ensure maximum information but strain memory capabilities (multiple testing). Another procedure may control memory strain but may be too time-consuming (single hypothesis testing).

When no information is available at the beginning of an assessment, the first thing one's strategy should do is narrow down the possibilities. Having a list of 11 pattern areas to be assessed is one aspect of a diagnostic strategy that does this. If these patterns are the focus of concern in nursing, then they circumscribe the important areas of assessment. Already, the universe is narrowed. Problem spaces are defined for retrieving clinical knowledge from memory. As data are collected broad questions and hypotheses give way to more specific diagnostic hypotheses.

Use of Pattern Sequence In addition to suggesting possible diagnostic hypotheses, assessing the health-perception–health-management pattern is a good starting point from the client's perspective. It is relevant, irrespective of the level of care or setting. As the reader may recall, defining the situation and learning how to manage are uppermost in the client's mind when seeking health care.

There has been no research about the relationship between the sequence in which patterns are assessed in the nursing history and the nurse's cognitive processing of the information obtained. Therefore it is not known whether or not nurses' utilization of information is facilitated by any certain sequence. As the pattern areas are used in the nursing specialties, a useful sequence may evolve.

There are a few ways of deciding what assessment sequence to use after the health-perception–health-management pattern has been assessed. For one thing, there should be a logical sequence from one content area to the next. For example, it seems logical to assess self-perception–self-concept, then role-relationships, and then the sexuality-reproductive pattern. One flows from the other. Similarly, the nutritional-metabolic and elimination patterns seem logically related.

From a psychological perspective, the value-belief pattern (including spirituality) and the sexuality-reproductive pattern may be considered highly personal areas. Most nurses would not assess these areas until rapport had been established and the client was at ease. Hence these patterns would be placed later in the sequence.

The sequence of pattern assessment can be related to individual situations. In a psychiatric setting, perhaps self-perception–self-concept or role-relationship patterns would be assessed early. In a medical or surgical setting, the nutritional-metabolic pattern might be the second area assessed, followed by the elimination pattern. With experience the clinician can develop an order that considers the client and situation and facilitates information processing in the history. For the first few nursing histories, try this sequence:

1 Health-perception–health-management pattern
2 Nutritional-metabolic pattern
3 Elimination pattern
4 Activity-exercise pattern
5 Sleep-rest pattern
6 Cognitive-perceptual pattern
7 Self-perception–self-concept pattern
8 Role-relationship pattern
9 Sexuality-reproductive pattern
10 Coping–stress tolerance pattern
11 Value-belief pattern

A problem can occur in one pattern and the etiological factors may be evident in other patterns. For example, the dietary and fluid pattern (nutritional-metabolic) may explain an intermittent constipation pattern (elimination pattern). Excess caloric intake (nutritional-metabolic pattern) and sedentary activity (activity-exercise pattern) may be etiological factors for a pattern of obesity (nutritional-metabolic pattern). Similarly, anxiety (self-perception–self-concept pattern) may be caused by a sleep pattern disturbance (sleep-rest pattern). The sequence of pattern-assessment permits integration of information. Interrelations among patterns suggest diagnostic and etiological hypotheses.

Use of the Client's Viewpoint   When hypotheses fail to "come to mind," it may be useful to obtain the client's viewpoint. Many nurses take the philosophical position that, as a general rule, clients should be involved in their problem identification and problem solving. In addition, the client's viewpoint may provide the nurse with hypotheses. One method of assessing problems from the client's perspective is to use the following set of questions (be sure to use a supporting, sincere manner during questioning, not challenging or an interrogation):

1 *Client's definition of the problem* (following description of signs and symptoms or a situation) "What do you think that means?" or "What do you think that is?"

2 *Client's definition of cause* "Why do you think that occurs (happens)?" or "I wonder what causes that?"

3 *Actions taken in response to the problems* "What do you do when that happens?" or "How do you handle that?" or "How have you managed that?"

4 *Effectiveness of action taken* "Did (does) that seem to help (work)?"

Clients' descriptions of their problems, their ideas about the causes of problems, and their responses and evaluations of actions taken provide a wealth of data on health perception, health management, coping patterns, as well as one measure of personal control and competency.

Use of Expectancies: Insight and Error   Background knowledge and experience stored in memory can be retrieved to *predict* events or *derive meaning* from assessment data. Stored knowledge used in this way forms the basis for *expectancies. An expectancy is a "ready-made" interpretation derived from memory.* The "norms" for evaluation previously discussed are expectancies. Also, expectancies can influence the aspects of the diagnostic process just discussed. Expectancies can influence:

1 Predictions that a particular problem or risk state may be present

2 Predictions about what a particular cue/cue cluster "means"

3 Inferences or diagnostic hypotheses that provide structure to isolated cues

As an example, most nurses would predict that the skin of an elderly client who is thin, immobile, and incontinent would break down. Having this expectation would suggest the diagnostic hypothesis of potential skin breakdown when these cues were present. Reasoning from insight and empathy would also suggest that the client may have fear (hospital procedures) and that the family may be ineffectively coping with the client's illness.

Generation of hypotheses on the basis of past knowledge of similar client situations can lead to *insights or errors.* To avoid errors, nurses should be aware of assumptions ("rules of thumb") underlying hypotheses and examine them for logical error. You may argue that this is unnecessary because hypotheses are tested by collecting further information—therefore, if they are wrong it will be evident in the lack of supporting data. This is true; but one common diagnostic error is holding hypotheses in the face of *disconfirming* evidence.

Basis for Expectancies: Reference Points   Let us consider points of reference, or expectancies, that can affect interpretations (inferences and hypotheses) about the meaning of data. These will include (1) contextual information, such as preencounter knowledge of the client and situation, (2) experience, (3) personal theories, (4) authority, and (5) initial impressions followed by a general summary.

1 INTERPRETATION: USE OF CONTEXTUAL INFORMATION   Information available prior to encountering a client can produce expectations that influence hypotheses during diagnosis. This information includes the type of setting, specialty area, medical diagnosis on the admitting sheet, previous records, and colleagues' comments. These are the contextual cues described in Chapter 6, both historical and current, that can be used to develop expectancies about the nursing diagnoses that might be present. For example, it is reasonable to assume that the level of care and setting, such as hospital, long-term care facility, or rehabilitation center influences the incidence of nursing diagnoses. Knowledge of high-incidence diagnoses can be used in generating hypotheses and anticipating high-risk problems. Expectations differ in different settings.

Specialty areas of practice can influence hypotheses. Before seeing clients, a nurse in a cardiac surgical unit expects them to have cardiac problems, surgery, and the nursing diagnoses that are commonly associated with these conditions. The use of expectations increases sensitivity to diagnostic cues. For example, in this specialty nurses would be sensitive to cues indicating ineffective coping with fear or anxiety regarding surgery and surgical prognosis, knowledge deficits regarding what will happen or how to do breathing exercises postoperatively, ineffective family coping, pain, activity intolerance, and other problems. These hypotheses are generated by cardiac surgical nurses from their knowledge and experience related to the co-occurrence of medical and nursing diagnoses in the specialty.

In addition to the practice setting, the nurse may draw upon information from other sources to generate hypotheses prior to seeing the client. A medical diagnosis of the present illness, records from previous hospitalizations or clinic visits, or referrals from community health nurses may create expectations. Nurses have learned that particular pathologies are associated with changes in certain functional patterns. Some textbooks specify the nursing diagnoses that co-occur with specific medical diseases (Carpenito, 1984; Doenges, Jeffries, and Moorhouse, 1984; Howe, Dickason, Jones, and Snider, 1984; Thompson, McFarland, Hirsch, Tucker, and Bowers, 1986). Use these only as "food for thought" about *possible* diagnostic hypotheses. There is insufficient research to predict which nursing diagnoses occur with each medical diagnosis. Some have a logical relationship to particular pathologies but it is unlikely that every client with the same medical diagnosis will have the same dysfunctional set of patterns (nursing diagnoses). Nursing and nursing diagnoses focus on the individuality of human responses. Validate through assessment the possibilities suggested in these textbooks.

Another source of diagnostic hypotheses is comments and observations of medical or nursing colleagues. A physician calls and says "I'm sending in a patient; she's been having a hard time with her husband over the surgery." Or another nurse may say: "I just saw him come in on the stretcher; he doesn't look good." Expectations start to form.

Contextual cues about the client's situation can also be a source of hypotheses. In a research study nurses used contextual cues to identify the most likely diagnostic hypotheses (Gordon, 1980). When given the task of determining the presence or absence of a set of surgical complications, the first information sought was *type of surgery performed* and *time lapse since surgery*. Even when information in the task was restricted, this was the first data collected rather than information about surgical complications. In actuality, their strategy was very efficient; the two contextual cues permitted them to predict the most likely hypotheses and quickly narrow the possibilities.

Preencounter hypotheses are formed before any interaction with the client and are confirmed or rejected during assessment. Expectancies or predictions may prove true or be totally inaccurate. Beware: they can also bias the diagnostician toward a particular hypothesis. Hold them, but not firmly. Wait for the assessment data and make sure hypotheses are supported by actual data.

2 INTERPRETATION: USE OF GENERALIZATIONS FROM EXPERIENCE Hypotheses that structure the data and interpret its possible meaning may be derived from experience. Generalizations derived from experience are based on the *recognition of similarities in repeated events*. When viewed as similar, repeated events are combined by *induction* to yield a generalization. The generalization may then be used in the next similar situation that occurs. Figure 7-5 depicts the formation of generalizations by induction. Various characteristics of client situations are used as a basis for induction.

For example, a nurse makes an observation: When one client in a unit gets very ill or dies other clients are anxious and upset. Repeated observations of this phenomenon are generalized to: *Critical illness or death on a unit produces anxiety in other clients on the unit.* Having acquired this knowledge from practice, the nurse may use it in the next similar situation encountered. (Notice that no data are used to indicate whether the clients are also anxious when the situation is absent! Herein lies the risk.) Application of the generalization stored in memory is depicted in Figure 7-5b. If this deduction is treated as just *one* hypothesis to direct cue search, then the risk is reduced. If the assumption, "Mr. J. is anxious because of Mr. B.'s cardiac arrest," is acted upon without further checking, risk of error is substantial.

The key to accuracy when generalizing from experience is not to rush into action before testing the hypothesis. Collecting information will determine the "truth" of the deduction. Unvalidated assumptions are risky; in this example, anxiety regarding Mr. B's arrest may not be the correct, nor the only, hypothesis to explain Mr. J's behavior. What explanations would have been proposed if

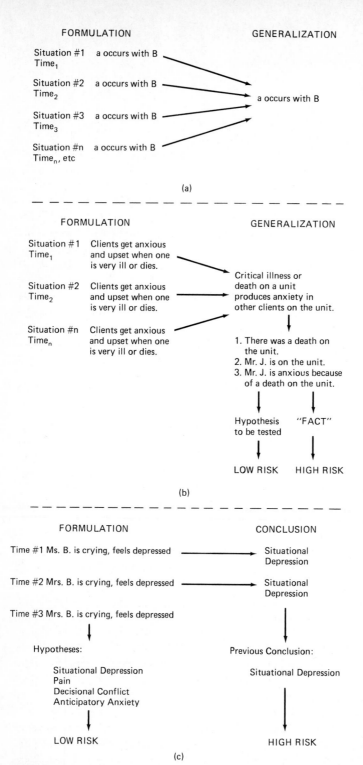

FIGURE 7-5
Examples of generalizations from experience (a) across situations (b) or time (c) and the risk involved in their use.

Mr. J was anxious and no cardiac arrest had occurred? Other hypotheses would have to be generated.

One can generalize not only from repeated experiences with a particular *situational context,* such as the cardiac arrest situation just discussed, but also from repeated similar experiences with the *same person or persons.* For example, the people in a community are resistant or hostile to developing needed health care services. The nurse *infers* that today the same reaction will occur (and perhaps responds to them as if it is occurring). Generalizations from past behavior to expectations of present or future behavior can be risky. When used as rigid assumptions, inferences may close out cues signalling *change.* Yet generalizations about a person's behavior can sensitize the nurse to important changes from base line. The key is to be open to cues and remember that most cues have an element of uncertainty.

Consider another example. A clinician, having cared for a number of families in a particular community health nursing district, noticed similarities in their knowledge of preventive health measures. He generalized about the neighborhood: Families in neighborhood A know of the need for immunizations for children. A young family that has lived in this small neighborhood for 10 years encounters some very complex health problems and is added to this nurse's caseload. He is very busy; what is his risk in inferring, versus assessing, their knowledge and practices regarding their small children's immunizations?

Generalizing from experience is useful if the relevant factors producing the similar events are identified. A risk is taken if (1) the new family does not have the same characteristics as the families on which the general proposition was built, (2) important factors producing the relationship are not identified, or (3) overgeneralization occurred initially. Living in the same neighborhood may be totally irrelevant to preventive health measures. On the other hand, it may be relevant because social interactions permit sharing of information about immunizations.

The use of induction from experience, as described above, requires that one have a grasp of the likelihood of events. Repeated experiences can suggest to the person making the inference (1) that things are about to change (the gambler's fallacy) or (2) that a "run" is occurring, that is, when a relationship between certain events has been observed ten times it is safe to infer that the same relationship will exist the eleventh time. Both rules can lead to error unless one is sensitive to the risks they entail.

People tend to *overestimate* the probability of *impressive events,* thinking more have occurred than was actually the case. For example, cardiac arrests produce an impression emotionally and cognitively. As a second example, when students begin the study of pathology they become impressed by the seriousness of some illnesses and begin to think they and their classmates have the symptoms. These examples describe *salient* (highly striking) experiences. The nurse in the first example may be more sensitive to cues because of the cardiac arrest experience. The students are sensitive to interpret symptoms using the new, impressive, readily accessible categories. In both cases there is increased readiness to infer because of experience.

Recall that anticipation facilitated sensitivity to cues and inferences. It can also lead to "systematic and predictable errors" (Tversky and Kahneman, 1974, p. 1131). Past impressive, salient events may be highly accessible in memory and because of this may appear to be more likely to recur than they actually are.

Generalizing from experience (inductive reasoning) is one reference point for deriving inferences. Sweeping generalities may be made, or sensitive reflections on multiple experiences and many years of practice may be the source of generalizations.

3 INTERPRETATION: GENERALIZATIONS FROM PERSONAL THEORIES In addition to single propositions, complex systems of propositions are sometimes constructed to interpret cues. Health care providers may have their own personal theories of health and disease and even an implicit theory of personality. This is particularly true in areas where science is "fuzzy." These personal theories can reflect reality or contain many illusions. Most have at least a portion of truth (Jones, 1977).

These so-called theories are constructed during social learning. They are based on experiences in living with other people. Generalizations can be made about human traits, dispositions, and actions. Jones states:

> One way to sensitize people to the existence of such beliefs is to pose a question such as "What do you think of a wise, cruel man?"—a jarring inconsistency for most people. For most people, wise men are generally kind, old, and perhaps jaded, but never cruel. (Jones, 1977, p. 3)

Implicit theories about what people are like, what personality characteristics go together, and what causes behavior can be firmly entrenched. In a study of nurses' inferences of suffering, Davitz and Davitz (1980) found differences between the inferences of Puerto Rican and American (white or black) nurses. The Americans inferred less suffering. In general the disease, age, and socioeconomic class of the portrayed patients influenced inferences of all the groups of nurses studied. Sociocultural learning was probably influential.

In brief encounters, a person's physical characteristics, a situation, or a patient's disease may be sufficient basis upon which to infer traits, dispositions, or secondary health problems. For example, "a high forehead goes with intelligence," "self-confidence predicts a successful and happy person," or "psychiatric patients will be violent" (Dion, Berscheid, and Walster, 1972). These stored "theories" and related propositional "knowledge" are implicit assumptions whose construction has been worked on since childhood. The tendency to make inferences without factual data is referred to as *bias* (Kaplan, 1973). It can influence interpretation of cues and even perception.

Beliefs about *groups of people* can also be incorporated into implicit theories (Jones, 1977, p. 52). The term *stereotype* describes an inference that all group members are alike. On the basis of one or two cues, a client is classified as a group member and then assumed to have all other attributes of the group stereotype. Stereotypic categorization ignores individual differences, as is evident in the group stereotypes about nurses, physicians, various cultures, races, and people of particular religions or nationalities.

Stereotypes are essentially expectations. They are constructed with minimal actual knowledge of the group and sometimes no experience with group members. Stereotypes generally are based on hearsay evidence that is culturally transmitted. Presumably they are not *directly* related to prejudice (negative attitudes toward a group of persons) (Jones, 1977, p. 61; Young and Powell, 1985).

A lack of information, a low degree of interest, and limited contact combine to increase anonymity and subsequent stereotypic classification (Berger and Luckmann, 1966, p. 33). Overemployment of stereotypes on the basis of insufficient information "appears to be a sign of rigidity, occasioned partly by lack of intelligence and insufficient familiarity" with persons (Sarbin, Taft, and Bailey, 1960, p. 196). (Nursing diagnoses meet the definition of stereotypic classification but are not used without valid, reliable, and sufficient data.)

Biases, errors, and misperceptions result if inferences derived from stereotypes are not subjected to validation. Stated differently, the use of stereotypes or attributions *as if they were observed data* ignores the uniqueness of the individual. A designation such as "the gallbladder in 321" encourages anonymity and extremely broad classification of the client.

When *negative* stereotypes are used without knowledge or rational thought, they can have unfortunate consequences. Merton defined these consequences as "self-fulfilling prophecy" (1957, p. 423). False definition of the situations can evoke new client behavior that makes the originally false conception come true. Simply, "if men define situations as real, they are real in their consequences" (Thomas and Thomas, 1928, p. 1104). Extreme caution has to be exercised not to draw negative inferences about clients and their behavior from propositions that have no basis in reality.

Consider an example of negative stereotyping (at least negative in terms of its social value): the *cancer-patient-as-terminal prophecy*. Future-oriented planning on the part of a "terminal" patient is sometimes labeled denial of terminal illness. With the great uncertainty in prognosis, many times there is no valid reason for the patient not to expect to survive for months or years. Hypotheses derived from pessimistic propositions or beliefs about death, coping, personal worth, and general ability to control events can be communicated unintentionally to clients during assessment. The potential then exists for the self-fulfilling prophecy to occur.

Another form of analogy, and by far the most commonly used, is *empathy*. One's own feelings and intentions are used to infer the feelings and intentions of a client. In using the self as a theoretical reference point, the nurse assumes that all (or many) people share *human* characteristics and behavior. Therefore the nurse's expectation is that he or she and the client will experience things similarly. The client's behavior is thought to be understood or predicted because it is the way the nurse would feel, behave, or act. Inner experiences of the self plus assumed similarity are the bases for the empathy (Sarbin et al., 1960, p. 15). In contrast to stereotyping without adequate information, empathy is a form of analogy that is highly valued.

In everyday conversation, people can understand each other because they share the meaning of the symbols (words) they use to communicate. Empathy, in contrast, depends on the shared meaning of reactions to human experiences. Empathy is a nonintellectual, nonlogical understanding of unspoken feelings resulting from active concern and involvement with another person. Empathy cannot be attained without personal concern and involvement.

Empathic understanding appears to be an ability closely related to imagination. It requires attention to situational cues and the *temporary* projection of oneself into the situation the client is experiencing. Resulting perceptions are used as hypotheses to direct cue search. Inferences generated by empathic understanding increase sensitivity to cues, particularly cues about feelings and intentions.

Bieri and his colleagues suggest that the use of the self as an analogy is more likely when one or more of the following are present: (1) similar beliefs, attitudes, and personality, (2) acceptance and liking of the person, and (3) similar social status (Bieri, Atkins, Briar, Leaman, Miller, and Tripoldi, 1966, p. 228). Considering these, it is understandable that one cannot use empathy to generate hypotheses about feelings when knowledge of the client and situation is scanty.

Sensitivity to the feelings of a person in distress depends heavily on the capacity to imagine how the person feels. Understanding is communicated when a clinician begins to inquire (test hypotheses) about feeling and intentions.

Care needs to be exercised that sharing empathic understanding is not influenced by a set to interpret events in a particular way. Consider two examples:

Surgical Nursing

Sue Jones, a 24-year-old primary nurse, has worked in a gynecological unit for 3 years since her graduation. She was married 2 years ago and has been trying to become pregnant. Today she is caring for Mrs. R. who is a 30 year old recovering from a hysterectomy (removal of the uterus). Mrs. R. says: "I feel so terrible today." Sue, without hesitation, says: "I know how you must feel but this hasn't affected your attractiveness and you have two lovely children." With a startled look, Mrs. R. replies: I mean the *pain* is terrible. . . ."

Sue learned (the hard way) from this experience. Putting herself in the client's situation caused her to assume that Mrs. R. felt "terrible" because she was unattractive as a woman after the hysterectomy and could not have any more children. She acted on her feeling of empathy rather than using it to generate hypotheses. Sue decided that she will (1) continue to be empathic, but (2) will check her impressions and consider alternative possibilities before she speaks. She realizes that because she thinks *she* would be less attractive to *her* husband after a hysterectomy and that *she* could not have the children *she* so desires, these personal feelings were projected to Mrs. R. Next time she will think that the cue, "feeling terrible," could mean any of the following conditions were present:

1 Perceived sexual identity disturbance
2 Grieving (loss of reproductive capacity)
3 Surgical pain
4 Postoperative fatigue

Rehabilitation Nursing

John Cari, a 28-year-old primary nurse in a rehabilitation clinic, was seeing Mr. D. who had been in a car accident in which he lost his leg. His wife was killed in the same accident. Mr. D. was being seen for follow-up on his gait and prosthesis. Initially, Mr. D. had experienced a severe body image disturbance after his amputation. This resolved after he learned to walk with the prosthesis and he returned to work. While doing a screening assessment of functional patterns, John observed that Mr. D. was exhibiting a disinterested manner and that he reported (1) "computer programming job was very demanding," (2) all he did was "work and sleep" and "sometimes sleep never comes . . . probably because I'm overtired," (3) didn't see that "life was ever going to be more than work and sleep with my job," and (4) "don't have the time to go out and meet new people."

John thought: Is there a reason for the choice of working so much? A body image disturbance could lead to focusing energy on work if he feels accepted there. His explanation for the sleep onset disturbance may be correct. If I was in *his* shoes with *his* history would I throw myself into my work for any other reasons? Maybe he has dysfunctional grieving over the loss of his wife and is using work as an escape from thoughts. I'll start with the sleep and see if it is more than being tired. Then I'll ask if he had considered changing jobs and why he doesn't get out more.

John said: "You mentioned that the difficulty getting to sleep was probably because you are overtired. Is there anything else that could be causing that?"
Mr. D.: "No, not that I can think of."
John: "All right, it's just that sometimes people start thinking about things and lie awake a long time."
Mr. D.: "Yea, I do that. When I'm overtired I keep reliving the accident and feeling I could have prevented it; I miss Angela so much and just can't seem to get on with my life. The leg isn't a problem now; it's the memories."

Personal theories develop as a result of experience in living. They can influence a data base by two routes: information collection and information interpretation. It is essential to be aware that this influence can occur. Although personal theories can lead to sensitivity to cues and the ability to generate hypotheses, a high risk is taken if hypotheses that are based on implicit theories, stereotypes, and empathic reference to the self are not tested and validated by data.

4 INTERPRETATION: GENERALIZATIONS FROM AUTHORITY Teachers, textbooks, research journals, and experienced colleagues are frequently used as reference points for inference. The propositions gleaned from these sources may be research conclusions, clinical lore, and experiential wisdom.

Inferences drawn from research conclusions are highly valid and useful if situations and clients are similar to the research subjects and setting. One has to be aware that conclusions are probabilistic, that is, they may be predicted to apply in 95 out of 100 cases. The risk is that a particular client may have a critically dissimilar characteristic or may be within the other 5 percent rather than the 95 percent to whom the research findings apply. Again it should be noted that information deduced from any propositions should be treated as constructions of the mind of the observer, not as clinical data. Validation in the real world is required if at all possible.

Other nurses also may provide a source of general propositions. Through a process of socialization and instruction, nurses share pooled experiences and probability estimates for certain signs and symptoms.

The orientation period for a new clinician provides opportunities for staff to communicate the nature of the client population in both formal and informal ways. New personnel are told—explicitly and implicitly—what cues are important; they are given feedback about their perceptions and socialized into the norms for assessment and diagnosis.

Socialization into a new role influences expectations. In turn, expectations activate categories and systems of propositions for identifying cues and interpreting data. By activating categories in memory and making them more accessible, socialization increases sensitivity to particular cues.

Bieri and colleagues suggest that the type of setting and type of clients influence perceptual sensitivity and cue search (Bieri et al., 1966, pp. 211–212). For example, if an increased heart rate and restlessness were encountered in a psychiatric nursing setting there might be a tendency to search for cues to self-concept or role-relationship problems. In contrast, the same signs in a surgical setting might influence the nurse to check the client's temperature, the dressing, and the perception of pain or discomfort. Would there not be greater sensitivity to parenting cues in pediatric and obstetrical settings than in medical-surgical nursing settings? Are not intensive care nurses highly sensitive to physiological cues? Indeed they should be, when physiological instability is the major factor requiring admission to this type of unit.

Soares has described an aspect of knowledge that is taken for granted in an intensive care unit; this research illustrates that certain norms exist among "inside nurses" (regular staff) and other norms among "outside nurses" (float staff):

> Inside staff nurses have been exposed to the informal rules of interaction within the particular unit, and they have learned the taken-for-granted meanings that are known to the members of the inside group. Since outside nurses do not appear to understand the meanings conveyed in the unit, as seen by the lack of response to action messages, it seems feasible that these messages and meanings are peculiar to this particular unit. (Soares, 1978, p. 203)

The degree to which the lore transmitted by nursing and medical colleagues influences an individual's thinking depends in part on that individual's professional confidence and experience. A high level of personal need to become part of the belief and value system of the group may be expected to facilitate acquisition of group norms. Studies of Tajfel (1969) and Schutz (1966) suggest that a person who is uncertain how to behave in a situation (possibly a new staff member or a new graduate) seeks information that can be used to respond in a "professionally appropriate" manner.

Caution must be exercised in accepting statements such as "Oh, yes, all the old people in this community act like that"; "We don't bother with that here; they're only in this unit for 3 days"; or "Just do a quickie assessment; the clients here are pretty healthy and don't have any problems." The key is to reflect on the expectancies and probabilities of events communicated by colleagues. Treat the information obtained as hypotheses, not facts. The information may contain gems of wisdom or may lead to perpetuation of errors. An "anchoring point" in theory, research, and one's own values is the best protection against unwisely adopting others' points of view.

Textbooks and teachers provide the most common anchoring point for generalizations and likelihood estimates about what occurs when and with what. Yet critical, logical examination of any reference point, including self-constructed propositions and ready-made inferences, is always in order. In this section we have considered research, colleagues, teachers, and books that may be perceived as authoritative. They can be, and generally should be, a source of propositional knowledge to use in deducing the possible meaning of cues. As with all other reference points, caution needs to be exercised. Hypotheses generated should be tested by collecting further information.

5 INTERPRETATION: GENERALIZATIONS FROM INITIAL IMPRESSIONS People, including clinicians, seem to need some overall reference point from which to begin to assess what a particular person or group is like. Why do they want to know? There are two reasons. The idealistic one is that in order to be very helpful one has to know the client as a person (or group) rather than as an object. One observes objects, but one interacts (or transacts) with people. The interpersonal relationship through which diagnostic information is obtained requires understanding of people as people, not assessment of functional patterns in isolation. The second reason is merely the other side of the coin. Realistically, to perform the clinician's role one must have some understanding of the feelings and intentions of the other.

An *initial impression* of a client and his or her general health and situation is formed early in an interaction.[5] It can influence assessment and diagnosis whether or not the nurse is aware of the influence. Therefore it is important to understand how people form initial impressions of others, what peculiarities of

---

[5]The client is probably also picking up an initial impression of the nurse. Frequently, this impression is generalized to all staff and the agency. Clients, like nurses, go beyond the information given to reach inferential conclusions: "She's nice"; "He's a considerate nurse"; "She'll know what to do if something happens."

practice influence impressions, and what suggestions can help one get around biased impressions. It should be noted that the following ideas apply particularly to cues about *personal attributes* and the *social inferences* that result from their interpretation. These are a "backdrop" which can color further assessments, diagnosis, and even intervention.

People learn through experience to make quick inferences about others' abilities, attitudes, interests, physical features, traits, and behavior. Category labels such as wholesome, friendly, cold, or hardworking are used to describe global impressions of people. Value-belief systems "explain" how these personal attributes are related and whether they are to be positively or negatively valued. (What is being described here is a form of implicit theory about personality and social interaction.)

An initial impression is formed when one meets a person or family or enters a community. Functionally, the initial impression or quick social evaluation permits one to choose one's words and behavior in an initial interaction. In addition, but related to the preceding discussion, people may have *general* tendencies to infer social characteristics of others. The extremes are the "Pollyanna syndrome" of extreme optimism and the negative disposition that "people are no darn good." In general, reports of impressions contain more positive than negative descriptors (Jones, 1977). Extreme dispositions to infer are usually modified, at least to some extent, by professional education. They do not disappear entirely, as is evident in studies of clinicians' dispositions toward judgments of maladjustment (Weiss, 1963) and judgments made in clinical assessments (Schmidt and Fonda, 1956). These global tendencies probably color initial impressions.

Nurses' initial impressions most likely are influenced also by the client's health state. If a health problem exists, the medical diagnosis may produce some social judgments as well as other impressions. For example, some conditions may be viewed as simply happening to a person (cancer) and other conditions may be thought of as the person's or family's fault (obesity or a child's growth delay). Impressions can be useful or can lead to erroneous conclusions. If they slip into the data base without validation, diagnostic errors can occur.

6 **SUMMARY** To summarize this section on reference points for inference, it may be said that people, diagnosticians included, interpret ambiguous uncertainty-based information by using both explicit and implicit generalizations. Their interpretations are sometimes colored by what they "know" is true or at least usually true.

Ordinarily people survive quite well on the basis of unexamined and, sometimes, untested inferences. Perception, as Neisser (1978) has said, is self-correcting in the long run. The difficulty in clinical nursing practice is that the "long run" may be too late. Harm or discomfort can occur from interventions that are based on unexamined and untested assumptions. Professionals need to set up a system of checks and balances.

Because at times information is insufficient, imagination fills in. The picture is clarified and gaps are filled. Inferences based on some data and some imagination are usually the fillers. Checks and balances have to be built in to avoid the risk of error; they can be summarized as follows:

1 If at all possible, inferences should be treated as hypotheses to be tested. Validate inferences with the client and recheck inferences about the social or physical environment.

2 The roots of inferences (expectations, assumptions, propositions, dispositions, and impressions) should reflect the likelihood of events in the world so that hypotheses are reasonable. Beware of overgeneralizing from experiences that are not representative. Ask for explanations and be curious so that a self-correcting process is established.

3 The process of inferring from incomplete data and previous knowledge should be checked for logical consistency. Avoid inferential leaps.

4 When inference and imagination are used in diagnosis, get feedback. Obtain this by further observation, follow-up, or colleague review. Always keep in mind the risk of acting with incomplete data. Build in safeguards.

5 Inferences tend to enter the data base used in diagnosis when the data base is incomplete. The more data, the less need for creating information by inference.

IMPORTANCE OF ALTERNATIVE HYPOTHESES

Explanations for cues that immediately "come to mind" are useful but always search memory for alternative hypotheses to explain the data, even when everything appears "obvious." Considering multiple hypotheses increases the chance that the correct diagnosis will be in the pool of hypotheses generated.

One idea for generating multiple diagnostic interpretations of data in a pattern area is to use knowledge stored in memory. Take a behavioral or environmental cue or set of cues, and explain their meaning from three familiar, knowledge frameworks:

1 Physiological framework
2 Psychological framework
3 Sociological framework

For example, consider a client who reports his heart is "jumping." A physiological framework would suggest hypotheses regarding cardiovascular function, such as palpitations associated with excess smoking or caffeine intake. A psychological framework might take into account the possibility of a subjective feeling of fear or anxiety. A sociological framework might suggest that something could have occurred during an interpersonal interaction that generated conflict or anger at a relative. Knowledge stored in memory and available cues lead to inferences; these are converted to hypotheses to guide the search for further cues.

The three areas—physiology, psychology, and sociology—are familiar. Many nurses' memory stores of basic knowledge are organized around the three.

Thus, the frameworks make a usable approach to analysis of information. *The application of different frameworks to clinical data will help the diagnostician overcome a psychological set to categorize data prematurely.* Alternative viewpoints prevent distortion of data by the *first* idea that "comes to mind." *The readiness to interpret information in habitual ways may yield (1) very accurate predictions because one has learned the real probability of events in practice, or (2) errors because one has forgotten that whenever people are involved cues have a degree of uncertainty and there is always an exception to generalizations. Reduce errors by always considering alternative explanations.*

Studies suggest that with previous education in nursing diagnosis nurses can use diagnostic terms (Appendix A) to describe the possibilities they are considering early in the diagnostic process (Craig, 1986; Gordon, 1986). This occurred when only one or two ambiguous diagnostic cues were present (Gordon, 1986). The advantage of this behavior may lie in the subsequent search for cues. For example, if the diagnostician thinks one possible meaning of an initial cue is *decreased self-esteem*, this hypothesis clearly structures further assessment. The search for cues is focused on the evaluation of self-esteem. In contrast a vague hypothesis such as *psychological problem* provides no clear focus for further assessment questions or observations.

There was a high percentage of agreement among the nurses that a particular set of diagnostic hypotheses should be investigated further; but the additional hypotheses they generated to explain initial cues indicated a great deal of variability. The results were similar to that found in "brainstorming" or divergent thinking exercises. Diagnosis commonly associated with the cues were suggested by a high percentage of subjects; the variability appeared in the "creative" alternatives that went beyond the diagnostic cues to less obvious possibilities. In this study of 160 baccalaureate staff nurses the average number of hypotheses generated per task was three (Gordon, 1986).

DETERMINING LIKELY HYPOTHESES

As determination of likely hypotheses is discussed, keep in mind that we are considering the point in assessment when the diagnostician has only a diagnostic cue or cue cluster in a pattern area (as for example when only data indicating restlessness is present) and three or four likely hypotheses have been generated to explain the meaning of the cue(s).

In the previous sections the reader was encouraged to think about all possible diagnoses that would explain a cue or initial cluster of cues. This was because *studies have shown that if the correct hypothesis is not within the pool of hypotheses, diagnostic errors occur* (Ciafrani, 1984, Gale and Marsden, 1983, pp. 111–113). Now the diagnostician has to determine the most likely possibilities for the individual client situation.

Why bother estimating which of the alternative hypotheses are most credible? Why not gather assessment data to test them all? The answer lies in efficiency, time conservation, and cognitive strain. It is more efficient and time saving to eliminate unlikely possibilities; (Of course, one should examine the unlikely possibilities if likely ones must be rejected.) Holding both high- and low-probability hypotheses in memory while collecting and interpreting data can strain cognitive capacities. Errors are the result. The reader may be thinking:

How do you know which of your hypotheses are the most probable explanations for the data?

The likelihood of a given hypothesis is determined by considering the data available in the client situation. These include:

1 Contextual cues such as age or developmental level, gender, culture, previous health history, and medical diagnoses, complications, and treatment. These factors may be used as *predictive cues.*

2 Functional assessment data already collected. For example, if some patterns have already been assessed, the data base may contain cues that can be used to estimate the likelihood of hypotheses generated to explain the data in subsequent patterns.

As you proceed through functional pattern assessment you gradually get a clearer, "individualized picture" of the client from a health perspective. This picture may help you to determine which current diagnostic hypotheses are most probable. *The key to estimating the likelihood of hypotheses is to learn the nursing diagnoses that are of high incidence with particular age or developmental levels, medical diagnoses, and the other factors specified above.* For example, there is a high incidence of social isolation in the frail elderly living alone without family ties or social support; there is also a high incidence of health management deficit in newly diagnosed diabetics with complex medication-exercise-diet regimens. Experts can quickly make associations between predictive cues and the probability of diagnostic hypotheses. Time and mental energy is not wasted investigating unlikely possibilities.

Predictive Hypothesis Testing: Use of Background Data

In some instances early cues point to only one or two hypotheses and these can be tested individually. If this is not the case, predictive hypothesis testing can be used to determine the most likely possibilities. *Predictive hypothesis testing is defined as the simultaneous testing of multiple hypotheses using contextual cues.* The objective is to (1) obtain a lot of information quickly, (2) estimate the probability of the multiple hypotheses in a set, and (3) reduce the number of hypotheses to avoid cognitive strain.

Frequently, the client's medical diagnosis provides a contextual cue to possible dysfunctional patterns. Consider a client who has experienced a cerebrovascular accident (stroke) involving the right side of the brain. Impaired verbal communication related to uncompensated aphasia (difficulty speaking) is less likely than if the left side of the brain was involved. The presence of a second diagnosis, such as cardiac or respiratory disease, serves as contextual data to increase the probability that self-care, mobility, and impaired home management will be present. Age, gender role responsibilities, and other data may make some hypotheses more credible and others less so.

Although not involving nursing diagnoses directly, an example drawn from research findings (Gordon, 1980) should further clarify predictive hypothesis testing. Nurses were given the task of determining whether or not a client was developing any postoperative complications (assessment task). All they were told was (1) that they could have any information they wanted by asking for it and stating why it would be useful, (2) the patient had general surgery, and (3) the list of conditions to be assessed (hypotheses) included thrombophlebitis, wound infection, atelectasis, urinary retention, hemorrhagic shock, and no post-operative complications. At this point which condition(s) do you think is present?

Obviously, if one knows only that the client has had general surgery, one hypothesis is as likely as the other. There are two options: search for cues to each hypothesis, one by one, or pick the most probable and test these first. If the most probable hypotheses can be determined quickly, information collection will be more efficient and less cognitive strain will occur. The information the nurses collected as a result of their first two questions indicated that predictive hypothesis testing was being used (testing multiple hypotheses simultaneously by collecting contextual data). Their first two questions were related to the *time lapse since surgery, and type of surgery performed.* These are historical, con-textual cues. They have nothing to do with the current state of the patient, as would blood pressure or urine output. Even when the nurses were limited to only 12 pieces of information in one of the tasks, these were the first two pieces of information requested. To know whether any surgical complication is present *now,* shouldn't one collect information on the current state of the client? Maybe so, but other information may be important *first.*

How shall we understand the efficiency of these nurses' approach?[6] In their first two questions they found that the patient had had gallbladder surgery and that it was done at "12 noon today" (in the second task, "11 a.m. yesterday").[7] For the experienced clinician this is meaningful information. Using a network of interrelationships stored in memory permits various problem-identification ac-tivities. One can restructure past events or predict future events. For example, *if* the cues *short time lapse since surgery* and *gallbladder surgery* are present, *then* hemorrhagic shock is probable. Or, in the second case, *if* the cues are *15 to 18 hours postsurgery* and *gallbladder surgery, then* atelectasis is highly probable.

The nurses' behavior indicated that they used contextual information to test several hypotheses simultaneously. That is, they used a predictive hypothesis-testing procedure. Contextual information about the client's situation made it

[6]Accuracy was very high when the information was limited and the correct judgment was hem-orrhagic shock. When information was unlimited and the correct judgment was atelectasis, 52 percent were inaccurate; errors were attributed to information overload and other aspects of their strategy (Gordon, 1980).

[7]The current time when they "did the assessment" was known to be between 2 and 5 p.m. Subtraction could be done to find how many hours had elapsed since surgery.

possible to set the probabilities of the surgical complications. By inferring the probability of each complication from the cues, the nurses were able to focus on the most likely ones and still have sufficient questions left to assess the *actual* presence of the complications.

Is this procedure useful only in the area of identifying surgical complications? Probably not. Logically it seems useful in all anticipatory diagnostic situations. The universe of possibilities cannot be tested, so events have to be forecast on the basis of likelihood estimates. Elstein, Schulman, and Sprafka (1978) have found that physicians dealing with uncertainty-based medical diagnoses also begin their task with predictive hypothesis testing.

Predictive Hypothesis Testing: Use of Diagnostic Groupings

When a diagnostic cue only points to a pattern area (e.g., sleep pattern) rather than a specific diagnosis, predictive hypothesis testing can be used. (Scan the groupings of currently identified nursing diagnoses within each pattern area in Appendix C. Each pattern can be used as a "problem space" and the diagnoses within the pattern as a pool of diagnostic hypotheses.) Consider the following example of determining likely hypotheses and then narrowing the possibilities. Before beginning the assessment the nurse has the following background information from the chart and from observation while entering the client's room.

Ms. B. is a 40 year old, alert, single, female executive who looks healthy but appears slightly overweight. Is sitting quietly near her bed. Third admission for gastric ulcer in two years.

At this point there are two cues: *slightly overweight* and *third admission in two years for gastric ulcer.* A health perception-health management problem and a nutritional-metabolic problem are possible. Let us use the diagnoses within the health perception-health management pattern as hypotheses first. They are:

1	Health Management Deficit (Total)	Not relevant
2	Health Management Deficit (specify)	Not relevant
3	Health Maintenance Alteration	Not relevant
4	Noncompliance (specify)	Not relevant
5	Potential Health Management Deficit	Likely
6	Potential Noncompliance	Likely
7	Potential for Infection	Hold; no data to predict
8	Potential for Physical Injury	Unlikely; alert 40 year old
9	Potential for Poisoning	Unlikely; alert 40 year old
10	Potential for Suffocation	Unlikely: alert 40 year old

Do you agree with the ratings in the right column? (Use just the data above.)

The initial data suggests two hypotheses that need to be investigated and one in which there is no data to predict. Some others are not relevant because the conditions cannot be diagnosed on the basis of historical cues and past behavior. Experts can analyze the likelihood of these hypotheses in milliseconds.

Let us begin the assessment of the client's health-perception–health-management pattern with a broad question that provides an introduction to the topic and to the client's viewpoint on her health situation. The first question posed could be: "How has your general health been the last few years?" Or the nurse might say: "I noticed from the doctor's note that you have been having problems with . . . (insert client's report); how has your *general* health been in the last few years?" The client's response provided the following:

Ms. B. has always perceived herself as "healthy;" no colds, infections; was thrown off her bicycle six months ago and now rides only on bicycle paths. "I get plenty of exercise and watch my diet. I don't know why the ulcer keeps acting up." In the last 5 months she gained weight from eating ice cream and drinking a lot of milk for an "acidy stomach;" says she looks "terrible" with the extra weight. Severe abdominal pain unrelieved by milk, cream, or antacids in the last week caused her to visit a physician; she was admitted on the same day due to a low hemoglobin and blood in her stool. She delayed seeking help because of her busy work schedule; stopped taking pills (name of medication not known) shortly after the last episode of bleeding because she felt better. "I guess women have to work twice as hard to succeed." States the doctor is going to try a regimen of "pills and antacids and see how I do for a few days."

Frequently at the beginning of assessment in a pattern area a broad question will produce considerable information on hypotheses. In this instance information decreased the probability of potential for infection and injury. The probability is high for a potential health management deficit (unless we find she has knowledge of medications, symptoms management, and diet). Further information has to be collected to test this hypothesis. She has provided some cues to possible job stress (busy work schedule; work twice as hard), pain management (episodes of severe pain), and body image disturbance (looks "terrible") but these can be noted and followed up during assessment of self-perception–self-concept and role-relationship patterns. Holding multiple hypotheses (ten) in working memory and inferring whether data tend to support or negate each hypothesis can produce cognitive strain. This is short-lived. The payoff is that assessment in this pattern area is now structured by one hypothesis. As will be seen in the next discussion, diagnosticians test the remaining hypotheses one by one, thereby reducing memory and inferential strain to the minimum.

To summarize, when a diagnostic cue or background data suggest a large number of possibilities, simultaneous testing of multiple hypotheses using contextual cues (predictive hypothesis testing) can usually help to determine the most probable hypotheses. This procedure reduces the number held in working memory. A useful approach to hypothesis generation and testing is

1 Use the routine screening questions suggested in Chapter 4. When a *diagnostic cue* is present consider alternative diagnostic hypotheses to explain the data; eliminate those that are unlikely in the *particular* client-situation; test the most likely possibilities first.

2 During assessment of a pattern area, keep in mind background contextual data related to developmental level or age, gender, medical diagnosis and treatment, and any relevant functional pattern data accumulated. Learning the relationship of nursing diagnoses to these data *and* being able to retrieve these associations from memory increases efficiency. Not all of the 70-plus nursing diagnoses have to be thoroughly assessed in every client if high-probability diagnoses can be predicted.

3 If contextual cues predict that the pattern may be dysfunctional, begin assessment in a pattern area with a broad, nondirective question to elicit maximum information on multiple hypotheses (see groupings in Appendix C). For example:

"How has your *general* health been lately?"
"How has your appetite and food intake been lately?"
"Do you find your energy level is sufficient for doing what you want to do or need to do?"
"How are working relationships in your job?"

Use the information to eliminate any unlikely diagnostic hypotheses from the pool.

4 Generating, testing, deleting, revising, and adding diagnostic hypotheses continues throughout functional pattern assessment.

After generating diagnostic hypotheses that would explain the initial cues to a dysfunctional pattern, the most likely hypotheses are tested. This requires branching questions, observations, or both. The end product of hypothesis testing is the statement of a nursing diagnosis.

As previously discussed, hypotheses may be vague or highly specific depending on the information available. Gale and Marsden (1983) refer to these as prediagnostic and diagnostic hypotheses. *Prediagnostic hypotheses* are the vague "educated" or "intuitive" guesses, such as "I think there is a relationship problem," "nutritional problem," or "She's not managing her disease well." If these early hypotheses survive, they become more specific *diagnostic hypotheses* that describe the problem and etiological factors: "weak mother-infant attachment/early separation" or "protein deficit/scarce financial resources." (The novice who is learning to use diagnostic categories may use a manual to translate "nutritional problem" and the assessment data available into specific diagnostic terminology.)

TESTING DIAGNOSTIC HYPOTHESES

Discussion in this section will center on strategies for testing hypotheses and the kind of data that increases confidence in diagnostic judgments. This will bring us to the subject of how to state a nursing diagnosis which will be the subject of the next chapter. Hypothesis testing takes the diagnostician beyond the routine assessment guidelines discussed in Chapter 4. Now questions and observations are focused on the high probability, diagnostic hypotheses under consideration. We are at the point where the most likely hypotheses for explaining an initial diagnostic cue or cluster of cues have been identified. Now the important question is: Does sufficient data exist to support the presence of any of the hypotheses? What is the best diagnostic category to explain the present data? *The answer is determined by a focused search for critical defining characteristics (diagnostic cues) specific to the diagnostic category represented in each hypothesis. Critical diagnostic cues are the signs or symptoms that are usually present if the diagnosis is present.* Cues to the client's health problem do not always match the "textbook picture" (see Chapter 6). Thus, a clinical judgment is required in order to say "This diagnosis best describes the cluster of signs and symptoms present."

Moving from vague "hunches" to specific diagnostic hypotheses during the diagnostic process requires a series of decisions about acquiring, retaining, and utilizing assessment information. The sequential set of decisions is called a *strategy. A diagnostic strategy includes decisions about what information to collect, in what sequence to collect it, and how to use the information* (Bruner et al., 1956, p. 51). Various hypothesis testing strategies can be employed to find out which of the possibilities best describes the client's health problem. The overall objectives of any strategy are efficiency, accuracy, and confidence in the diagnosis attained. To meet these objectives,

1 Know what information would be present if the health problem described by a hypothesis was present.

2 Rely on highly valid and reliable cues so that confidence will be sufficiently high to use the final diagnostic judgment as a basis for planning intervention.

3 Prevent "thinking" errors by controlling cognitive strain during information collection and processing.

This section will answer questions the reader has probably raised from the above description of hypothesis testing strategies:

What strategy shall I use and how do I prevent "thinking" errors?

How do you know what information would be present if a diagnosis was present?

Perhaps the best way to discuss hypothesis testing is through examples. Cues or cue clusters and diagnostic hypotheses will be presented and then we will examine how the hypotheses are tested:

CASE 1: INITIAL DATA

Billy Smith, a premature baby, is 4 weeks old and weighs 6 pounds. He is transferred to a medical center 10 miles from his home for treatment of a congenital defect in his heart. He has progressed well since birth and does not require an incubator at this time. Billy is the third child of 26-year-old parents; the two other children are 3 and 5 years old. During visiting hours the parents stand viewing their baby at the nursery window. Only after the nurse's aide offers do they say they would like to hold their baby. Mrs. Smith holds the baby on her lap with the child facing Mr. Smith. They continue to talk to each other. No inquiries are made about the baby's condition. During the second visit that day the same behavior is repeated. When the baby cries, Mrs. Smith rocks him on her knee.

CASE 1: EARLY HYPOTHESIS GENERATION

Observations and background data contained diagnostic cues. These cues suggested hypotheses that could structure the diagnostic task. The following hypotheses were generated, in an order of most to least likely (see manual for defining characteristics):

Weak parent-infant attachment
Early separation reaction
Fear (attachment to sick infant)
Reactive situational depression
Knowledge deficit (baby care skills)
Postpartum depression

The initial behavioral cues suggested that the parents' attachment to their baby was weak; early separation can produce this condition. On the other hand the baby's cardiac condition may be viewed as life threatening and the parents' reaction might be fear of bonding to an infant that they think is going to die. A reactive situational depression is also plausible, if they think the baby is going to die. The cues may be explained by a postpartum depression but the frequency of this is low. Knowledge deficit (baby care skills) is a possibility but unlikely when the parents have two other children. The major cues of concern are the lack of inquiry regarding the baby's condition and the parent-baby interaction. Lack of inquiry alone may not be significant, as the parents may have consulted with the physician. Yet, when this cue is combined with the interaction cues both gain significance.

CASE 1: DETERMINING THE MOST LIKELY HYPOTHESES

The nurse, in a friendly way, introduces herself and asks the parents how they are managing. The response to this broad question should elicit cues to estimate the likelihood of hypotheses in the set. The cues listed on page 250 would have to be present if the conditions were present (look up defining characteristics of the remaining diagnostic categories in the Manual of Nursing Diagnosis, Gordon, 1986):

Hold in mind the diagnostic hypotheses and use each piece of the following data to estimate their probability (high, medium, low). Consider the response of the parents to the nurse's question and her accepting, attentive manner:

Parents responded (rather hesitantly at first) that they "have this feeling that this is not our baby, but know that it really is"; "it's a strange thing to have these feelings

Hypothesis	Focused cue search	Cues supporting DX
Weak parent-infant attachment	Facial expression, talking to baby, eye contact, kissing, holding position, comforting measures used, inquiries regarding baby's feeding, care, physical condition	Minimal smiling, close contact, enfolding and talking to baby; does not assume "en face" position; low eye-to-eye contact; minimal kissing; continues unsuccessful comforting measures; infrequent inquiries regarding baby's condition.
Early parent-infant separation	Time lapse; postpartum parent-baby interaction; frequency of interaction and caring activities	Separation of baby and parents postpartum or low-frequency contact for holding, cuddling, feeding, caring activities
Reactive situational depression	Mood state; degree of hope; current life situation and perception of situation	Expressed feelings of sadness, hopelessness, or despair; crying; feelings of failure or powerlessness; perception of current situation as crisis, stress, unmanageable

occurring; the baby is cute." (Estimate the probabilities of the previously listed hypotheses with each piece of data; watch how they change or remain the same.)

The nurse asks why they think these feelings are occurring. (She is thinking about weak parent-infant attachment and fear of attachment. If depression exists it probably is a secondary reaction to the other conditions.) The parents respond that the baby was premature and had a heart condition. They couldn't touch or hold the baby "because of the incubator and tubes." Stated that it was "so devastating that they began to visit less frequently." "We had trouble handling the news about the cardiac condition but the doctors say the baby will do fine. . . . Don't know why but sometimes it seems to me (mother) like we are giving our love to the other children and can't seem to have any left for this one." I feel sad about this but really think it will be better now that they let me touch the baby; we really wanted a boy, seeing we had two girls. No mention here of fear of losing the baby (thus, fear of attachment is reduced in probability for the moment). During this interaction Mrs. Smith is holding the baby as described above. The nurse asks her if she is comfortable holding the baby this way and if Mr. Smith wanted to hold the baby. The mother replied: "I didn't even realize how I was holding him; see that's an example of my not feeling close; I know how to hold a baby!" Nurse suggests she let Mr. Smith hold Billy and that she guide him in how to hold the baby.

CASE 1: FORMULATING A WORKING DIAGNOSIS

At this point a diagnostic judgment is to be made. When the problem is as complex as this one, thinking about the diagnostic judgment as a "working diagnosis may be useful." Which of the hypotheses is supported by the data, that is, *which cluster of signs and symptoms from the Manual most closely correspond to the cluster of signs and symptoms collected from questions and observations thus far?* You may wish to write down each hypothesis and underneath list supporting and nonsupporting data. Then see which hypothesis has sufficient support in the data. State your conclusion: the problem and what is contributing to the problem (etiology). Following this, look at footnote 8 at the bottom of the page.[8] Consider another example:

CASE 2: INITIAL DATA

Mr. W. is an alert, 75-year-old, retired teacher who was admitted for removal of rectal polyps. A secondary diagnosis was chronic arthritis. Assessment of his *cognitive-perceptual pattern* revealed: Hearing-aid left ear; perceives whisper with aid. Glasses for reading; checked 1 year ago; reads newsprint. No recent change in memory; keeps pills in kitchen near coffee so he is reminded to take these in the a.m. Reports no difficulty in making decisions; balances check book for his daughter. No reported sensory changes in extremities. Complains of periodic aching pain in left hip joint, especially in the a.m. after arising. Arthritis diagnosed 10 years ago. Pain getting progressively worse in last two years; takes buffered aspirin 4X per day, one tab (not sure of dose). Grimacing noted when arising from sitting to standing position.

CASE 2: EARLY HYPOTHESIS GENERATION

When assessment revealed a diagnostic cue (pain in hip joint), the nurse switched from the routine assessment format of the nursing history to the diagnostic process. The diagnosis of pain is clear. The critical diagnostic criterion that has to be present is: verbal report of pain or pain descriptors. Pain can signify serious conditions. In this case the order of likelihood is:

Arthritic pain
Post-hip fracture
Other bone pathology

Further checking revealed no history of injury to the hip and the physician's examination revealed minimal osteoporosis. The nurse concluded that the pain was associated with the documented medical diagnosis *chronic arthritis*. The

---

[8]The nurse believed she had sufficient data to support the diagnosis of weak parent-infant attachment/early separation reaction.

client's report of periodic pain and its character will be noted in the chart for the physician. Consultation with the physician will be necessary in order to discuss the drug regimen. Having referred the pain cues to the physician, the nurse began to consider how nursing may be able to help this man. From a nursing perspective what would be a useful way of thinking about this problem?

The diagnostic hypothesis that guided further data collection was *chronic pain self-management deficit.* Cues to *chronic pain* were present, but was there a *self-management deficit?* If this condition was present, the following additional cues would have to be present: (1) lack of use of pain management techniques appropriate to type of pain and (2) physical and cognitive ability to manage pain.

CASE 2: HYPOTHESIS TESTING

Further assessment revealed that Mr. W. did not know ways to manage arthritic pain. This information, plus the previous data on his cognitive and physical abilities met the criteria stated above. At this point the nurse had to think about what was contributing to this problem (etiological factors). Those considered were

Arthritis
Insufficient knowledge (management techniques)

In general, focusing on the medical diagnosis as an etiological factor is not useful. Recall that etiological factors are used to plan the definitive *nursing* interventions. What definitive treatment will the nurse provide for arthritis, a medical diagnosis? None; the definitive treatment plan for the pathophysiology of arthritis is within the physician's domain of practice.

CASE 2: FORMULATING A WORKING DIAGNOSIS

For now, the nurse decided to formulate the diagnosis as *chronic pain self-management deficit/insufficient knowledge (management techniques).* She then continued her admission assessment. When the assessment was completed she began to review the dysfunctional patterns that she had diagnosed. This is a step that must not be missed. During a final review of findings, judgments will be made in regard to interrelationships among problems. Earlier in the assessment, the nurse had diagnosed impaired mobility on the basis of Mr. W.'s report (1) that he did not walk much any more (maybe once a week) because of the progressively increasing joint pain and (2) the presence of some limitation in range of motion (15 degrees right hip; 25 degrees left hip). The nurse reasoned that if he could be helped to manage his pain (by drugs and other techniques), this would improve his mobility. Then he could be started on an exercise program and daily walks which would improve his general health and feeling of well-being. These thoughts led her to revise her diagnosis. The nursing diagnosis was formulated as *impaired mobility (level II)/chronic pain self-management deficit.* The treatment plan was focused on the *chronic pain self-management deficit.* The daily evaluation focused on the problem *impaired mobility.* Two additional points need to be discussed in regard to the formulation of Mr. W.'s problem. First, the nurse could have missed the interrelationship between the activity-exercise and cognitive-perceptual dysfunctional patterns *if final review of data and diagnoses was not done.* Second, note that *two of the diagnostic categories listed in Appendix A were used to describe the problem.*

DIAGNOSTIC STRATEGIES

Having discussed hypothesis generation and testing as the "route" to formulating nursing diagnoses, let us now consider two strategies that were mentioned during the discussion: multiple and single hypothesis testing. The terms mean that either a single diagnostic hypothesis is tested, such as sleep onset disturbance, or multiple hypotheses are tested simultaneously, such as sleep onset disturbance, early awakening pattern, sleep pattern reversal, and other disturbances. These two major hypothesis testing strategies, identified originally by Bruner and his colleagues (1956), influence

1 *Information intake.* This refers to the amount of information that is obtained from a question or observation. If three hypotheses are being tested simultaneously and the diagnostician uses the information in evaluating the three hypotheses, then the information *value* is tripled. If only one hypothesis is being tested, the information intake is one bit.

2 *Cognitive strain.* The major cognitive processes involved in diagnosis are memory and inference (retrieval of knowledge from memory, holding new and retrieved information in working memory, and deductive and inductive inference). Memory and inference requirements are greater when multiple hypotheses are tested with each question or observation. Thus, the cognitive strain is greater.

3 *Risk regulation.* Strategies can control the risk of (*a*) not getting sufficient information to make a diagnosis with confidence and (*b*) errors in processing because of overwhelming the cognitive capacity of the diagnostician.

Multiple Hypothesis Testing

The multiple hypothesis testing procedure is useful if (1) a number of hypotheses (possibilities) have been generated, such as occurs early in assessment of a pattern area or (2) diagnoses represented in the hypotheses share the same cue but different values. A clinically significant change in blood pressure, for example, is a critical cue in hypertension and hemorrhagic shock. The value for blood pressure is elevated in hypertension but considerably reduced in shock.

Cognitive requirements are high when multiple hypotheses are tested simultaneously. This is because the number of hypotheses to which information has to be related increases. Inductive and deductive inferences are required to relate the cues obtained to each hypothesis being tested and to increase or decrease hypothesis probabilities as a result of the information obtained. Yet, unlikely diagnoses are eliminated and the memory and inferential strain is reduced quickly.

Cognitive strain can occur if memory and inferential requirements exceed the diagnostician's capacity. Strain on cognitive capacities is manifested by forgetting information and by inferential errors. One reason for cognitive strain is prolonged holding of a large initial pool of hypotheses because of poor selection of predictive cues. To identify highly probable diagnostic hypotheses quickly requires clinical knowledge of predictors and optimal decisions about the sequence of information collection.

A second, but related, reason for cognitive strain is prolonged multiple testing of hypotheses. Highly valid predictors may have been collected but the diagnostician attempts to further reduce uncertainty. Usually the continued search for predictive cues is due to a lack of understanding of the probabilistic nature of clinical information. Recognize that uncertainty in prediction cannot be totally eliminated. Rely on good predictive cues and begin to test likely diagnostic hypotheses; one can always return to the unlikely possibilities if necessary.

Multiple hypothesis testing can be expected to decrease or be absent after (1) the most probable diagnoses to explain a dysfunctional pattern have been identified and (2) values of defining characteristics shared by two or more diagnoses have been obtained. After possibilities are generated and an estimate of the probability of each hypothesis is made, a decided shift in procedure is required (Gordon, 1972, 1980). Thereafter, the data sought are specific to the remaining hypotheses and each is tested, one by one.

Collecting information that differentiates among the remaining hypotheses requires a search for diagnostic cues. These are the critical cues that define and differentiate among diagnoses. Single hypothesis testing is appropriate at this point.

Single Hypothesis Testing

A *single-hypothesis–testing procedure* involves assessing a client or situation to test one hypothesis at a time. This is a reasonable approach when critical, differentiating cues apply to only one diagnosis. Moreover, if only one or two hypotheses remain, they can be tested one by one. The main advantage of testing hypotheses one by one is that *memory strain* and *inferential strain* are not increased over the basal level. This ease is welcomed if the generation of hypotheses, predictive testing, and testing of overlapping cues were prolonged early in the assessment of the pattern area. Another advantage is that the potential for forgetting or inferential errors is low when only a few hypotheses exist. The use of cues to test single hypotheses one by one ensures accuracy. No risk is taken, because *all* hypotheses in the set are tested. For this reason, confidence in the results of assessment should be high.

To use single hypothesis testing exclusively throughout the entire admission assessment would be an inefficient diagnostic strategy. Maximum information is not obtained from each question with this procedure. If only one hypothesis is generated and tested at a time, information relevant to other possibilities is lost. On the other hand, the information could be held in memory; but this approach removes one of the major advantages of this procedure, which is low memory strain.

Single testing is a costly procedure if used exclusively. It increases total time for assessment. In addition it would require repetitious questioning and observation, which would create the impression of disorganization. Yet when memory and inferential strain are high and when time and resources for testing are unlimited, this procedure is useful. If the assessment situation is problem focused, as occurs after diagnoses are established, the procedure is certainly ideal. The successive investigation of single hypotheses is a "safe but slow" way of proceeding (Bruner et al., 1956).

The major shift to a single-hypothesis–testing procedure within a strategy appears to occur when the diagnostician is confident (for the moment) that the most probable tentative diagnoses have been identified. Consider an example. The sleep-rest pattern of a 40-year-old client is being assessed. A question has been posed and the client has responded that she has not been sleeping too well. This cue indicates a sleep pattern disturbance; a diagnostic strategy for investigating the cue is needed. The change to a dysfunctional pattern occurred about 2 weeks before hospital admission. Background information and the pattern areas already assessed suggest one etiological cue: This client has realistic health concerns; about 2 weeks ago she was told she may have cancer.

The diagnostic hypotheses generated were (1) sleep onset disturbance, (2) sleep pattern disturbance—early awakening, (3) sleep pattern interruption, and (4) sleep pattern reversal. Interventions for these four are different; thus it is important to identify which is the problem. The only causal hypothesis at the moment is broad and vague: health concerns—cancer.

A cue to predict the probabilities of the multiple hypotheses generated was sought. The client was asked for a specific description of her sleep pattern. Simultaneous testing of the four diagnostic hypotheses revealed that sleep onset disturbance and early awakening disturbance were most likely. Data about the hours she was sleeping did not support either hypothesis 3 or 4. The client sleeps 3–4 hours per night. The etiological hypothesis (concern about having cancer) and two of the four hypotheses about the problem remain at this point. A focused single hypothesis-testing procedure is appropriate. Sleep onset disturbance and early awakening disturbance are the diagnoses still under consideration. Now the critical differentiating cues must be obtained. Early awakening decreases in probability when the nurse asks a clarifying question: The client says the reason she awakens early is that the whole household always retires at 10 p.m. and arises at 5 a.m. The next question asked is designed to elicit data to support or reject the remaining diagnostic possibility, sleep onset disturbance.

What type of data should be collected to test this single hypothesis?

The cues diagnostic of a sleep onset disturbance are: (1) perception of difficulty falling asleep, (2) a 15-minute or longer sleep delay after attempts to go to sleep, and (3) consecutive episodes of delayed sleep onset (Schwartz and Aaron, 1979, p. 27). Knowing this, the nurse can formulate questions to elicit the pertinent data. As previously discussed, measures of client characteristics must be reliable and valid. Which of the following would elicit the most reliable and valid data:

1 When you have difficulty getting to sleep, how many minutes would you estimate it takes to fall asleep? Does this occur frequently?

2 When you have difficulty getting to sleep, how long do you lie awake? Is this every night?

The first option focuses in on the data needed, whereas the second is less specific—the client could respond, "A long time." A time-consuming second question would then have to be asked. Moreover, the question about consecutive episodes is leading the client to a particular response in the second option. As experience is gained in formulating good questions, the time required for assessment decreases. In this case, the client responded that most nights it takes 3 or 4 hours to fall deeply asleep. The diagnostic hypothesis of sleep onset disturbance is supported. Now the probable cause of this sleep problem has to be determined.

In summary, hypothesis testing procedures differ from hypothesis generation procedures. This appears to be the case in both actual and potential problem identification as well as in identification of etiological factors. After likely diagnoses have been identified, procedures within a strategy shift. The most probable diagnostic hypotheses become the bases for a focused cue search. Unless diagnostic cues overlap (have differing values that distinguish one diagnosis from another), the procedure of choice is to investigate the remaining hypotheses one by one.

A single-hypothesis-testing procedure is useful when only a few hypotheses are being considered or when there are no overlapping cues. The type of data sought is specific to each diagnostic hypothesis. These data are the diagnostic cues that constitute the critical defining signs and symptoms of each nursing diagnosis. Without the presence of these specific cues, the diagnostic category name should not be used. (As previously stated work is in progress to identify critical signs and symptoms.) Critical diagnostic cues are usually few in number and differentiate one diagnosis from another. Supporting data may also be sought. Supporting data influence confidence in a diagnosis when cues are uncertainty-based or available measures are only partially reliable.

Summary: Interpretation of Data and Initial Clustering

This section was concerned with the interpretation of data and their initial clustering. Although the focus was on nursing diagnoses, the diagnostic process is also applicable in the collaborative realm of nursing practice. Tentative diagnostic judgments for purposes of referral, such as diabetic ketoacidosis, heart failure, extension of a blood clot in the brain, or wound infection, are made in the same way. The difference lies in the specificity with which the problem and etiological factors are identified. With nursing diagnoses, specificity is required as a treatment plan has to be developed. With referral, the physician has responsibility for exact diagnosis and treatment.

It was stressed in this section that meaning does not come with clinical data but has to be derived through analysis and interpretation of the data by a clinician. After any needed clarification and verification, the diagnostic work begins. Cues are evaluated against norms, simple inferences are made, and selective, focused attention is paid to diagnostic cues. Sometimes a diagnostic cue is clear and points to only one or two health problems (nursing diagnoses). At other times, deriving the possible diagnostic meaning (hypotheses) of a cue requires cognitive work. Some helpful hints were given for generating possible diagnostic hypotheses that might explain the initial cues and give some structure to the diagnostic task. These included the use of pattern areas, pattern assessment sequence, client's viewpoint, and expectancies derived from contextual information, and related knowledge stored in memory.

In a typical history and examination the nurse is presented with hundreds of elementary findings. It is impossible for any human being to process this amount of information at one time. The objective is to reduce the information by combining interrelated cues in a cluster (chunking) under a set of tentative hypotheses that gives them meaning. After considering background data and initial data, some diagnostic hypotheses will be eliminated from the mental list of possibilities. This further reduces the information that has to be held in working memory while hypotheses are tested.

Cue clusters differ from diagnoses. Only a few, initial cues comprise the patterns that are recognized in tentative diagnostic hypotheses. Hypotheses about diagnostic meaning of cues are created in the mind of the clinician to structure the search for cues. It is when they are tested by further information collection that their validity is revealed. Always be conscious of the fact that we *create* diagnostic hypotheses and, subsequently nursing diagnoses; only the human behaviors upon which they are based are close to reality. Keeping this in mind will increase the chance that *hypotheses or diagnoses that have no support will be modified or discarded.*

Some checkpoints for hypothesis generation and testing can be outlined as follows (specific guidelines are found in the discussion):[9]

1 Have I clarified and verified information as necessary so that I understand the client's reports and have confidence in my observations?

2 Have I paid attention to diagnostic cues in the data?

3 Have I interpreted what client reports mean or signify? Norms? In the context of other data?

4 Have I considered alternative explanations for the cues? Eliminated those not applicable in this client situation?

---

[9]If just beginning to learn nursing diagnosis, the reader may wish to photocopy these checkpoints and refer to them before recording nursing diagnoses on the chart and Kardex.

5 Have I recalled all the critical, diagnostic characteristics for the hypotheses I am testing and assessed for these characteristics? (See Manual of Nursing Diagnoses; Gordon, 1986.)

6 In my best (unbiased) judgment, do I have sufficient data to support the diagnostic hypothesis that I am about to formulate as a nursing diagnosis?

INFORMATION CLUSTERING

Hypotheses permit cues to be related and clustered as they are collected. This clustering process goes on in short-term, or working, memory. Simultaneously, data under each pattern area are recorded on paper. Going from no information to a well-supported diagnosis is not always a smooth process. Inconsistencies and conflicts in the data are sometimes observed. How to resolve these, and the process of weighting information to make judgments, will be topics considered in the next section.

During hypothesis testing, cues are clustered. To do this, one must make decisions about how information is to be combined. Does *this* cue support a possible diagnosis? Does *that* cue suggest the problem is not present? Frequently these are not simple judgments to make. Inconsistencies among cues have to be resolved. In discussion of information clustering it will be seen that one cue can influence the interpretation of other cues in the cluster and that some cues influence judgment more than others. Like collecting and interpreting information and naming, information clustering is continuous throughout the process of nursing diagnosis.

This section will discuss how to resolve inconsistencies and conflicts in data as the data accumulate. Weighting of clinical cues in making diagnostic judgments will also be discussed. *Weighting* refers to the power of a cue to influence judgment. The respective weight given a cue by a diagnostician influences which information gets clustered under a diagnostic hypothesis and which information is discounted as not useful.

Resolving Inconsistencies

Previous information, irrespective of its source, sets up expectations for new information. Expectations are based on the nurse's past knowledge and experience or previous data from the client. When new information conflicts with expectations, one becomes aware of inconsistency. To inquisitive clinicians, such inconsistency creates a dilemma. They know that ignoring inconsistencies increases the risk of diagnostic error and can also result in harm to the client. Attention has to be paid to resolving the dilemma. Through expectations we "know" how things *should* appear, come about, or be related. Inconsistencies represent an inability to fit data together. To recognize inconsistencies, first a comparison is made between what was expected and what has been observed. Then the nurse reasons deductively using "If . . . then . . ." statements. For example, *if* a client reports not eating much, *then* obesity should not be present.

When "things don't turn out as they should" the question of why arises. Resolution of inconsistencies must take into account possible sources for the apparent conflict: measurement error, expectations, and conflicting or unreliable reports.

Inconsistencies Caused by Measurement Error   When inconsistencies arise, a measurement error should be considered. During a nursing history, verbal reports of the client can be misunderstood. At times this occurs because of inattentive listening. Misunderstanding can also result from lack of clarity in a client's communication. If there is any doubt as to whether a client's statement was heard correctly, the client should be asked to validate or repeat the information. Care must be exercised to explain the reason for the repetition, because rephrasing or requesting repetition is also a technique for confronting a person or focusing attention on statements.

During examination of a client, measurement errors can produce apparent inconsistencies. Observations should be repeated if doubt exists. Instruments, for example, sphygmomanometers, should be checked, as well as the technique used to obtain the blood pressure measurement.

Inconsistencies Caused by Expectations   What appear to be inconsistencies in data may be merely a nurse's incorrect expectations. Inadequate knowledge or inexperience can produce faulty expectations. In addition, expectations are based on interpretations; thus errors in previous or current reasoning may be the basis for apparent inconsistencies. Sometimes an understanding of the client's personal intentions, values, or beliefs provides a logical interpretation of the client's behavior and resolves what had seemed to be inconsistencies in the data. This is in contrast to viewing behavioral data from one's own inferences and perspective.

Inconsistencies Caused by Conflicting Reports   Clients' and families' verbal reports may conflict. This produces apparent inconsistencies among various people's reports. Or the same person may give inconsistent reports at different times.

It is not uncommon for conflicting or contradictory reports to be given by a client and family member, by different members of a family, or by different groups within a community. The question arises, Whose information is to be taken into account and whose discounted? A number of hypotheses can be raised. Do biases or cognitive deficits explain the conflicting reports? Is it a matter of different perspectives, such as objective (others') versus subjective (client's) points of view?

Resolving conflicting reports requires caution and tact. The strategy has to be well thought through. Direct confrontation may serve only to induce guilt or defensiveness. If conflicting reports are discussed only with one party, interpersonal conflict between the two parties could arise later when they become aware of differing reports. In some instances it may be wise to discuss the differences in perceptions with both parties together. A major factor in the decision is the current mental or physical health of the people involved.

Conflicts may also be apparent when a client's previous and current verbal reports differ. For example, a client may report an event or set of symptoms that is not consistent with the report the client gave to another health care provider or at another time. Temporary memory lapse, the interpersonal milieu in which the client felt the need to report things differently, or the way questions were formulated may explain the conflict in data. The client can be asked in a gentle manner about the apparent inconsistency.

Inconsistencies Caused by Unreliable Reports   A client's verbal reports during a nursing history may be judged unreliable. Extreme caution must be exercised in making this judgment if errors are to be avoided, because information considered to be unreliable will be discounted and therefore given minimal weight in diagnostic judgments. Assumed incompetency is one reason verbal reports are judged unreliable. The presence of cognitive or sensory deficits can suggest to the care provider that verbal reports should be used cautiously. Yet errors can result if a client's reliability has been incorrectly assessed. For example, many times elderly clients are stereotyped as incompetent or cognitively deficient because they look old, whereas in fact no deficit may exist.

A well-publicized case of psychiatric stereotyping was reported by Rosenhan (1973); it dealt with "being sane in insane places." Behavior of a group of persons was interpreted as manifesting psychosis because psychotic behavior was what was expected in the setting, a psychiatric hospital.

Concluding that information is biased is a second reason for discounting it as unreliable. Situations can occur wherein clients or family members consciously or unconsciously provide biased reports. For example, a strong motivation, and perhaps a realistic need, to leave the hospital may influence a client to bias reports of his or her health state. Moreover, family members may overemphasize or underemphasize certain symptoms because of basic anxieties or needs. These situations are usually easily recognized because the reported information is inconsistent with other observations. The nurse needs to focus on discovering the underlying problem.

A third reason that some observers discount information as unreliable is their prior classification of the character, or personality type, of a client or relative. Consider the following client classifications: drug addict, alcoholic, hospitalized prisoner, hypochondriac, malingerer, sociopath. These negatively valued client classifications may predispose health care providers to question clients' verbal reports and can lead to very serious error.

Reasonable and respectful consideration should be given to any client report without discrimination on the basis of character stereotypes. Health care providers may infer that five instances of complaint without a basis predict that the sixth complaint is of the same type. Sometimes this is the instance when the appendix ruptures or the client acts in desperation.

Resolving, as opposed to ignoring, inconsistencies decreases the risk of error. Awareness of inconsistencies prevents fitting the data to hypotheses. Rather, hypotheses should be generated to fit the data actually present.

Weighting Cues in Judgment

Much research and rhetoric has occurred in order to explain how clinicians put information together. Do they add one cue to another, or are cues weighted? Some resolve this controversy by demonstrating that clinicians can do either (Anderson, 1972; Elstein, 1976).

When cues are added together to make a diagnostic judgment (Dx) the procedure is merely $a + b + c + d = Dx$. The whole (Dx) is merely a sum. For example, the following cues could be added together:

1 Two-centimeter-wide break in skin over coccyx
2 Demarcated border
3 White and glossy lesion
4 Minimal depth
5 Redness at borders and in adjacent skin
6 History of long periods of lying on back
7 Verbalized pain and discomfort
8 Left-sided paralysis

The problem would be decubitus ulcer. (Etiological factors will be ignored for the moment.) Do you think all pieces of information should be weighted exactly the same? In the above list, are some cues not as important for *diagnosis* as others?

The highest weighting would be given to *two-centimeter-wide break in skin over coccyx.* This is an ulcer. The term *decubitus* refers to lying down; the cue *history of long periods of lying on back* should be given weight equal to the skin break in diagnosis of a decubitus ulcer. *White and glossy lesion, minimal depth,* and *red at borders and in adjacent skin* are cues to severity (grading) of the lesion. They permit a finer discrimination and would be of equal value in judging severity. The cue, *demarcated border* would be weighted and valued lower; it is not as influential in judgment. *Verbalized pain and discomfort* is of low diagnostic value; it supports the observation, but the diagnostic judgment could be made without it. The verbal cue would not be available if the patient was comatose. (Actually, this cue points to another problem, that of pain management.)

Consider another example in which the judgment is not as clear. The setting is a community clinic. The client is being treated for hypertension. These cues are present:

1 Tense posture
2 Flat, low tone; slowed speech; dull, depressed facial expression
3 Lost job (company closed plant)
4 Depressed thoughts but no thought of suicide

 5 Perceived himself as self-made success in past
 6 Perceives self as self-made failure now
 7 Wife is poorly controlled diabetic
 8 Cannot discuss problems with friends: "They would think I was a failure."
 9 Does not know what to do: "The job market is so bad"; "I just sit all day";
This never happened to me before."

Considering the above cues, which of the following is the best diagnostic judgment?

- Self-concept disturbance/role change
- Ineffective coping/role change
- Potential for suicide
- Situational depression/role change

The selection of self-concept disturbance/role change suggests that cues 5 and 6 were weighted most heavily in judgment. Cues 8 and 9 may have been most impressive to some readers, who would then have chosen ineffective coping/role change. Cues 2, 4, 7, and 9 may have been most influential, thus leading to the conclusion that situational depression/role change was present. Selecting potential for suicide suggests that the reader discounted the cue *but no thought of suicide;* this verbal report must have been weighted very low or considered unreliable as a predictor.

Now let us see whether adding two other cues can influence judgment. One is a situational cue and the other is historical information. The clinic is a community mental health clinic and the client has a history of suicide attempts. Did these additional cues influence your weighting of previous cues?

The example demonstrates that different people can be influenced differently by information. This is especially true when data are uncertain, as clinical data are. Second, the example suggests that pieces of information are not always judged independently of one another. One cue can influence the weighting of another. Weighting and clustering information differently is probably the reason experts may differ in their diagnoses.

A third point demonstrated was that information can be discounted in making a diagnostic judgment. Care providers make an estimate of the quality of information. Their estimates can be affected by other information or inferences about the client and situation.

Case Example

The following case will illustrate topics in this chapter and the diagnostic process used in problem formulation. The setting is a hospital. As you read the *nursing* assessment and take notes, attempt to cluster the cues that signify actual or potential health problems.

Before making this assessment the nurse had background information from the physician's history and physical examination. The client, Mr. K., had a 5-

year history of "slightly elevated blood pressure." *One year ago* he had experienced an episode of dizziness for 12 hours. *At that time* he started taking medication for his blood pressure. *Six months ago* he had discontinued medication when he felt better. In the *last 6 months* before his admission, two other episodes of dizziness occurred, lasting 1 to 2 hours and being relieved by rest. Frequent headaches were also reported.

Mr. K's father, now deceased, had had diabetes and hypertension. The client's mother, who died one year ago of a stroke, had also had hypertension. His wife and two children (14 and 10 years old) are well.

An episode of dizziness and numbness of his left arm brought Mr. K to the emergency room. The physician described him as a 55-year-old obese Caucasian male who was head of a Spanish center in a large southern city. The medical diagnosis at admission was hypertension and transient ischemic attack. This diagnosis and his family history placed Mr. K at risk for a stroke.

When the nurse began the nursing history and assessment, Mr. K's dizziness and numbness had gone. The background information suggested the possibility of problems in his health-perception–health-management pattern. The following assessment data were collected; the main diagnostic hypotheses the nurse raised while doing the assessment are added in italics.

NURSING HISTORY AND EXAMINATION

First hospital admission of 55-year-old married, obese, white male administrator of a Spanish center. Sitting upright in bed, tense posture and expression (*fear; obesity*).

Health-perception–health-management pattern Viewed health as good until 1 year ago when diagnosed as "having high blood pressure." States job "stressful" "but the people need me" (*job stress*). Had headaches for last 6 months and two episodes of dizziness (one at work and one at home) lasting about 2 hours. Rested and symptoms went away. Delayed seeking care because was "too busy" (*job stress*). Thought dizziness was caused by "overwork," not blood pressure (*job stress*). Discontinued blood pressure medication and M.D. visits about 6 months ago "when blood pressure came down and I felt better"; states medicine caused impotence (*potential noncompliance/disease management*). To emergency room today because of left arm numbness and fear of stroke. Mother died of "stroke" 15 months ago. Concerned that he hasn't been taking care of himself; states, "I need to learn about what to do." Wants to know "everything" (*fear of stroke or death*). Asked if OK to do some job-related paper work if someone brought it in (*job stress*). Takes no medicines currently except Alka-Seltzer and laxative; doesn't smoke; social drinking.

During introductions and while stating the purpose of the interview, the nurse's first impression was of a person in fear. Mr. K was sitting upright in bed; his posture and facial expression were tense. It was inferred that he had been very frightened by the loss of feeling in his arm. Was he interpreting his symptoms in the context of his past experience (mother's stroke and death)? The hypothesis of fear influenced the conduct of the interview. It was important to establish trust in care providers and to provide some reassurance.

The hypothesis of obesity was also generated from the initial impression. The nurse planned to follow up this topic when nutritional and activity patterns were assessed.

Review of the client's health-perception pattern indicated a change. He had thought his health was good until 1 year ago, when high blood pressure was diagnosed. Although blood pressure had been "slightly elevated" for 5 years, the change in health perception had probably occurred with the first episode of dizziness and start of medication. This was also about the time of his mother's death.

Six months after beginning treatment, Mr. K perceived that his "blood pressure came down" and he "felt better." Sexual impotence had occurred (impotence is common with certain blood pressure medications) and he discontinued medication and medical care. Further symptoms occurred and the client's action was to rest. This action was consistent with his previous interpretation of the cause of symptoms, "overwork" and being "too busy." There seems to have been delay in seeking health care, but today the loss of sensation in his arm could not be ignored.

Previously there may have been denial of change in health state or vulnerability. In addition the client may not have had knowledge to interpret the physical signs. What should the present data suggest to a nurse? One, the present symptoms have had an impact. Two, the client wants to "learn what to do." Yet knowledge deficit may not be the only reason for his past behavior.

The tentative diagnostic hypothesis, potential noncompliance, served to cluster early cues and inferences—past history of not attending to symptoms, discontinuation of medication and care, misinterpretation of symptoms, and possible conflict between his health management and work-related activities. Knowledge deficit may be *one* risk factor, but the cue of "too busy" suggests motivational or time-management factors. The need to "learn what to do" is suggestive; yet readiness for learning and actual knowledge deficiencies need further assessment. Moreover, the client does not yet have medical recommendations for future care, so teaching about self-care in compliance with the medical regimen will have to be deferred.

Mr. K's asking whether he may do job-related paper work could have meaning. Does he need to take his mind off his concerns, need diversion, have guilt about being away from his responsibilities, or need to maintain the self-perception of being well enough to do work?

"Wants to know everything" was tentatively interpreted as either fear, need for control, or motivation toward better health management. This and the cues to dysfunctional patterns cited previously were underlined during note taking for follow-up as other patterns were assessed.

The nurse suggested to Mr. K that he seemed to want and need more information to help him plan how he could take care of himself. Then a smooth transition was made to the next area discussed which was his nutritional-metabolic pattern.

> *Nutritional-metabolic pattern* Mr. K's diet history revealed adequate protein, excess carbohydrate and fat, minimal high-roughage foods (fruits and vegetables), approximately 3 cups of coffee per day, but a fluid intake of 700–800 ml/day (*constipation pattern*). No history of lesions in mouth corners or mucous membranes. Has gained weight gradually last 15 years (*exogenous obesity*); dieting unsuccessful; problem is "probably the stress of my job; I get home and eat a big supper and snacks in the evening"; no food dislikes (*caloric excess*). Takes lunch (sandwich and cake) to work and eats at desk. Restaurants in area not good. Some indigestion and heartburn after lunch attributed to days with multiple stressors (*job stress*); takes Alka-Seltzer.

At this point the nurse reevaluated Mr. K's emotional state. He had begun to relax his body and facial muscles.

Unsuccessful dieting, excessive intake of carbohydrate and fat, "big supper and snacks," minimal high-roughage foods, report of gradual weight gain last 15 years, and the absence of an endocrine disease (medical assessment data) suggested that probable cause of obesity was caloric intake. Intake of both fluid and high-roughage food was low. These cues will have to be followed up when Mr. K's elimination pattern is assessed. The cues "days with multiple problems" and "stress of job" supported the previous hypothesis of job stress. This stress will have to be further assessed. It is influencing hypertension management and the client's nutritional pattern. The nurse then assessed the elimination pattern.

> *Elimination pattern* Daily bowel movement pattern with 2 or 3 episodes per month of constipation (hard stools and straining) lasting 2 days; laxatives used when constipation occurs (*intermittent constipation pattern/dietary habits*). Attributes constipation to his diet; knows he should eat better.

The data about this pattern supported the hypothesis of intermittent constipation pattern. Was the constipation related to dietary habits (low fluid intake, minimal high-roughage foods) previously reported? Job stress may be a contributing factor. In this pattern there is again evidence of health-management deficit. A picture of conflict between health practices and work "responsibilities" seems to be emerging.

> *Activity-exercise pattern* Spectator sports, uses car, minimal walking due to time schedule, sedentary job, considers self too old for exercise. Increasing fatigue last few weeks, less energy during the 2 months before admission; no self-care deficit (*decreased activity tolerance* and *knowledge deficit: age-exercise*). Recreation consists of reading novels, watching TV, dining with other couples. Lives in first floor apartment in city and drives 3/4 mile to work (*exogenous obesity/caloric intake–energy expenditure imbalance*).

Activities (work and leisure) suggested a sedentary pattern with minimal exercise. The perception of having less energy was not attributable to anemia (laboratory tests) or heart failure (physician's examination). Yet the perceptions of fatigue and less energy were real; the hypothesis was descriptive of the functional problem, decreased activity tolerance. Again, there was further indication that a busy schedule was conflicting with health management. Knowledge deficit existed regarding age and exercise. Also, note the revision of the hypothesis about obesity; information from two pattern areas was clustered and exogenous obesity/caloric intake–energy expenditure imbalance was formulated.

Sleep pattern Averages 4 to 6 hours of sleep per night, quiet atmosphere, own room with wife, double bed, uses bed board. Presleep activities include watching TV or completing paper work from job; difficulty with sleep onset 1 month; awakens many mornings thinking about job-related problems (*sleep pattern disturbance/presleep activities; job stress*).

A sleep pattern existed. This may have been contributing to the increasing fatigue. A probable cause lay in the presleep activity (paper work from job). Comments about awakening with thoughts of job-related problems supported the nurse's supposition that job stress was an influential factor for this client. Cues were clustered under this etiological hypothesis.

Cognitive-perceptual pattern Sight corrected with glasses, changed 1 year ago; no change in hearing, taste, smell. No perceived change in memory; "I couldn't take it if I started losing my mind, like with a stroke" (*fear of stroke*). Learning ability: sees self as somewhat slower than in college, alert manner, grasps questions easily. Takes no sedatives, tranquilizers, other drugs. No headache at present.

Again during discussion of this pattern there was mention of stroke. Fear (stroke) was further supported.

Self-perception–self-concept pattern Sees self as needing to do things well (job, father role, husband role); "Sometimes I don't think I'm doing well with my family, having them live in this area, but in my job you have to be near when people need help" (*role conflict*). "It will be just great [sarcasm] if I get sick and they have to take care of me instead of me taking care of them" (*fear of dependency*).

Conflict between sense of responsibility to family and to job seemed to be present. Now he will have three responsibilities to balance: family, job, and responsibility to self (health). Fear (stroke) was changed to fear (dependency). The cue "just great if I get sick and they have to take care of me . . ." influenced this modification.

Role-relationship pattern Describes family as happy and understanding of his job commitments; wife former social worker; "kids good." "But I know we'll have trouble as Joe [10 years old] gets older"; "Maybe I should move out of [lower socioeconomic neighborhood]"; 10-year-old assaulted 4 months ago; 14-year-old boy interested in sports and "keeps out of trouble, so far" (*family concerns*). Family usually "sits down together" to handle problems. Social relationships confined to "a few other couples"; finds this sufficient. Job demanding 9 to 10 hours per day; "always trying to get money to keep the center solvent" (*job stress*). Assistant taking over while in hospital. Enjoys job and helping people; coworkers are "good to work with." Wife states the two of them are close; worried about husband's health; states he is more concerned with other people than himself; she admires him for this. Wife able to handle home responsibilities during hospitalization. States she and children had physical exam recently; no health problems; no elevation in blood pressure.

The family relationships elicited were positive and supportive. Concern and indecision were voiced regarding the environment (assault, "know we'll have trouble," and "maybe I should move"). The neighborhood environment could be a source of worry and stress in addition to the job problems (center's financial solvency).

A picture of his work was emerging: indigestion and heartburn on "days with multiple problems"; "stress of job"; "job was cause of high blood pressure"; "too busy"; "overwork"; wants to do job-related paper work in hospital; sedentary job; awakens thinking of job-related problems; financial solvency; presleep activities sometimes job-related; and job demands 9 to 10 hours per day. These data were clustered as job stress. Is he saying that although his work is stressful he enjoys it and his coworkers?

Concern expressed by Mr. K's wife was expected under the circumstances. She and the children were managing, so at present there was no evidence of family coping problems. How did her comment about the client's concern for others fit into the picture? Is this a value that the client and his wife hold?

Sexual-reproductive pattern Two children; states impotent when on BP medication. When BP "went down," stopped meds; potency returned (*potential noncompliance*). No problems perceived in sexual relationship.

These data generated no new hypotheses. The information about impotency related to blood pressure medication would be a useful aid to the physician in his or her choice of medication.

Coping–stress-tolerance pattern Feels tense at work (*job stress*); has tried relaxation exercises with some alleviation; doesn't always have time. States the best way to deal with problems is to "attack them." Afraid of having a stroke and being dependent: "This thing today has really scared me" (*fear of dependency*). "I have too many things to think about at work and at home, and now this blood pressure thing" (*role conflict*). Life changes: father died 3 years ago; mother died of stroke 15 months ago; took job at Spanish center 2 years ago to be near mother who "was getting old." Pleased he did this and feels good about it.

The previous mention of job and family stressors led naturally to a discussion of the coping–stress-tolerance pattern. "Attacking" problems seemed to be the predominant coping pattern expressed. The continuing theme of job stress was evident. Job stress was not interpreted as the factor receiving the "blame" for his state of affairs.

Further support for the fear (dependency) hypothesis was found in the cue "This thing . . . really scared me." The tentative hypothesis of conflict received support from the cue "Too many things to think about, and now this. . . ." Questions regarding his mother's death elicited no verbal or nonverbal cues to un-resolved grieving.

The life changes as well as the assault on his child placed considerable strain on coping patterns. Yet there were indications of support (family relationships) and a disposition toward finding a solution for present problems.

> *Value-belief pattern* "Life has been good to me"; feels deeply about "injustices in society" and wants to do something about them (*value conflict*). States family is important to him. Religion (Catholic) important to him; would like to be active in church affairs.

In response to a question about things important to him, "injustices" and family were mentioned. These data prompted a change in the earlier hypothesis of role conflict. A value conflict is more likely present. This hypothesis revision was supported by cues about (1) family concerns and perceived responsibilities, (2) the valuing of the needs of others, and (3) time available.

The nurse performed an examination following the history. The above hypotheses were kept in mind. There was also an openness to further cues.

EXAMINATION

Vital signs BP 205/118; T 37.6°C (99.8°F); P 80, regular and strong; R 18.
Nutritional-metabolic pattern:

Skin No redness over bony prominences; no lesions. Dryness, calluses on feet with discomfort when touched.

Oral mucous membranes Moist, no lesions.

Height and weight 180 cm (5 ft 11 in); 104 kg (230 lb) actual weight; 99.8 kg (220 lb) reported weight.

Activity-exercise pattern:

Gait. Steady.

Posture. Well balanced.

Muscle tone, strength, and coordination Hand grip firm left and right; lifts legs; can pick up pencil; tenseness in neck and shoulder muscles.

Range of motion (joints) Within normal limits.

Prosthesis and assistive devices None.

Absence of body part No.

Cognitive-perceptual pattern:

Perception Hears whisper; reads newsprint with glasses.

Cognition Language—English; grasps ideas, both abstract and concrete; speech clear; attention span good.

Self-perception–self-conception pattern:

General appearance Well groomed, evidences good hygiene.

Nervous or relaxed Tense; some relaxation during history taking.

Eye contact Yes.

Attention span Good.

Role-relationship pattern:
Interactions Communications with wife supportive, both somewhat tense; children not present.

Obesity was further confirmed by the height and weight measurements. Tenseness of neck muscles was clustered with other cues to Fear (dependency). Numbness had disappeared. Calluses are relevant to his exercise pattern.

The nursing history and examination provide a beginning understanding of the client's health patterns. The history and examination also demonstrate the individuality of clients and show how assessment can identify clients' problems. Diagnostic hypotheses in Mr. K's situation were added, deleted and revised as follows:

Fear → fear (stroke; death) → fear (stroke) → fear (dependency)
Obesity → exogenous obesity → exogenous obesity/caloric intake–energy expenditure imbalance
Job stress → (delete; incorporated under value conflict and responsibilities)
Potential noncompliance (health management)
Constipation → intermittent constipation pattern/dietary pattern → intermittent constipation pattern/dietary and exercise pattern
Caloric excess → (delete; incorporated as etiology of obesity)
Decreased activity tolerance (to be evaluated further after medical treatment)
Knowledge deficit (age and exercise) → (incorporated under health management)
Sleep pattern disturbance/presleep activity, job stress
Family concerns → (delete; incorporated under value conflict and responsibilities)
Role conflict → (delete; incorporated under value conflict and responsibilities)
Value conflict → value conflict/perceived job and family responsibilities

A final review of findings produced further revision. The following nursing diagnoses, supported by data, were recorded (a slash separates the problem and etiological factors):

Exogenous obesity/caloric intake–energy expenditure imbalance
Intermittent constipation pattern/dietary and exercise pattern
Sleep pattern disturbance/presleep activity, perceived responsibilities
Fear (dependency)/perceived risk of stroke
Potential health management deficit
Value conflict/perceived job and family responsibilities

The diagnoses related to obesity, sleep, and constipation became more specific as data accumulated. It can be noted that these represent a problem in one pattern area and etiological factors in other pattern areas.

Fear (dependency) was probably related to the perceived risk of a stroke. A care plan that emphasized developing a feeling of personal control through reduction of risk factors might help this client.

Potential health management deficit was used to describe the history of noncompliance with medication and follow-up care and the client's general neglect of health. The diagnosis *potential noncompliance* could have been used. Yet no evidence was present to suggest there was previous intention to comply.[10] In addition, there were data to support an interest in learning "what to do." The care plan would emphasize teaching and counseling for general health promotion. Special emphasis would be given to correcting misinformation about age and exercise. A podiatry referral will be recommended to Mr. K to relieve his calluses which may cause sufficient discomfort to prevent walking and other forms of exercise. Specific teaching would be provided about hypertension and other areas of risk factor management.

A conflict in values existed. Mr. K's family was important to him. Also important was his contribution to resolving "injustices" through his work. A sense of responsibility "to do things well" in both areas produced conflict. The cues were: "need to be near when people need help," "maybe I should move . . . ," "sometimes I don't think I'm doing well with my family . . . ," more concerned with others than himself, enjoys job and helping people, and multiple references to demanding responsibilities in his job. The cues were clustered and described as value conflict related to perceived job and family responsibilities.

From the nurse's perspective, the problem is more complex. The client's value system (hence his conflict) should also include responsibility to himself, to protect his own health. A serious illness will not permit Mr. K to realize either set of values or carry out the responsibilities he has chosen to assume. Yet at this time there are few cues that his conflict includes health-maintenance responsibilities to self. The nursing diagnosis has to describe the conflict that exists, not the conflict that *should* exist.

Nursing care will focus first on helping the client to examine the possibility of balancing his life. First, things important to him will be discussed, that is, his perceived job and family responsibilities. It is expected that current health concerns will come to be perceived as a third area of conflict. This insight can then lead to an examination of how a balance of responsibilities can be attained. The nurse must exercise caution during these explorations of Mr. K's personal values and lifestyle, since clients have a right to choose how to conduct their lives. The nursing responsibility is to help them look at alternatives that include health promotion. In the end, the client chooses.

The case of Mr. K illustrates the broad life pattern that was previously discussed as an overriding pattern that encompasses all diagnoses. For example, *all* of Mr. K's health problems seem to be related to the choices he has made and the responsibilities he has chosen, and not chosen, to assume. In fact, a nursing diagnosis could be stated as: health management deficit related to value-choice pattern. Currently, some nurses intuitively grasp clients' life pattern problems and intervene at this broad level. But questions remain. Is this level

---

[10]*Noncompliance* is defined as failure to participate in carrying out the plan of care *after indicating initial intention to comply.*

of problem identification useful for planning intervention? Are both broad and specific levels of diagnosis needed? Could this broad pattern be identified without going through the step of identifying specific diagnoses, such as exogenous obesity, sleep pattern disturbance and the other diagnoses in this case?

The first step toward answering these questions is to have nursing diagnosis an integral part of nursing practice. Then it will be possible to see at what level diagnoses should be formulated. Facilitation of care planning will always be an important criterion by which nursing diagnosis is further developed, and decisions about level of diagnosis will be made in accordance with that criterion.

SUMMARY

Discussion in this chapter has focused on how to analyze and interpret diagnostic cues during assessment. As previously summarized, first the clarity of the data is evaluated. Following this, the meaning of cues is interpreted and structured by hypotheses (possibilities). The most likely alternative hypotheses provide a focused search for cues. Data that should be present if the condition is present are collected, evaluated, and clustered under the appropriate hypothesis. When psychological confidence in the "best" working hypothesis is present, a nursing diagnosis is stated. This provides a focus for projecting outcomes and planning treatment until a "better" hypothesis is generated. Note that this last statement suggests an attitude toward diagnosis that will prevent some of the errors discussed in Chapter 8.

BIBLIOGRAPHY

Anderson, N. H. (1972). Looking for configurality in clinical judgment. *Psychological Bulletin,* 78: 93–102.

Asch, A. E. (1946). Forming impressions of personality. *Journal of Abnormal and Social Psychology,* 41: 258–290.

Aspinall, M. J. (1979). Use of a decision tree to improve accuracy of diagnosis. *Nursing Research,* 28: 182–185.

Berger, P. L., & Luckmann, T. (1966). *The social construction of reality.* Garden City, NY: Anchor.

Bruner, J. S., Goodnow, J. J., & Austin, G. A. (1956). *A study of thinking.* New York: Wiley.

Bieri, J., Atkins, A., Briar, S., Leaman, R., Miller, H., & Tripoldi, T. (1966). *Clinical and social judgment.* New York: Wiley.

Carnevali, D. L., Mitchell, P., Woods, N., & Tanner, C. (1984). *Diagnostic reasoning in nursing.* Philadelphia: Lippincott.

Carpenito, L. J. (1984). *Nursing diagnosis: Application to clinical practice.* Philadelphia: Lippincott.

Ciafrani, K. L. (1984). The influence of amounts and relevance of data on identifying health problems. In M. J. Kim, G. McFarland, & A. McLane (Eds.), *Classification of nursing diagnoses: Proceedings of the fifth national conference.* St. Louis: Mosby.

Craig, J (1986). Types of statements made by nurses as first impressions of patient problems. In M. Hurley (Ed.), *Classification of nursing diagnoses: Proceedings of the sixth conference.* St. Louis: Mosby.

Davitz, L., & Davitz, J. (1980). *Inference of patient's pain and psychological distress.* New York: Springer.

Dion, K., Berscheid, E., & Walster, E. (1972). What is beautiful is good. *Journal of Personality and Social Psychology,* 24: 285–290.

Doenges, M., Jeffries, M. F., & Moorhouse, M. (1985). *Nursing care plans: Nursing diagnoses in planning patient care.* New York: Davis.

Elstein, A. S., Schulman, L. S., & Sprafka, S. A. (1978). *Medical problem solving: An analysis of clinical reasoning.* Cambridge, MA: Harvard University Press.

Elstein, A. S. (1976). Clinical judgment: Psychological research and medical practice. *Science,* 194: 696–700.

Friedlander, M., & Phillips, S. (1985). Preventing anchoring errors in clinical judgment. *Journal of Counseling and Clinical Psychology,* 52:366–371.

Gale, J., & Marsden, P. (1983). *Medical diagnosis: From student to clinician.* New York: Oxford University Press.

Goffman, E. (1965). *Stigma: Notes on the management of spoiled identity.* Englewood Cliffs, NJ: Prentice-Hall.

Gordon, M. (1980). Predictive strategies in diagnostic tasks. *Nursing Research,* 29:39–46.

Gordon, M. (1972). *Probabilistic concept attainment: A study of nursing diagnosis.* Unpublished doctoral dissertation. Boston College.

Hamilton, D. L., & Huffman, L. J. (1971). Generality of impression formation process for evaluative and non-evaluative judgments. *Journal of Personality and Social Psychology,* 20:200–207.

Howe, J., Dickason, E. J., Jones, D. A., & Snider, M. J. (1984). *The handbook of nursing.* New York: Wiley.

Jones, R. A. (1977). *Self-fulfilling prophecies: Social, psychological and physiological effects of expectancies.* Hillsdale, NJ: Erlbaum.

Kaplan, M. F., (1973). Stimulus inconsistency and response dispositions in forming judgments of other persons. *Journal of Personality and Social Psychology,* 25: 58–64.

Levine, M. (1975). *A cognitive theory of learning.* Hillsdale, NJ: Erlbaum.

Levine, M. E. (1973). *Introduction to clinical nursing.* (2d ed.) Philadelphia: Davis.

Merton, R. K. (1957). *Social theory and social structure* (rev. ed.) New York: Free Press.

Neisser, U. (1978). Perceiving, anticipating, imagining. In G. W. Savage. (Ed.) *Perception and cognition, Minnesota studies in the philosophy of science* (Vol. 9). Minneapolis: University of Minnesota Press.

Newell, A., & Simon, H. (1972) *Human problem solving.* Englewood Cliffs, NJ: Prentice-Hall.

Rosenhan, D.L. (1973). On being sane in insane places. *Science,* 179: 250–258.

Sarbin, T. R., Taft, R., & Bailey, D. E. (1960). *Clinical inference and cognitive theory.* New York: Holt, Rinehart and Winston.

Schmidt, H. O., & Fonda, C. P. (1956). Reliability of psychiatric diagnosis: A new look. *Journal of Abnormal and Social Psychology,* 52: 262–268.

Schutz, W. C. (1966). Interpersonal underworld. In W. G. Bennis, K. D. Benne, & R. Chin (Eds.), *The planning of change.* New York: Holt, Rinehart and Winston.

Schwartz, A. K., & Aaron, N. S. (1979). *Somniquest.* New York: Berkeley Books.

Soares, C. (1978). Low verbal usage and status maintenance among intensive care nurses. In N. L. Chaska (Ed.), *The nursing profession: Views through the mist.* New York: McGraw-Hill.

Tajfel, H. (1969). Social and cultural factors in perception. In G. Lindzey and E. Aronson (Eds.), *Handbook of social psychology.* Reading, MA: Addison Wesley.

Thomas, W. O., and Thomas, D. S. (1928). *The child in America.* New York: Knopf.

Thompson, J. M., McFarland, G. K., Hirsch, J. E., Tucker, S. M., & Bowers, A. C. (1986). *Clinical nursing.* St. Louis: Mosby.

Thyne, J. M. (1966). *Psychology of learning and techniques of teaching.* London: University of London Press.

Tversky, A., & Kahneman, D. (1974). Judgment under uncertainty: Heuristics and biases. *Science,* 185: 1124–1131.

Weiss, J. H. (1963). Effect of professional training and amount of accuracy of information on behavioral prediction. *Journal of Consulting Psychology,* 27: 257–262.

Young, L., & Powell, B. (1985). Effects of obesity on the clinical judgement of mental health professionals. *Journal of Health and Social Behavior,* 26: 233–246.

274

CHAPTER 8

DIAGNOSTIC STATEMENTS AND DIAGNOSTIC ERRORS

It will be recalled from Chapter 1 that *nursing diagnosis* was defined as a category label for a dysfunctional or potentially dysfunctional pattern and as a process (reasoning and judgment). This chapter focuses on using diagnostic categories to describe judgments and the potential for errors in nursing diagnosis. At the point a diagnosis is stated, confidence exists in the diagnostic judgment. The diagnostician is ready to make the judgment public (charting) and to use the diagnostic statement (problem and etiological or related factors) to design a treatment plan. To facilitate the use of nursing diagnosis in nursing process the diagnostic statement has to be precise, clear, and sufficiently supported by critical defining characteristics.

Stating the diagnosis is the endpoint in the process of problem formulation. Actually, *when the first diagnostic cue was noticed, problem formulation began.* This is an important point to remember. Errors can result if one thinks information collection and diagnosis can be separated in time (diagnose after all information is collected) and space (back at the desk or community agency office). This chapter will emphasize how to state a precise nursing diagnosis and how to deal with the uncertainty and dilemmas inherent in making diagnostic judgments. Continued validation of the diagnosis during treatment will be considered as well as ways to avoid the major diagnostic errors that can occur.

REVIEW OF ASSESSMENT FINDINGS

When learning nursing diagnosis it is difficult to follow the advice in Chapter 6 (p. 175) that is, to review the health problems identified with the client at the end of the assessment. Time to think is needed and all that can be expected is a vague statement, such as "I think while you're here, I can help you with some of the things you have mentioned . . . " (Insert things that seemed important to the client, such as how to take medications, helping to relax, information about the surgery). For the novice this is better than leaping in and stating health problems that one later regrets. As experience and confidence accumulates, diagnoses and plans can be discussed at the end of assessment.

Kelly (1985, p. 28) makes an important point in regard to reviewing findings with the client. She points out that the medical diagnosis of disease does not require involvement of the client except as a reporter of symptoms. Nursing diagnoses focus on human responses and require inclusion of the client and his or her subjective perspective. The nurse's interpretation of the significance of behavior may change when the client's view of a situation is obtained and the client's understanding may shift when the nurse's professional knowledge and experience is shared.

The client's situation as a whole is the basis for all behavior observed during history and examination. Pattern areas are only a way of organizing data and coping with the complexity of the human situation. Therefore a review of findings is necessary to ensure that diagnostic judgments are not made in isolation. Interaction and interdependence of pattern areas have to be considered. *Each problem identified is reviewed in the context of the whole client situation (environment).*

FORMULATING THE DIAGNOSTIC STATEMENT

As the reader will already have learned, a diagnostic statement consists of a problem and etiological or related factor(s). In this section some guidelines will be offered about how to state the problem, the etiological factors, and, lastly, the relationship between problem and etiology that comprises the nursing diagnosis.

Problem Statements

The problem describes the state of the client at the time the diagnosis is made. If the critical diagnostic criteria for a category listed in Appendix A match the cluster of cues observed, then the category name is applied. Stating the problem in a nursing diagnosis is not merely labeling. It has to be kept in mind that the nurse will use the problem statement to project outcomes which describe the desired state the client wishes to attain (or when necessary acting on behalf of the client, which is the desired state the nursing treatment will attain). The following are characteristics of useful problem statements:

1 It is a phenomenon of concern to nurses.
2 It is a condition that the client, nurse, or both agree(s) requires changing. (See qualifier above regarding nurse-determined outcome.) It is a problem, a potential problem, or a condition where there is potential for growth in a health-related area.

3 The name given to the cluster of observed signs and symptoms is an accepted diagnostic label (unless none of the current labels apply). (This applies mostly to the learner; experts may wish to experiment with new diagnostic category labels.)

4 The diagnostic category label is clear and concise.

5 A sufficient cluster of signs and/or symptoms can be documented to justify the diagnosis. Critical diagnostic criteria are included in the cluster.

Precision in Diagnostic Labeling   *Precision* refers to specificity. If a problem statement is to be used to project outcomes and measure the effectiveness of nursing care, it must be specific. (As will be seen in the next chapter diagnoses are also being used for staffing, reimbursement, and health statistics.) For example, *alterations in parenting* is not specific; *total self-care deficit* is specific. When considering alterations in parenting, the question arises: What type of alteration? In contrast, by definition *total self-care deficit* means feeding, bathing, toileting, dressing, and grooming (Hurley, 1986; McLane, 1987).

Specific Focus or Level   A second factor that increases precision is the term *specify* that follows certain diagnostic categories (Appendix A). This requires that the diagnostician include the focus or level of the problem. For example, "fear" and "noncompliance" are *nonspecific. Fear (anesthesia), noncompliance (follow-up care), skill deficit (insulin administration), activity intolerance (level I), total self-care deficit (level IV)* are specific. In the case of *self-care deficit,* diagnosing the level provides a very useful specification. The definition of *level IV* is: dependent and does not participate in self-care (Hurley, 1986; McLane, 1987). When a diagnostic category requires specification, assessment has to continue until focus or level is determined.

Specific Modifiers   Some diagnostic categories require that the level of acuity be determined. This specification clarifies the description of the client's state; in some instances acuity can be used to prioritize diagnoses. *Anxiety* is not a specific formulation; *mild anxiety* is. *Grieving* is nonspecific but *acute dysfunctional grieving* is a useful formulation.

Further refinement of diagnostic categories will establish the cluster of cues that represents each acuity or risk level. Until this occurs, try to identify levels that influence treatment decisions and continue assessment until the level can be specified.

Tentative Diagnostic Hypotheses   In some instances the cluster of cues is insufficient for identifying a problem. Only tentative diagnostic hypotheses are suggested by the data and further data collection is not possible at the time. As will be discussed in the next chapter this situation is followed by a diagnostic plan and further assessment. Some authors (Carpinito, 1983; Iyer, Taptich, and Bernocchi-Losey, 1986) suggest describing the cluster of cues as a "possible problem," such as "possible body image disturbance." This would communicate that *some diagnostic cues are present but they are not sufficient to justify a* *diagnosis.* Presumably, this means that the most likely hypothesis is chosen to be labeled *possible.* From a clinical reasoning perspective, this may encourage premature closure. It is more advisable to *record the cluster of cues.* As will be recommended in Chapter 9, a cluster of cues requiring further investigation are to be recorded as such and a diagnostic plan written; tentative hypotheses are included in the diagnostic plan for further investigation.

Etiological Factors

Dysfunctional client-environment patterns can contribute to the development and maintenance of problems. They are used in the identification of nursing treatments and are currently referred to as *etiological or related factors,* the probable causes of a problem. As will be seen below, many of the characteristics of clinically useful etiological factors are the same as those listed for problems. *This is because etiological factors are dysfunctional patterns. When the problem-etiology link is established by the diagnostician the pattern is then referred to as an etiological factor.*

To understand this statement we must consider the process of clinical reasoning and the minimal nursing research–based data on the links between particular problems and etiological factors. Assessment may support the judgment that *dysfunctional patterns exist when data are compared to expectations, norms, or the client's baseline* (Chapter 7). This is the first judgment made by the diagnostician: a dysfunctional pattern. It is a second-level diagnostic judgment to say that one dysfunctional pattern is the problem and another is the reason for the problem. This requires application of theory, research, experience or a combination of these. The *problem-etiology link is an inference;* the link cannot be observed during assessment. For example, can you *observe* that a particular client's activity intolerance is the major factor causing self-care deficit (level II)? No; but you can provide observational data that supports the presence

FIGURE 8-1
Formulation of problem-etiological/related factors linkage.

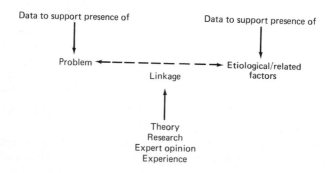

of activity intolerance *and* self-care deficit (level II). As illustrated in Figure 8-1, the linkage of these two dysfunctional patterns (problem-etiology) can be logically argued from theory, mostly nonnursing research, expert opinion, and experience. At the present time the problem-etiology linkages for most nursing diagnoses have to be based on clinical judgment. Recognize this when you use the "related to" statement or the problem/etiological format. Be prepared to justify the "causal" reasoning that underlies the problem-etiology link you propose.

Etiological factors should meet the same requirements for precision as problem statements discussed above. Characteristics of the dysfunctional patterns designated as etiological factors are

1 Nursing treatment can usually resolve the pattern or factor; thus a nurse can assume responsibility for the outcomes.

2 It is a pattern or factor that the client, nurse, or both agree(s) could be one reason for the problem.

3 The name given to the pattern or factor is clear and concise. (Diagnostic categories in Appendix A are used to describe etiological factors when possible, e.g., sleep-onset disturbance/anxiety.)

4 A sufficient cluster of signs and/or symptoms, including diagnostic criteria, can be documented to justify the presence of the pattern or factor. (It is recognized that currently most of the etiological or related factors listed in manuals and by the North American Nursing Diagnosis Association (NANDA) are not defined nor do they have diagnostic criteria listed. The exceptions are when diagnostic categories in Appendix A are used to describe these factors.)

A number of views have been expressed regarding the concept of etiology and the reader may wish to review these: Forsythe, 1984; Halfmann and Pigg, 1984; Ziegler, 1984; McLane and Fehring, 1984; Dederian, 1987; Fitzpatrick, 1987.

Potential Problems

As was discussed in Chapter 5, potential problems alert the nurse to the need for preventive intervention. Although the word *potential* is currently used to describe a risk state, by definition this term is nonspecific: it can refer to high or low risk. It may be useful to consider the format used by the American Nurses' Association–American Association of Neuroscience Nurses (1985). In their format, risk states such as potential for infection and potential fluid volume deficit would be labeled *high risk for infection* and *high-risk fluid volume deficit.* On one hand it could be argued that only high-risk states should be identified and addressed by a specific treatment plan. Yet, the counterargument is that if treatment begins before the risk for a problem becomes high, less aggressive treatment may be necessary. Even more specificity can be achieved by modifiers. High risk for wound infection would be an example. The "high-risk" format and modifiers for labeling a set of risk factors should be clinically tested and evaluated before these changes in format are applied to all the potential problems in Appendix A.

It is useful to note that if etiological factors contribute to the development and maintenance of an actual problem, then logically they are major risk factors for a potential problem. For example, when a person has one or more of the following, they are usually not able to independently manage the treatment for a complex disease or their health promotion activities (health management deficit):

1 Activity intolerance (level IV)
2 Uncompensated cognitive impairment
3 Uncompensated visual or hearing loss
4 Impaired reality testing
5 Depression

These conditions are major etiological factors in health management deficit. Now shift thinking; if you had a client with one or more of the five conditions above, wouldn't the client be at risk for health management deficit? When the need exists to state a potential problem and no labels are available, review the etiological factors for the actual problem.

Even with all the guidelines that books offer for formulating the diagnostic statement, difficulties will arise. In the next section we will try to anticipate some of the dilemmas.

POSTASSESSMENT DILEMMAS

Any of the following prediagnostic situations, or combinations of situations, may exist at the end of an admission assessment for both the novice and expert: (1) no cues or cue clusters, (2) cluster of dysfunctional cues with no idea of the problem, (3) nothing fits the cues, (4) cues with a broad problem formulated, (5) a list of problems but no idea of what goes with what in the problem/etiology format, (6) imprecise problem formulated with or without etiological factors identified, (7) problem formulated but is it a nursing diagnosis? Let us consider the way out of each of these wicked dilemmas.

No Diagnostic Cues or Cue Clusters

After a functional pattern assessment it is difficult to face the fact that there are no cues or cue clusters that point to a diagnosis. This can be a dilemma for a student who believes the instructor assigned the patient so diagnosis could be practiced or the staff nurse who believes the client must have one.

Possibility No. 1   There are no nursing diagnoses; the client is healthy and even with a disease, is managing well.

Action   Provide feedback to ensure that the client realizes that health practices being employed are beneficial. If the setting is appropriate see if there is potential for growth to higher levels of functional well-being.

Possibility No. 2   The assessment was superficial; therefore cues were missed.

Action   Check the screening assessment in Appendix E (or Appendix F if client is a child). Were the items assessed and attention paid to client reports and observations? See Chapters 4–6.

Possibility No. 3   The assessment was adequate but diagnostic meaning of cues was not derived. Hypothesis were not generated to guide branching questions and observations.

Action   See Chapter 7.

Cluster of Cues; No Idea of Problem

A dilemma exists if assessment resulted in a set of dysfunctional cues and there is no idea of how to formulate the problem. Yet, this is more positive than the situation above where information collection and first level interpretation skills may be missing. Cues but no problem formulation is usually expressed as "I didn't know what to call it!"

Possibility No. 1   Knowledge of diagnostic categories, labels, and critical cues (diagnostic criteria) is insufficient. This is an example:

> States becomes fatigued about midday after minimal activity; feels heart thumping and some shortness of breath after "getting breakfast and doing the morning dishes." *Medical diagnosis:* Congestive heart failure, arteriosclerosis.

If it can be assumed that cue evaluation was correct and diagnostic cues *are* present (as in the example above) the difficulty lies in placing the appropriate diagnostic label on the cluster.

Action   If in a clinical situation think why even a broad dysfunctional pattern was not identified, such as activity problem. To solve the immediate need, look up the *alphabetical* index in the *Manual of Nursing Diagnosis* (Gordon, 1987) or Appendix A and see if a few category labels seem applicable. Go to the pages listing applicable diagnoses and read the defining characteristics. Do any match the assessment data? In the future, modify information collection procedure by collecting and organizing data under each pattern area. Diagnostic cues will then be under a pattern and will indicate the *general area* of a problem. Then look at the diagnoses under the pattern in your *Manual* (Appendix C here). See if the cluster of cues matches any of the diagnostic categories within the pattern area and their defining characteristics. The data above should have suggested activity intolerance.

Possibility No. 2   The cluster of cues under consideration includes more than one set of diagnostic cues. The difficulty lies in trying to make one diagnosis when more than one is present. For example:

> Thin, lanky 16 year old during check of an arm cast states: "Those guys (parents) are always making me feel like a kid; come in by 10:00, clean the room, get better

grades; wish they'd leave me alone. I can't wait till I finish school and can live on my own. States that mother checks cast every day but "now she's working and is never home when I get home from school like she used to be." Reports he comes home after school and "gets some junk food out of refrigerator" and then doesn't eat supper. States that doesn't prepare a lunch for school, gets food out of the machines. "She yells at me for that too."

Action Recognize that the nurse, not the client, organizes the information into clusters of cues that go together; the nurse has to be sensitive to the different meanings in a communication and organize the data under the patterns. This will help in processing the data. The client probably has a nutritional deficit and also may be having some developmental independence/dependence conflict that requires more investigation.

Nothing Fits the Cues

A dilemma exists when none of the current diagnostic categories can be applied and a diagnosis needs to be made to guide care planning. A number of explanations exist.

Possibility No. 1 There is a cluster of cues but none are the critical defining characteristics. This is associated with lack of confidence in applying *any* diagnostic category.

Action Try focusing on hypothesis generation while assessing. Diagnostic hypotheses direct you beyond the routine questions to the assessment of critical cues. See Chapter 7. Also learn the critical cues for common diagnoses.

Possibility No. 2 The cues signify a disease, complication of a disease, or adverse effect of medical therapy. For example, a client with bladder cancer may report blood in her urine.

Action This is an important cue to be reported immediately to the physician if the condition is not already documented on the chart. Avoid creating a label such as, "alteration in urinary elimination: bleeding" when you record this observation. The physician will never find the data recorded under this label; use the medical diagnosis on the chart to which the data applies.

Possibility No. 3 There is no current diagnostic category that describes the information collected.

Action After checking the current listing carefully, try to come up with a concise category label and check it out with the instructor/clinical specialist. Chapter 11 will provide some guidelines for creating new diagnostic category labels. Never use a category that doesn't fit the clinical "picture" described by the data. That would be a forced classification.

A Lot of Problems Formulated

This situation is typical of the advanced beginner who can derive meaning from cues, cluster the data, and identify dysfunctional patterns (perhaps a list of six to ten) but has difficulty in knowing what goes with what. When this happens frequently the difficulty may be expressed as "Today, I really don't feel like working up more than three or four!" (Said by student who has to chart and also write lengthy recordings or staff nurse who has two other admission assessments to do).

Possibility No. 1   The client-environment situation is complex and there *are* a lot of problems and etiological factors. This can occur in long-term care or with multiproblem families.

Action   Check to see if some problems do not require immediate treatment. Are they low priority today (e.g., discharge preparation in a preoperative client)? Record them; do the treatment plan tomorrow. Make sure good judgment is exercised (e.g., that the client isn't going home tomorrow).

Possibility No. 2   The six to ten "problems" *are* dysfunctional patterns. However, a final synthesis of the assessment data was not done. If the causal links or relationships among problems was determined there may only be three or four.

Action   Always remember to do a final review of the findings; this provides a holistic look at the client's health. Learn to "put things together" as you move from assessment of one pattern to another by thinking while assessing. Possibility No. 2 is a typical difficulty; the following is a list of patterns that were not reviewed at the end of an assessment (75-year-old female, two days post-fractured hip, concussion):

1 Sleep onset disturbance
2 Self-care deficit (level II)
3 Potential for impaired home maintenance management
4 Ineffective airway clearance
5 Anticipatory fear (future loss of independence)
6 Impaired bed mobility (level II)
7 Viscous secretions, pain in hip with cough

Reviewing the findings made it clear that relationships existed among these problems. Rather than trying to do a care plan for each, the nurse examined dysfunctional patterns for causal links. Some were seen as the problem and others as the probable cause; the problem/etiological factors format was used, thereby reducing the number of diagnoses and providing a useful focus for treatment planning:

1 Sleep Onset Disturbance/Anticipatory Fear (Loss of Independence)
2 Self-Care Deficit (Level II)/Impaired Bed Mobility (Level II)
3 Ineffective Airway Clearance/Viscous Secretions, Pain in Hip With Cough
4 Potential for Impaired Home Maintenance Management

Imprecise Problem Formulation

At times novice diagnosticians get feedback that their diagnoses are vague and imprecise. It is a dilemma when the reasons cannot be found. Precise diagnoses are important because they facilitate treatment planning and communication among care providers.

Possibility No. 1 Insufficient assessment. The diagnosis is made but lacks specificity. Certain diagnoses require specification of the acuity, level, or focus. Examples are

Self-Care Deficit (Specify Level)
Pain (Acute, Chronic)
Knowledge Deficit (Specify)
Health Management Deficit (Specify)

Action Continue assessment after the problem is identified. Include specifications as in

Self-Care Deficit (Level III)
Knowledge Deficit (Medication Regimen)
Acute Lower Back Pain
Health Management Deficit (Follow-up Care)

Possibility No. 2 Affirming a causal relationship between the whole and component parts. A diagnosis is imprecise when the problem-etiological factors merely communicate the relationship between the whole and its parts or divisions. Imprecise diagnoses would be: "alterations in parenting related to weak parent-infant attachment" or "self-care deficit related to bathing deficit." *Self-care deficit* represents the "whole" diagnostic class and has components: feeding, bathing, dressing, and toileting. Thus bathing deficit is not a contributing or etiological factor but rather a component. Treatment is directed toward factors contributing to the problem; thus whole-part formulations are not useful clinically. It would be comparable to the physician writing a medical diagnosis such as "cardiac disease related to rheumatic fever."

Action Use the specific, not the general classification category. Try to determine the major contributing factors. For example:

Self-Bathing Deficit (Level III) related to Uncompensated Sensory-Motor Loss

Weak Parent-Infant Attachment related to Separation

When terms such as *alterations in* or *impairment of* come to mind, assess further to determine the *specific* alteration or impairment and the etiological or related factors.

Possibility No. 3 The diagnostic category requires refinement. The novice cannot be blamed for using "accepted" nursing diagnoses that are imprecise. (See Appendix A.) Diagnostic categories are in the process of development by staff nurses, specialists, faculty, researchers, and theoreticians. All agree that the classifications will be much more precise 50 years from now.

Action Learn what precision means (see section above) and obtain help when tempted to use broad categories. As diagnostic abilities increase, (1) think of all the types of "alterations in . . ." that are encountered, (2) refine the diagnostic category and clinically test the specific categories, and (3) submit to NANDA for review and incorporation into the taxonomy (Appendixes L and N).

Problem Formulated—Is it a Nursing Diagnosis?

The way a diagnostic statement is structured can be elegant but it may not represent a condition amenable to nursing intervention. A dilemma exists if the condition is recorded as a nursing diagnosis and it isn't one. The primary nurse may not be able to assume accountability for the outcomes.

Possibility No. 1 Unclear understanding of the nursing diagnosis–treatment realm of practice as opposed to the collaborative practice domain. The possibility exists that the "obvious" is focused upon and problem formulation is superficial. For example, the medical diagnosis is very "obvious" in acute care settings. Some may assume that everything has to be tied to the medical diagnosis or it will "get lost." Such incorrect diagnoses as the following may result (problem/etiological factors format): activity intolerance/chronic obstructive pulmonary disease (COPD) or body image disturbance/hysterectomy. Etiological factors are supposed to focus the nursing treatment plan; but nurses don't assume independent responsibility for treating diseases (COPD) or surgical procedures. Thus, *chronic obstructive pulmonary disease* and *hysterectomy* are not useful as etiological factors. A more useful formulation would be *situational depression/body image disturbance*.

A second reason given for the possible "loss" of the medical diagnosis in the suggested format is that nurses treating situational depression/body image disturbance will not realize that the client had a hysterectomy. How could this occur? Errors result if *any* diagnosis is treated out of context of the whole client-environment situation.

Action When inclined to view the medical diagnosis as the etiology of a problem, (1) consider looking deeper into the situation, (2) assess for etiological factors that will respond to nursing treatment, and (3) formulate the diagnosis in nursing terms. As one author frequently states, Florence Nightingale cautioned that we should not mix nursing and medicine, it confuses them both (Halloran, 1987). Understand the independent and interdependent (collaborative) areas of nursing practice; this leads to a clear view of responsibility and accountability in each area of clinical judgment (see Chapters 1, 2, and 9). *Also always consider the possibility that the "problem" may, in fact, be the etiology. Consider activity intolerance/COPD. Now ask the question: If a person had activity intolerance, what problems might it produce?* The diagnosis, *from a nursing perspective,* may be impaired home maintenance management/activity intolerance or self-care deficit (level III)/activity intolerance.

Possibility No. 2 Nursing diagnosis is defined by the diagnostician as *both* independent and interdependent (collaborative) practice. Not all nurses agree that nursing diagnosis should only describe conditions within the independent area of nursing practice. They suggest, for example, that activity intolerance/decreased cardiac output is a nursing diagnosis. Some accept body image disturbance/hysterectomy as a diagnosis.

Action Consider the pro and con arguments (Chapters 1, 5, and 9), take a position, and test its clinical usefulness in practice and in your work with physicians or other care providers.

CONSISTENCY AMONG CARE PROVIDERS' DIAGNOSES

Some would argue that nursing diagnoses should be consistent with medical diagnoses or those of other care providers (American Nurses' Association, 1973). *Consistency* by definition means compatible, noncontradictory, or conforming to some principle or course of action.

The first point to be made is that there may be no medical diagnoses. Thus consistency is unattainable. The second point presents more difficulty. Problems diagnosed by physicians, nurses, or social workers are in three different domains: disease, functional patterns, and personal-social matters. Clients can have various problems in each area and in many combinations. Is a nursing diagnosis of *unresolved grieving/loss of wife* consistent with a medical diagnosis of *appendicitis*? A client could have both of these diagnoses, yet neither consistently predicts the other.

Apparent inconsistencies may arise in regard to assessment data collected by different professionals. Although used in different ways, many of the same data are gathered by the various health care providers. If the data are inconsistent, discussion among the professionals and reassessment can usually resolve any contradictions. If apparent inconsistency occurs at the level of diagnosis, disagreement on a diagnosis that is *well supported by data* is also resolved by discussion. The opinion of that care provider who is expert in the problem area and most knowledgeable about the client should be weighted most heavily.

SOURCES OF DIAGNOSTIC ERRORS

Diagnostic errors lead to undertreatment or overtreatment of clients. If a problem is not diagnosed, harm may result or quality of life may be impaired. This failure to diagnose an existing problem is an error of *omission.* Harm and impairment of the quality of a client's life can also result from overdiagnosing, or diagnosing nonexistent problems. These diagnoses would be errors of *commission.* Both errors can occur during data collection, data interpretation, and data clustering. Discussion in this section will focus on potential errors in these areas and how to prevent them. It will be seen that clinical knowledge, inferential reasoning, and the ability to put information together are major influences on diagnostic accuracy.

Is it more serious to diagnose a problem when no problem exists or to judge the client "healthy" when a problem is present? In nursing diagnosis, uncertainty and doubt will arise. It is usually said that clinicians must avoid errors. Because of the probabilistic nature of the information upon which diagnoses are made, it is more realistic to say that the error rate in diagnosis should be kept very low. To return to the question, Are certain errors more tolerable than others in doubtful situations?

Perhaps errors of omission and commission are not equally tolerated by clients, colleagues, and society. To determine which error is more serious, we need to look at the values practitioners hold and the social factors that influence values. On the basis of certain values, professions develop implicit but persuasive ways of dealing with uncertainty in judgments. Let us first discuss sources of error in nursing diagnosis and then consider how to prevent them.

Data Collection Errors

The information collected during assessment influences the *entire* diagnostic process. If data are omitted, diagnoses can be missed. If large amounts of data are collected in an unorganized manner, cognitive processes can be overwhelmed. Irrelevant data can produce the same effect. Thoroughness is important. Yet data must be relevant to areas of nursing concern if the purpose of data collection is nursing diagnosis.

Interviewing and examination skills are critical factors in perceptual accuracy. Data are generated by the things the nurse does. These activities include inquiries, supportive replies, silence, touching, and examination. Characteristics such as physical attributes of the head, face, shoulders, arms and posture of a client in bed are observable. Actions are required to elicit data about less readily apparent characteristics. If these actions are not taken, not chosen wisely, or not performed correctly, the nurse's perceptual accuracy suffers.

To maintain a low rate of error in data collection, think of what the data collection process involves: (1) perceptual accuracy, (2) organization, and (3) interviewing and examination skills. First, consider *perceptual accuracy*. What may influence this? Clinical knowledge is one factor. People may at times observe without perceiving. Many errors in perception result from not having available categories for classifying sensory information. These categories are based on clinical knowledge. The nurse must be curious and question what is observed; this is how knowledge develops and errors are avoided for both the novice and expert diagnostician.

Perception is a neuropsychological phenomenon. Thus it is influenced by health states, fatigue, and boredom or routine. It is particularly important for perceptual alertness that nurses maintain their own functional health patterns, particularly sleep and rest. One could surmise that extended work shifts may tax perceptual-cognitive processes, perhaps especially in settings where continuous alertness is critical.

Neglecting to collect critical data is another source of potential error. The nurse may overlook critical cues because of distraction, lack of organization, or inadequate clinical knowledge. For example, lack of knowledge about coping deficits or about risk factors in potential skin breakdown can lead one to miss cues. Too narrow a concept of nursing may cause one to exclude some material for assessment (for example, coping patterns). Data collection errors result.

Failure to obtain client reports in areas about which the client's subjective information is critical is another source of inaccuracies. Similarly, relying on only predictive (contextual) data and inferences increases the rate of error; current data about the state of the client are also needed. Sometimes data are collected but not considered in analysis. Ignoring a critical cue that should have been pursued leads to errors of omission.

Overload of data can also lead the diagnostician astray. When large quantities of irrelevant data are collected, cognitive capacities for processing information can be overloaded. For example, questions may be irrelevant or clients may ramble.

Methodological errors can be caused by inaccuracies in measurement of a client characteristic. Questions asked during history taking may lead the client to say what seems to be expected. Or the nurse may not listen attentively. Perceptual errors, such as underestimating the depth of respirations, or faulty equipment can also be a source of measurement error.

A second factor related to data collection errors is *organization.* There are two aspects: (1) preorganization and (2) organization during assessment. *Preassessment organization* has been emphasized in previous discussions. Briefly, one must know one's conceptual focus and the pattern areas. The critical areas for data collection within patterns should be listed. In addition, one must decide how to begin and select a possible sequence.

As data collection begins, *concurrent organization* is needed: that is, as the assessment proceeds, the nurse has to organize the data by generating hypotheses that permit clustering of data. (This has to be supplemented by also recording the data under pattern areas.) The human mind cannot handle large amounts of unorganized data. Some method of keeping track of what has gone before is needed because previous data and hypotheses influence what questions are asked in branching. One of the major reasons for missing critical cues is lack of concurrent organization of data during history taking and examination.

Data Interpretation Errors

If the meaning of cues is inaccurately interpreted, diagnostic errors result. Cues signifying a dysfunctional pattern may not be interpreted as dysfunctional; an error of omission will result. Overdiagnosing occurs when a functional pattern is interpreted as dysfunctional. Usually the diagnostic errors occur because of inadequate clinical knowledge. Not taking developmental or individual norms into account also contributes to errors of interpretation.

Another source of error in data interpretation is overgeneralizing from one observation of client behavior. The behavioral sample can be inadequate (too few observations, or atypical ones) or interpreted outside the context of the situation in which the behavior took place. One episode of hostility does not mean the client is a hostile person. Remember that assessment relies on patterns of behavior, not isolated events.

To maintain a low rate of error the nurse must validate his or her inferences. Errors occur if hypotheses are not treated as tentative and subject to revision. Furthermore, generating hypotheses early does not mean that early ideas are the only ones considered. Additional data may require additional hypotheses.

When judgments have an element of uncertainty, probabilities have to be taken into account. Errors can result from incorrect notions about the likelihood of diagnoses. As described, an element of forecasting or prediction enters into diagnosis. Adequate testing of hypotheses helps to control errors in prediction.

One technique for examining interpretations of data is *reframing* (Clark, 1977). This is a process of shifting perspectives. A familiar example is looking at the sky and deciding the day is partly cloudy; from another perspective the day is partly sunny.

Behavior can have so many meanings that it is well to consider alternative explanations. Reframing can be applied to one or two cues, a tentative hypothesis, or a cluster of cues in a diagnosis. Try to reframe the following cues:

> This behavior is familiar to nurses who work in pediatric, public health, or school settings with "shy" children. A child who clings to his mother, withdraws, and does not play with other children is apt to make a lasting impression on a nurse. There is a tendency to call this "separation anxiety." (Clark, 1977, p. 840).

After attempting to look at these cues in a different way, read the following. Note that Clark reinterprets data from the perspective of the child's thinking:

> Reframing will enable the nurse to pick out the adaptive portions of the child's behavior from his point of view. The child does not know what the new experience holds. He only knows he has been taken to a strange place for some unclear purpose. He is actually to be commended for sticking close to the one familiar object in the environment, his mother, until he can figure out what is happening. In this sense, the child's behavior is quite adaptive, since it allows for some stability through closeness to mother until information can be gathered on what action is appropriate. (Clark, 1977, p. 840)

The earlier interpretation of separation anxiety may be realistic if the behavior continues. If separation anxiety is ultimately diagnosed, having considered adaptation as an alternative should increase the nurse's confidence that error has been avoided.

Try another example adapted from Clark (1977). For medical reasons a client requires complete bed rest. He is not to get out of bed. This activity restriction has been discussed with him and he acknowledges the need for it. Repeatedly the nurse observes the client out of bed. Obviously, the problem is noncompliance with activity prescription! What might be the reasons for this behavior? Is there a deeper problem? Here is how Clark reframed this data:

> To reframe the patients' behavior from his point of view, staying in bed may seem like an attempt to force him into a dependent, helpless position, and getting out of bed may be an adaptive maneuver. A patient who refuses to accept the "sick role" may harm himself physically in the short term, but he may be taking steps to preserve his long-term self-image. In other words, refusing to accept the "sick role" can be adaptive. (Clark, 1977, p. 840)

Reframing is similar to branching. It is an important concept in reducing errors. Try to see the world from the client's eyes when interpreting cues. Also, as previously recommended, obtain the client's perception of the health problem, its probable cause, and any action that has been taken to remedy the problem. A total reformulation or rejection of a hypothesis may result.

Data Clustering Errors

Clustering, it may be recalled, is the combination of cues. Three kinds of errors can occur in clustering: A nursing diagnosis may be made prematurely, incorrectly, or not at all.

Premature closure is a common error. A diagnostic judgment is reached before all critical information has been considered or even before all information has been collected. The observations that have been made are inadequate supporting data.

One of the reasons a new charting system, the problem-oriented method, was introduced in hospitals around the country was to prevent premature closure. Problem-oriented recording requires the diagnostician to list the subjective and objective data for each problem. Clearly this form of charting forces the clinician to specify the data base for each diagnostic judgment. Having recorded the cues used in making each judgment, the clinician can examine whether or not sufficient supporting evidence is available. More will be said about this charting system in the next chapter.

Incorrect clustering of cues can occur in formulating the problem, in identifying the etiology, or in combining the problem and etiology. The result of incorrect clustering is that data supposedly supporting the diagnosis clearly contradict it (Voytovich, Rippey, and Suffredini, 1985). This error is usually related to inadequate knowledge of critical signs and symptoms. It is similar to labeling a chair as a table. The rules for using any language apply also to diagnostic "language."

Lack of standardization of diagnostic categories used in nursing diagnosis contributes to this type of error. If the difference between a chair and table was not specified in dictionaries, errors in use of the terms would occur. The situation is similar in nursing diagnosis. Try to use currently identified signs, symptoms, and category definitions. The potential for errors will be reduced but probably not eliminated until precise definitions are standardized.

Not synthesizing (not combining cues) obviously leads to errors of omission. Whereas some nurses tend to close prematurely, others delay diagnostic judgment. This delay may represent an attempt to reach absolute certainty when in reality the situation is inevitably based on some degree of uncertainty. Think of a nursing diagnosis as the best hypothesis of the moment; be open to new information that can reject or further confirm judgments: These are the keys to working with uncertainty-based data and judgments.

Attribution Errors

Errors can occur if the reasons (etiological factors) for a problem are attributed to the client's behavior, when in fact the reason lies in the situation or in client-environment interaction. This type of error has a direct effect on intervention because a treatment plan is based on etiological or related factors. Obtain the client's viewpoint regarding probable causes of the problem and consider these in formulating etiological factors. Abraham's review of causal attribution research (in press) suggests that clinicians are more apt to attribute cause to the client's behavior under specific circumstances, whereas clients are more apt to see the source of a problem in their situation or environment.

IMPLICIT RULES

In an interesting article about unwritten rules for making decisions, Scheff (1963) examined differences in tolerance for certain errors of judgment. The following synopsis of his ideas will serve as a basis for considering what implicit rules might influence nursing diagnosis.

In a court of law, a person is innocent until proven guilty. The rule is "when in doubt, acquit." Underlying this rule are the assumptions that (1) conviction will do irreversible harm to a person's reputation, (2) the person is weak and defenseless relative to society, and (3) society can sustain some errors without serious consequences.

Note the dilemma. A legal judgment of guilty when innocent has serious consequences for the individual. Yet a judgment of innocent when guilty can have serious consequences for society. An acquitted offender may commit further crimes. Western society resolves the dilemma in favor of the individual; in fact the assumption of innocence is stated in legal codes and accepted by jurists.

What is actually occurring? There are two types of errors a jury could make:

Type I error. The accused is *actually guilty,* but the hypothesis of *not guilty* is accepted.

Type II error. The accused is *actually innocent,* but the hypothesis of *guilty* is accepted.

Before receiving data from witnesses and the interpretations of lawyers, juries are instructed to avoid a type II error. Society does not tolerate convicting the innocent; if doubt exists, acquit.

In the profession of medicine, the same types of errors are possible when clinical data are ambiguous:

Type I error. The client *actually has a disease,* but the hypothesis of *no disease* is accepted.

Type II error. The client is *actually disease-free,* but the hypothesis of *disease* is accepted.

Colleagues, clients, and the general society generally do not tolerate a type I error. What implicit rule is followed by practitioners of medicine?

According to Scheff (1963), the rule is not always explicitly stated or as rigid in medicine as in law. Yet it does exist: "When in doubt, diagnose disease." This bias can influence medical assessment. It encourages the physician to consider symptoms as possibly signifying illness until disease is ruled out. When in doubt, it is far more important to continue to suspect illness than to suspect health.

The assumptions that underlie this implicit rule are: (1) undetected disease will have serious consequences, (2) diagnoses are not considered irreversible, and (3) society expects disease, if present, to be diagnosed. Physicians are aware that a malpractice legal decision can result from a type I error. That is, a client may sue if dismissed as healthy when in fact disease was present and subsequently produced harm. Furthermore, if a client remains in society with untreated infectious disease or behavior harmful to others, there may be serious consequences.

A dilemma accompanies the rule "When in doubt diagnose or suspect illness." Calling clients' attention to their bodily state can produce physiological and psychological changes. The client may alter many aspects of life and assume the sick role in work, family, and social situations (Haynes, Sackett, Taylor, Gibson, and Johnson, 1978). Furthermore, psychiatric as well as some medical disease labels carry social stigma. Type II errors are costly to individuals or society, and many people question whether unnecessary surgical and psychiatric treatment is occurring. Yet the implicit rule of "Better safe than sorry" prevails (Scheff, 1963, p. 100).

Scheff suggests that personal biases toward type I or type II errors are influenced by the disease characteristics, the physician, the client, and the health care setting in which diagnoses are made. He raises a number of possibilities that are relevant to nursing as well as medical diagnosis:

> Physicians who generally *favor active intervention* probably make more type II errors than physicians who view their treatments only as assistance for natural bodily reactions to disease. The physician's *perception of the personality of the patient* may also be relevant; type II errors are less likely if the physician defines the patient as a "crock," a person who ignores or denies disease.
>
> The organizational setting is relevant to the extent that it influences the relationship

between the doctor and the patient. In some contexts, as in medical practice in organizations such as the military or industrial setting, the physician is not as likely to *feel personal responsibility* for the patient as he would in others, such as private practice. This may be due in part to the conditions of financial remuneration, and perhaps equally important, the sheer volume of patients dependent on the doctor's time. Cultural or class differences may also affect the amount of social distance between doctor and patient, and therefore the amount of responsibility which the doctor feels for the patient. Whatever the sources, the more the physician feels personally responsible for the patient, the more likely he is to make a type II error. (Scheff, 1963, p. 104)

It is also interesting to think about whether nurses are influenced by their perception of the personality of the client for example, in the initial impression. Does perception of personal responsibility for a client versus perception of team responsibility influence diagnostic errors? Do nurses who view nursing as assisting the client make fewer type II errors than nurses who view nursing as doing things for the client? Answers are not available, but the questions provoke thought.

No research has been published about nursing diagnostic errors. One could imagine that there are rules that bias practitioners toward either of the following errors:

Type I error. The client actually *has a functional health problem,* but the hypothesis of *no problem* is accepted.

Type II error. The client is *actually problem-free,* but the hypothesis of *functional problem* is accepted.

In doubtful situations are the rules in nursing similar to those of the courtroom? When in doubt, assume health. Or are nurses' implicit rules and assumptions similar to those of their colleagues in medicine? When in doubt, diagnose a problem (or continue to suspect a problem).

Many comments are heard admonishing nurses *not* to be problem-focused. It is said that the client's strengths, not problems, should be emphasized. This is quite true in *treatment.* Focusing on strength—areas of wellness and capabilities—is an approach that mobilizes the client's resources. In *diagnosis,* a bias toward recognition of health rather than of problematic states can result in diagnostic errors of omission, type I errors. If symptoms signifying a nursing diagnosis are not investigated, problems can be missed.

With regard to observing signs and symptoms of disease, nurses are told that when in doubt they should assume these signify complications and call a physician. As Hammond (1966, p. 29) has suggested, nurses have to think for themselves as well as think "as" the doctor thinks; when observing disease states and carrying out medical treatment the nurse is under the "cognitive control of the doctor." Within this cognitive set may be the rule "When in doubt, diagnose or suspect disease complications." Is it difficult to shift to an opposite rule in nursing diagnosis? This question would make an interesting clinical study.

Legal as well as moral responsibilities argue for avoiding errors of omission.

It is understandable that one may not wish to diagnose potential for injury or trauma when cues are uncertain. This diagnosis, for example, might necessitate cautioning the truck driver with uncontrolled seizures not to drive although his employment would be interrupted by following that recommendation. Values enter into any judgment. The best thing is to be aware of the potential consequences of diagnosis and treatment when symptoms are doubtful.

Also, be aware of the consequences of delay in diagnosis and treatment. If delay is the action of choice, continue to collect data and attempt to resolve ambiguities. Learn the technique of discussing observations with clients in a nonthreatening, nonanxiety-producing manner. It is important not to reinforce the sick role but instead help clients to *feel capable* of handling any health problems diagnosed.

In addition to errors of omission (type I) and errors of commission (type II) there is an "error of the third kind," solving the *wrong* problem (Mitroff and Featheringham, 1974). Preparing a care plan for the wrong problem wastes nursing time. Most importantly, the real problem can cause client discomfort if allowed to progress.

Diagnosing and treating the wrong problem can usually be avoided if the meaning of client behavior is explored. The only way to understand the behavior of the client is to ask. It is as simple as that. Inferences made without checking the client's viewpoint can lead to completely erroneous problem formulations and ineffective care plans.

RETROSPECTIVE EVALUATION OF DIAGNOSES

When uncertainty in diagnosis can be reduced but not eliminated it is helpful to have ways of checking judgments. Checking that critical defining cues are present is one way of validating a diagnosis before intervention begins. A second way is to evaluate change in signs and symptoms of the problem after problem-specific intervention has been initiated. This second check involves retrospective evaluation of a diagnostic judgment.

Nursing care is directed at the probable cause of a problem and effectiveness of care is measured by client outcomes. If the outcome of nursing care is a positive change in the status of the problem, then the nurse may assume that the previously identified etiological factors were at least one probable cause. This procedure of evaluating the correctness of the etiological factors by observing the effectiveness of the intervention is a *retrospective test* of the cause of a problem.

Consider an example. If (1) knowledge deficit is *correctly* viewed as the predominant factor causing noncompliance and (2) the intervention is designed to increase the client's knowledge, then (3) the outcome assessment should indicate a change from noncompliance to compliance. What if this expected outcome does not occur, as shown in Table 8-1?

As seen in Table 8-1, one cannot make clear-cut assumptions about etio-

TABLE 8-1
OUTCOME EVALUATION OF THE PROBLEM—ETIOLOGICAL FACTORS IDENTIFIED

Outcome evaluation	Considerations
I Change in problem status not as predicted (e.g., signs and symptoms of problem still present)	1 Were the assumed etiological factors (cause) not correct? 2 Were other unidentified factors, etiological or otherwise, operating? 3 Was the intervention inadequate to produce change in the problem? 4 Were the intervention methods applied correctly?
II Change in problem state as predicted (e.g., signs and symptoms of problem not present)	1 Are there any other explanations for the change in the problem? 2 Was the intervention influencing only the assumed etiological factors or others also?

logical factors from outcome data. If there is no change in signs and symptoms, several possible reasons have to be considered. Returning to the example about knowledge deficit, let us assume the intervention was the best possible for the diagnosis. Four questions can then be raised. Was knowledge deficit the correct etiology? Could there have been other, unidentified etiological factors? Were some events or situational factors overlooked? Was noncompliance just a sign of another problem? These are possible reasons why nursing care did not produce a change.

Now let us assume that the etiology is correct but the intervention was ineffective. As can be seen in Table 8-1, either the choice of intervention or its implementation (or both) may not have been correct. Knowledge deficit may indeed have been the predominant etiological factor, but teaching methods may have been ineffective—maybe the client's readiness for learning new information was not considered. It is useful to think about intervention as a test of the accuracy of nursing diagnosis.

The questions for consideration when the expected outcomes *are* attained (again see Table 8-1) will benefit future clients. Asking these questions enables the nurse to learn from practice experiences. For example, was knowledge deficit the predominate cause of the client's noncompliance? Could it be that the human concern and rapport established during teaching influenced the client's *motivation,* and that motivation, rather than learning, produced change? Perhaps the intervention influenced other unspecified factors as well and the combined effect produced the result.

Unless these questions are considered, the previously effective combination of problem, etiological factor, and intervention, when applied in a future situation, may not produce the outcome. Why? Mainly because a *group* of factors may be operating, not just the one or more that have been identified (in the present example, knowledge deficit). By chance, the intervention dealt with these unrecognized factors and hence produced the desired outcome.

Conclusions from unexamined judgments cannot be applied to future clients' problems. The kind of reflection just discussed is necessary. Essentially, this is called "learning from practice." Future clients benefit from the nurse's past experience. (This is probably why employment advertisements specify "experience required"; the implicit assumption is that past experience has been used to increase clinical judgment and skill.)

SUMMARY

The focus of this chapter was on formulating nursing diagnoses. It was pointed out that diagnoses begin to be formulated when attention is paid to a diagnostic cue. Guidelines were provided for stating problems, etiological factors, and potential problems. Precision in stating the diagnosis was stressed in the discussion because the nursing diagnosis is used to project outcomes, design a treatment plan, and evaluate outcomes. A number of postassessment dilemmas reported by learners were discussed and suggested actions outlined. It was pointed out that the criterion of logical consistency among care providers' diagnoses was probably not relevant. Different domains of diagnostic focus will, in many instances, result in unrelated diagnoses.

Sources of diagnostic error and some implicit rules that may apply were considered. The potential for errors in nursing diagnosis lies in data collection, interpretation, clustering, and the attribution of cause. Retrospective tests of diagnostic formulations were suggested. It was seen that if anticipated outcomes do not occur, both diagnoses and interventions should be examined for error. Perhaps the most important way to self-monitor diagnostic accuracy is to be open to new information, recognize that biases can enter the diagnostic thinking process, and treat nursing diagnoses as tentative judgments. Although diagnoses represent the clinician's best judgment, based on the available data, they may not represent the actual health problem. There is always room for error.

BIBLIOGRAPHY

Abraham, I. L. (In press). Diagnostic discrepancy and clinical inference. In *Genetic, social, and general psychology.*

American Nurses' Association–American Association of Neuroscience Nurses (1985). *Process and outcome standards for nursing diagnoses.* Kansas City, MO.

American Nurses' Association (1973). *Standards for nursing practice.* Kansas City, MO.

Carpinito, L. J. (1983). *Nursing diagnosis: Application to clinical practice.* New York: Lippincott.

Clark, N. (1977). Reframing. *American Journal of Nursing*, 77:840–841.

Dederian, A. (1987). Etiology: Practical relevance. In A. McLane, (ed.), *Classification of nursing diagnoses: Proceedings of the seventh conference.* St. Louis: Mosby.

Fitzpatrick, J. (1987). Etiology: Conceptual concerns. In A. McLane, (ed.), *Classification of nursing diagnoses: Proceedings of the seventh conference.* St. Louis: Mosby.

Forsythe, G. (1984). Etiology: In what sense and of what value? In M. J. Kim, A. McLane, & G. McFarland, (eds)., *Classification of nursing diagnoses: Proceedings of the fifth conference.* St. Louis: Mosby, pp. 63–72.

Halfman, T. M., & Pigg, J. S. (1984). Nurses' perceptions of rheumatic disease patient problems as evidenced in nursing diagnoses, etiologies, defining characteristics, expected outcomes and interventions. In M. J. Kim, A. McLane, & G. McFarland, (eds)., *Classification of nursing diagnoses: Proceedings of the fifth conference.* St. Louis: Mosby.

Halloran, E. (1987). Nursing complexity, the DRG, and length of stay. In A. McLane, (ed.), *Classification of nursing diagnoses: Proceedings of the seventh conference.* St. Louis: Mosby.

Hammond, K. R. (1966). Clinical inference in nursing: A psychologist's viewpoint. *Nursing Research* 15:27–38.

Haynes, R. B., Sackett, D. L., Taylor, D. W., Gibson, E. S., & Johnson, A. L. (1978). Increased absenteeism from work after detection and labeling of hypertensive patients. *New England Journal of Medicine*, 299:741–744.

Hurley, M. (ed.). (1986). *Classification of nursing diagnoses: Proceedings of the sixth conference.* St. Louis: Mosby.

Iyer, P., Taptich, B., & Bernocchi-Losey, D. (1986). *Nursing process and nursing diagnosis.* Philadelphia: Saunders.

Kelly, M. A. (1985). *Nursing diagnosis source book.* Norwalk, CT: Appleton-Century-Crofts.

McLane, A. (ed.). (1987). *Classification of nursing diagnoses: Proceedings of the seventh conference.* St. Louis: Mosby.

McLane, A., & Fehring, R. (1984). Nursing diagnosis: A review of the literature. In M. J. Kim, A. McLane, & G. McFarland, (eds),*Classification of nursing diagnoses: Proceedings of the fifth conference.* St. Louis, MO: Mosby, pp. 526–527.

Mitroff, I., & Featheringham, T. (1974). On systematic problem solving and the error of the third kind. *Behavioral Science,* 19:383–393.

Scheff, T. J. (1963). Decision rules, types of error, and their consequences in medical diagnosis. *Behavioral Science,* 8:97–107.

Voytovich, A., Rippey, R., & Suffredini, A. (1985). Premature conclusions in diagnostic reasoning. *Journal of Medical Education,* 60:302–307.

Ziegler, S. M. (1984). Nursing diagnosis: The state of the art as reflected in graduate students' work. In M. J. Kim, A. McLane, & G. McFarland, (eds.), *Classification of nursing diagnoses: Proceedings of the fifth conference.* St. Louis, MO: Mosby, pp. 199–208.

NURSING DIAGNOSIS IN NURSING PROCESSES
  Guiding Values
  Guiding Concepts and Theory
  Guiding Standards
NURSING DIAGNOSIS IN CARE PLANNING
  Projected Outcomes
  Interventions
  Generating Alternative Interventions
  Individualizing Interventions
  Predicting Effectiveness of Interventions
  Priority Setting
  Implementation and Evaluation
NURSING PROCESS IN DISEASE-RELATED CARE
  Treatment Coordination
NURSING DIAGNOSIS AND COMMUNICATION
  Verbal Communication
  Written Communication
  Computer-Based Communication
FORMATS FOR DOCUMENTATION
  Problem-Oriented Recording
    Documentation: Admission Assessment
    Documentation: Nursing Diagnoses/Treatment Plans
    Documentation: Progress Notes
    Documentation: Discharge Summary/Referrals
    Documentation: Disease-Related Care
  Kardex Care Plans: Nursing and Medical Diagnoses
NURSING DIAGNOSIS AND DISCHARGE PLANNING
  Predischarge Planning
  Referral Decisions
  Communication of Plans
NURSING DIAGNOSIS AND THE LAW
  Element of Duty
  Breach of Duty
  Cause and Effect
  Harm or Injury
  Legal Decisions
DIAGNOSTIC RESPONSIBILITY
  Legal Considerations
  Professional Considerations
  Educational Considerations
  Process Considerations
  Situational Considerations
  Experiential Considerations
SUMMARY
BIBLIOGRAPHY

298

CHAPTER 9

USE OF NURSING DIAGNOSIS IN DIRECT CARE ACTIVITIES

The previous chapters have defined nursing diagnosis and attempted to lay before the reader the process of diagnostic judgment. This earlier discussion has been to one end: application of diagnosis to client care.

In a profession with a social responsibility, thinking and reasoning skills have to be applied, not just learned for abstract, theoretical purposes. In fact, it is questionable whether true learning about concepts like diagnosis can occur without application in the real world. The test of an idea is its usefulness in practice: Does nursing diagnosis facilitate direct client care activities? If nursing diagnosis is merely an intellectual exercise, a status symbol, or an ivory tower idea, why learn it?

The reader would not have been led through eight chapters if nursing diagnosis had no clinical relevance. In this chapter it will become clear that the effort spent in formulating diagnoses greatly facilitates the planning of effective nursing care. First we shall consider the rightful place of diagnosis, that is, within the nursing process. It will be demonstrated that diagnosis is used as a focus for decisions about the care that is needed to attain the desired outcomes.

Verbal and written communications are an integral part of direct care activities. How nursing diagnoses enhance the transfer of information about a client's condition and nursing care needs will be a second topic. Examples will demonstrate that diagnoses organize thoughts for purposes of communication.

A third topic, discharge planning, builds on the understanding of nursing diagnosis in nursing process and in communication. The process of care planning is taken beyond a daily activity to planning of continuity between settings and care providers. Again, examples will illustrate how nursing diagnoses are the basis for making and communicating discharge plans. A fourth topic, resource allocation, will include a consideration of the cost of nursing process and how a nurse's time is allocated on the basis of the decisions made about client's diagnoses and their treatment.

Diagnosis and the nurse's legal responsibilities and risks are interrelated. We shall consider a way in which diagnostic judgments might enter into cases of alleged professional negligence. By a case example it will be made clear that diagnostic judgments are a "duty" in the legal sense; not diagnosing can be as serious as misdiagnosing. This will lead us to the last topic of this chapter, who should diagnose.

NURSING DIAGNOSIS IN NURSING PROCESS

As currently conceived, nursing process is a problem identification and problem-solving approach to client care. It is the way in which a helping relationship, characterized by knowledge, reason, and caring is established. The art of caring for human beings involves the application of clinical judgment, nursing science, intuition, empathy, and technical skills. Structurally, nursing process is adapted from the scientific approach to solving problems; the knowledge and judgment used identifies the process as nursing.

Previous chapters have emphasized the problem-identification phase of nursing process. We have seen that the diagnostic process is used in this phase to identify problems if any are present, and label these problems with nursing diagnoses. *When a sufficient understanding of the client's health problems is gained, a nurse shifts from a diagnostic to a problem-solving process.*

Within the problem-solving phase of nursing process, outcomes are projected, plans for reaching the outcomes are determined, actions are implemented, and progress is evaluated. The components of problem identification and problem solving can be summarized as follows:

  I *Problem identification using diagnostic process*
   A Data collection
   B Diagnostic judgment
   C Diagnostic labeling of actual and potential problems
 II *Problem solving using problem-solving process*
   A Outcome projection
   B Care planning
   C Intervention
   D Outcome evaluation

The elegance of this approach lies in its broad applicability to reasoning in any domain. Yet clearly the skeletal structure needs to be clothed. Nursing process becomes a process of nursing when the above components are attired in *values, concepts,* and *standards* of nursing.

Guiding Values

The way problem identification and problem solving are carried out depends on a nurse's values and beliefs about human nature and helping. Some nurses believe that clients should diagnose their own problems. Others advocate having the nurse act as diagnostician and expert decision maker. Neither approach is applicable to *all* nursing situations. This will become evident as we examine two extremes.

At one extreme a nurse may believe that a client comes to a health care provider for help. What is sought is clinical expertise in the identification and solution of health problems or potential problems the client cannot identify and solve. The nurse serves the client as resource and expert. Strategies for implementing nursing process require that the nurse collect data, diagnose, and intervene. The client provides information and then things are done to improve his or her health.

This belief system and strategy for using nursing process are useful if the client is unconscious or feels too weak to participate; but if applied to all clients and situations this becomes an authoritarian approach.

At the opposite extreme is the position that all nurse-client interactions should promote growth toward a realization of human potential. The nursing role is "helper, assistant, and colleague in a cooperative search" for health (Combs, Avila, and Purkey, 1971, p. 214).

The second philosophy leads to a strategy in which a client is considered the expert in assessing situations, diagnosing problems, and arriving at effective solutions. Nurses operating under this philosophy accept responsibility for creating conditions in which the client carries out these activities, not for identifying problems and solutions. This procedure is similar to the problem-solving method of social work practice discussed earlier.

This approach to nursing process requires that the client have both energy and inclination to develop insight into problems and to engage in problem solving. It is applicable in situations in which change in the client's perceptions and behavior has to occur in order to facilitate healthy functional patterns. The nurse retains responsibility for labeling health problems the client identifies. The strategy associated with this form of helping requires expert diagnostic and problem-solving skills because conditions must be created in which the client develops insight, considers options, and makes choices.

Values that guide nurses' decisions and actions within nursing process are derived from their philosophical beliefs about human beings and human interaction. One particular set of professional values is in the area of ethics. These values, as will be seen in the section on standards, are expressed in a code of ethics that guide professional conduct.

Guiding Concepts and Theory

Problem identification and problem solving are guided by a set of *abstract concepts* and *practice theory*. The abstract concepts provide a way of thinking about the following:

1 The health problems that are of concern to nurses
2 The kinds of solutions (outcomes) sought
3 The types of interventions to be used to attain outcomes

This triad will be recognized, from the discussion in Chapter 3, as a framework for nursing. Suppose, for instance, that actual and potential self-care deficits were the focus of concern. The diagnosis nutritional deficit/food selection would be thought of as a discrepancy between self-care agency and self-care demand. An educative and supportive system of care would be designed to assist the client in learning about food selection (Orem, 1980).

A conceptual framework is necessary to guide thinking. Within the self-care agency framework a nurse would think of problem identification as identification of self-care agency deficits. Problem solving would focus on the design of a nursing system of care. Goals, or outcomes, would be expressed in terms of independent self-care management. Other frameworks, such as the adaptation, life process, or behavioral systems previously discussed, provide different concepts to guide nursing process.

Practice theories, facts, and principles are the body of knowledge within nursing science. Recall the discussion of deriving meaning from cues in Chapter 7 (simple, inferential, and diagnostic meaning) and the discussion of etiological factors that describe the probable causes of a problem. The knowledge used to derive meaning from cues, make diagnoses, and identify probable causes rests on practice theory learned in the classroom, from books, and from experience. Similarly the knowledge to predict that certain nursing actions will resolve certain nursing diagnoses is based on practice theories. For example, does providing information about what is going to happen during the surgical experience reduce fear of the experience? Practice theory suggests it does (if fear is due to insufficient information), and this theory is the basis for nursing intervention. Why would you say that taking in insufficient fluids and a low-roughage diet would contribute to constipation? What are the arguments for a causal relationship between fluids, diet, and constipation? You have just stated a practice theory!

Guiding Standards

A profession derives its authority to practice from society. In return it has a responsibility to be mindful of the public trust. Standards are developed by a profession to guide and evaluate practice and demonstrate accountability to society. Two types of standards are relevant to nursing process:

1 Standards for nursing process that decribe areas of professional accountability to consumers of nursing
2 Standards for conduct in nurse-client relationships

Standards represent a consensus of the profession and are published by the professional organization, the American Nurses' Association (ANA). Practice standards and the assurance of quality care is relatively new; standards for conduct expressed in a code of ethics are not.

Standards for Practice   Traditionally, the quality of practice has been monitored by colleagues and state licensing boards. In recent years public pressure for assurance that quality care is being delivered has prompted professions to develop standards of practice. In 1973 the Congress on Practice of the ANA published basic standards for professional nursing practice in any setting. These may be seen in Table 9–1. Since that time other councils and specialty groups have published their specific standards using the original standards as a model. The question may be asked: Why are standards important and what do they have to do with nursing diagnosis?

Standards are valued and achievable criteria for nursing performance, against which actual performance can be judged (Bloch, 1977). For example, suppose

TABLE 9-1
AMERICAN NURSES' ASSOCIATION STANDARDS OF NURSING PRACTICE

Standard I
The collection of data about the health status of the client/patient is systematic and continuous. The data are accessible, communicated, and recorded.
Standard II
Nursing diagnoses are derived from health status data.
Standard III
The plan of nursing care includes goals derived from the nursing diagnoses.
Standard IV
The plan of nursing care includes priorities and the prescribed nursing approaches or measures to achieve the goals derived from the nursing diagnoses.
Standard V
Nursing actions provide for client/patient participation in health promotion, maintenance, and restoration.
Standard VI
Nursing actions assist the client/patient to maximize his health capabilities.
Standard VII
The client's/patient's progress or lack of progress toward goal achievement is determined by the client/patient and the nurse.
Standard VIII
The client's/patient's progress or lack of progress toward goal achievement directs reassessment, reordering of priorities, new goal setting, and revision of the plan of nursing care.

Source: American Nurses' Association (1973).

a registered nurse wishes to know whether the way he or she practices is at least satisfactory. A comparison between personal practice and the national standards for practice could be made. Or suppose a nursing student wants to evaluate the progress he or she is making toward professionally accepted nursing standards. The student could make the same comparison, knowing that by the time of graduation the standards should be met.

Standard II is of particular interest in this discussion. It states that nursing diagnoses are derived from health status data. The fact that this standard exists means that nurses have stated a criterion for satisfactory professional practice in the area of nursing diagnosis. Thus consumers can expect nursing diagnoses to be made if they are getting an acceptable quality of care. *Professional nurses have a responsibility to ensure that standards of care are met for clients, since many cannot ensure this for themselves.*

Problem identification and problem solving, nursing process, and standards of practice have many similarities. The resemblance is evident in the comparisons presented in Table 9–2. The *collection of health status data* (Standard I) is referred to as assessment in the nursing process. In problem solving, it is referred to as observation and data collection. *Nursing diagnosis* is specified in both the standards (Standard II) and nursing process; it is synonymous with problem identification. The *nursing plan* is described more specifically in the standards than in nursing process, but is the same as designing methods and stating goals and outcomes in the problem-solving model.

Clearly, both the standards and nursing process are similar and both are based on problem identification and problem solving. It is well to appreciate

TABLE 9-2
COMPARISON OF NURSING STANDARDS, NURSING PROCESS, AND THE PROBLEM-SOLVING MODEL

Nursing standards*	Nursing process	Problem-solving model
Collection of health status data (I)	Assessment	Observation, data collection
Nursing diagnosis (II)	Diagnosis	Problem identification
Plan, goals (III)		
Priorities (IV)	Outcome projection	Problem solving
Client/patient participation (V)	Planning	(methods, goals, outcomes)
Actions (VI)	Implementation (intervention)	Problem-solving actions
Progress determination (VII)	Evaluation	Evaluation
Reassessment; revision (VIII)		

*Roman numerals refer to particular standards listed in full in Table 9-1.

these similarities and not to think three different things are being referred to when the different labels are encountered.

To supplement the general process standards the ANA Councils and the specialty organizations, such as the Neuroscience Nursing Association, are currently writing standards for nursing diagnoses. Discussion and examples of these specific standards will be included in the next chapter in the section on assurance of quality care.

Ethical Standards   Standards for ethical conduct are presented in Table 9–3; they are called the *Code of Ethics* for professional practice. They represent areas of *moral accountability* to the consumer of nursing. Standards of this type are monitored by colleagues and professional organizations. State nurses' associations are the disciplinary body if members violate the code.

The interpretative statements that accompany the Code (ANA, 1985) are quite explicit in items 4 and 6, which relate to nursing diagnosis. The major

TABLE 9-3
AMERICAN NURSES' ASSOCIATION CODE OF ETHICS

1. The nurse provides services with respect for human dignity and the uniqueness of the client, unrestricted by considerations of social or economic status, personal attributes, or the nature of health problems.
2. The nurse safeguards the client's right to privacy by judiciously protecting information of a confidential nature.
3. The nurse acts to safeguard the client and the public when health care and safety are affected by the incompetent, unethical, or illegal practice of any person.
4. The nurse assumes responsibility and accountability for individual nursing judgments and actions.
5. The nurse maintains competence in nursing.
6. The nurse exercises informed judgment and uses individual competence and qualifications as criteria in seeking consultation, accepting responsibilities, and delegating nursing activities to others.
7. The nurse participates in activities that contribute to the ongoing development of the profession's body of knowledge.
8. The nurse participates in the profession's efforts to implement and improve standards of nursing.
9. The nurse participates in the profession's efforts to establish and maintain conditions of employment conducive to high quality nursing care.
10. The nurse participates in the profession's effort to protect the public from misinformation and misrepresentation and to maintain the integrity of nursing.
11. The nurse collaborates with members of the health professions and other citizens in promoting community and national efforts to meet the health needs of the public.

Source: Reprinted with permission: American Nurses' Association (1985). *Code for nurses with interpretive statements.* Kansas City: MO.

points regarding ethical/moral responsibility are excerpted in the following (italics are the author's):

1 The *regulation and control of nursing practice by nurses* demand that individual practitioners of professional nursing must bear primary *responsibility* for the nursing care clients receive and must be *individually accountable for their own practice.*

2 Nursing obligations are reflected in the ANA publications *Nursing: A Social Policy Statement* (1980) and *Standards of Nursing Practice* (1975). (See Chapter 2 and Table 9–1.)

3 In order to be *accountable,* nurses act under a code of ethical conduct that is grounded in the moral principles of *fidelity and respect for the dignity, worth, and self-determination of clients.*

4 Nurses are *accountable for judgments made and actions* taken in the course of nursing practice. *Neither physician's orders nor the employing agency's policies relieve the nurse of accountability for actions taken and judgments made.*

5 Inasmuch as the nurse is responsible for the continuous care of patients in health care settings, the nurse is frequently called upon to carry out components of care delegated by other health professionals as part of the client's treatment regimen. The nurse *should not accept these interdependent functions if they are so extensive as to prevent the nurse from fulfilling the responsibility to provide appropriate nursing care to clients.* (ANA, 1985, pp. 7–11.)

Beliefs about helping relationships, concepts, theories, and standards guide the use of nursing process and its component, nursing diagnosis. Previous chapters have demonstrated how diagnostic categories are used in problem identification. In the following sections the relevance of nursing diagnoses to care delivery will become clear. The objective will not be an in-depth discussion of problem-solving activities; rather the emphasis will be on how to use nursing diagnoses in these activities.

NURSING DIAGNOSIS IN CARE PLANNING

The nurse's desire to change the course of events gives nursing care planning its momentum. A health problem may have dire consequence if left to run its course. It also may cause great discomfort even if natural resolution occurs. Nurses attempt to alter these possibilities by thinking ahead, making decisions, and formulating nursing care plans.

Once the client's health problems and contributing factors are recognized and labeled as nursing diagnoses, responsibility for treatment arises and decisions are required. The decisions to be made in the treatment of any nursing diagnosis are:

1 What are the desired outcomes?
2 What plan of nursing care is needed to reach the outcomes?

3 After implementation of nursing care, were the desired outcomes actually reached?

Nursing diagnosis is merely an intellectual exercise unless used in making these therapeutic judgments.

Let us consider the way nursing diagnoses can help in decision making. During the discussion the nurse will be viewed as the decision maker. If the process is understood and practiced, the important ideas can then be modified for application to situations in which clients are guided to do their own decision making and planning. The first step is to decide what health outcome is desired and attainable.

Projected Outcomes

Suppose you wish to be in San Francisco on Tuesday to meet a friend. Deciding this before starting a trip increases the probability that you will get there. Otherwise, on Tuesday you may be in Louisiana. This failure to specify what outcome is desired can produce inconvenience, additional cost, distress, and delay.

The reasoning is similar in nursing. Being in San Francisco on Tuesday would be called the desired outcome. In health care an *outcome* is a valued health state, condition, or behavior exhibited by a client. It may be, for example, a client's verbalized intention to take some particular health-promoting action, or it may be a behavior or condition observed by a nurse.

Other, similar terms are in use, such as *objectives* and *goals. Outcomes* is synonymous with *behavioral objective;* both specify observable behaviors of the client. Goals are usually broader statements that require further specification. Measurable outcomes that indicate goal attainment have to be identified.

Adding the term *projected*—projected outcome—means that a prediction, or forecast, of a future behavior has been made. Outcomes are projected in order to guide decisions about care; later they are measured to evaluate the effectiveness of the care that has been given. *Projecting outcomes permits the nurse to know when the problem is resolved.*

Outcomes are projected before nursing actions are planned or carried out. There are two reasons for this:

1 The health problem describes the present health state of the client; the projected outcome describes the desired health state. When the discrepancy between present and desired state is consciously examined, the treatment focus becomes evident and nursing actions can be considered. The actions most likely to lead to desired outcomes are selected and implemented.

2 Outcomes precede plans and actions because they are the basis for deciding when actions should cease. When outcomes are attained the client is discharged from care. During implementation of the nursing plan, projected outcomes are used to evaluate daily progress toward attainment.

Of what relevance to outcome projection is a nursing diagnosis? Without a diagnosis that describes the health problem it would be difficult even to attempt to specify outcomes. Projected outcomes describe the state of a client after, or at some stage of, problem resolution. Thus, the health problem is the basis for outcome projection.

Consider an example of a hospitalized client:

> Mr. Jones is a 25-year-old with paralysis of the lower half of his body as a result of a car accident in which his spinal cord was severely damaged. A number of risk factors predispose him to reduced circulation to tissues over the bony prominences of his body. The nursing diagnosis was potential skin breakdown.

Given this diagnosis, what desired outcome of nursing care would you wish to observe at the time of the client's discharge from the acute care setting? Obviously the valued outcome is *skin intact at discharge.* Notice what has occurred. The diagnosis of potential skin breakdown was made, and then the reverse of breakdown, intact skin, was stated as the desired outcome of nursing care.

Converting the diagnosis into a desired health state is a quick method for projecting outcomes. The critical signs and symptoms that define a diagnosis are useful in the transformation. Logically, their opposites define the resolution of the problem. Even positive changes in symptoms would indicate progress toward problem resolution. The "rule" to remember is:

Outcomes are derived from the problem statement which is a part of the nursing diagnosis.

Consider another problem. A client with heart failure is unable to bathe; whenever she tries, shortness of breath and fatigue occur. The nursing diagnosis is self-bathing deficit, level II (requires assistance) and the probable cause is decreased activity tolerance. Mentally transforming the problem into a desired functional state permits outcome projection. In this case the outcome would be self-bathing.[1]

Notice that outcomes in the previous examples are *stated concisely and definitely.* Specificity is necessary to guide planning; vague words and statements make it difficult to know exactly where one is going. Furthermore, only with specific outcomes does one know when the nursing goal has been reached. For example, "good skin color" or "good knowledge of . . ." are difficult to measure. How is "good" to be recognized?

Consider the following diagnoses and outcomes; which of these are useful for planning care and evaluating progress (diagnoses are written in the problem/etiological factor format)?

---

[1] The diagnostic category of self-bathing/hygiene deficit has four levels. These levels (Chapter 5) can be used to state progress toward independence.

1 Exogenous obesity/caloric intake—energy expenditure imbalance
Outcome: weight loss 10 pounds; 5-week visit
2 Ineffective airway clearance/decreased energy
Outcome: breath (lung) sounds clear; day 2
3 Low mother-infant bonding/separation
Outcome: parental attachment behaviors present; 3-week visit

In the above examples, numbers 1 and 2 are measurable outcomes that can be used in planning care and evaluating the effectiveness of nursing intervention. The third statement is too broad. What attachment behaviors are to be present? What should be expected in 3 weeks?

Value-Laden Decisions Outcomes are value decisions. In the example above it can be inferred that having intact skin and bathing independently are highly valued by most people. The arguments are numerous: (1) bathing removes dirt, dead skin, and secretions; (2) intact skin prevents infection; and (3) independence is "better" than dependence. Most adults probably would agree. Yet in essence writing an outcome is stating a personal value—the profession's value or a social value. The desirability of intact skin would raise little if any controversy, but with many other diagnoses the situation is not as clear.

The client has the right to choose outcomes. In their enthusiasm to promote health, nurses can easily unconsciously impose their own personal or social values on others. Outcomes for problems related to cognition, beliefs, self-perception, or relationships require choices that are best made by the client or in collaboration with the client. *Philosophically, if the nurse believes clients should participate in actions to solve their problems, it follows that clients must be involved in deciding outcomes. From a practical perspective, participation in setting outcomes increases motivation toward achieving those outcomes.*

In many instances the client says what he or she wishes remedied; listening can enable the nurse to know what that is. On the other hand, clients may not know what outcomes are possible. Additionally, they may have difficulty coping with an event or may be in conflict about making a choice. Their ability to use their problem-solving capacities may be lowered. In these situations a nurse may suggest alternatives.

A 65-year-old woman had a nursing diagnosis of social isolation related to altered body image and fear of rejection. After having a leg amputation and being fitted with an artificial limb, she stayed in her apartment. She told most close friends that she was unable to have visitors and avoided other tenants. The desired outcome for the health problem was: resumes previous level of social relationships.

The nurse took an indirect approach because of the high degree of stress the woman was experiencing. Yet the client was given an opportunity to reject the outcome. In essence, here is how the diagnosis and projected outcome were translated to the client: "You mentioned before that you are trying to avoid your friends because you think they would be disgusted by someone with a leg off. Could we think about how they would react and how you could handle this if you did decide to invite them?"

The nurse paused for the client's reactions to the subtly introduced outcome of inviting friends to her apartment. The client looked down and said, "I do miss having people in." The nurse interpreted the statement as a wish to resume previous social contacts. At that time the client could not more directly agree to the outcome because of her fear of rejection by friends.

Some have advocated written, signed contracts for outcomes. It has been demonstrated that contracts with clients have some effect on compliance with needed behavior changes, such as dieting. But contracts produce a formalism in the nurse-client relationship that many nurses reject.

In order to introduce the idea of projecting outcomes by using nursing diagnoses, the concept of problem resolution has been somewhat oversimplified. Transforming indicators of a problem (signs and symptoms) to positive health behaviors is easier to do "in the head" than "in the world of reality." The final resolution of a client's health problem may require steps rather than one leap.

If short-term resolution of a diagnosis is not possible, outcomes representing progress toward resolution are stated. For example, outcomes may be projected for accomplishment by the date of hospital discharge *and* for 3 months, 6 months, or longer if the client is under continuing care.

Time, resources, and costs are factors to be considered in projecting outcomes. Before one can specify individualized outcomes within a realistic time frame for outcome attainment one must know what interventions will be used. What is done (nursing and client actions) influences the client's progress toward resolution of the health problem. Yet what is done is influenced by clients' choices, capabilities, and resources.

Interventions

Thinking of ideal outcomes such as being in San Francisco on Tuesday motivates a person to find a way of getting there. Realistically, the traveler would have to consider wardrobe, packing, transportation schedules, and finances. With these considerations in mind, outcome attainment may be set for Tuesday 3 years hence! Similarly, in care planning the current state of the client and highly valued outcome are considered first, and then the way of getting "from here to there."

Interventions are the actions taken to help the client move from a present state to the state described in the projected outcomes. They may involve doing for, doing with, or enabling a client to do something to influence or resolve the health problem. The type of intervention selected depends on the nursing diagnosis and outcomes. As Figure 9–1 shows, specific interventions for individual clients depend on the choices, capabilities, and resources of the client, the creativity of the nurse, and research findings.

FIGURE 9-1
From diagnosis to outcome.

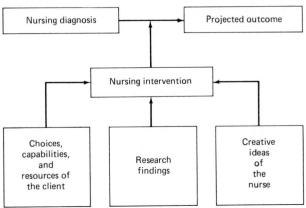

Focus for Interventions   A nursing diagnosis provides a focus for thinking about what interventions may resolve a problem. The alternative approach would be to treat isolated or unorganized signs and symptoms such as frequent crying spells, difficulty in breathing, or inability to bathe self. Interventions based on symptoms may help for the moment but rarely resolve the underlying problem. If the truth of this last statement is not apparent, try to identify interventions by using the above signs and symptoms as a focus. Contrast those interventions with the ones you would use for the diagnoses stated in the following paragraph.

Using a diagnosis and projected outcome as a focus increases the probability of selecting effective nursing interventions. For example, each of the previously listed signs (crying spells, difficult breathing, and inability to bathe) was investigated and clustered with other signs and symptoms. The problem and etiology were formulated in each case and labeled as follows: (1) the crying client's diagnosis was ineffective coping/perceived incompetence (parenting); (2) ineffective airway clearance/thick secretions was the statement formulated for the client with dyspnea; and (3) self-bathing deficit (level III)/activity intolerance suggested many more specific interventions than did the sign *inability to bathe self.* In the third situation, bathing the client might solve the immediate need, but helping the client to increase activity tolerance gets at the essence of the problem.

Trial and error is a common approach if isolated signs and symptoms are used as a focus for care planning. This method is wasteful of nursing time. It also can prolong the client's discomfort, allow problems to become more severe, and lead to adverse effects. Trial and error is used either because meaning has not been derived from the unclustered signs and symptoms or because possible meanings have not been validated. Think of the multiple meanings of the sign *crying*. Each is associated with a different intervention.

Diagnoses are concepts from which a knowledgeable nurse can revive meaning. Consider the diagnosis *ineffective airway clearance/thick secretions*. Biopsychosocial theories and research about airway obstruction, secretions, and client responses can be used as a framework to determine an approach to care. Specifically, theories provide help in understanding a problem, designing possible interventions, and calculating when intervention may be effective. Thus identifying problems facilitates memory or textbook search for theory. This in turn provides meaning and ideas that guide care-planning decisions.

Focusing on the nursing diagnosis and on the available theoretical knowledge is similar to what occurred in the generation of diagnostic hypotheses during problem identification. The right problem space opened up multiple possibilities. In problem solving, this occurs when a problem space in memory or a textbook index is searched for alternative interventions.

Although on the surface a routine intervention may appear sufficient, clients deserve thoughtful planning of their care. This requires *thinking of alternative methods, their consequences, and the probability that they will be effective* for the particular client and situation.

Generating Alternative Interventions   When searching textbooks or memory stores for possible interventions, keep the problem in mind but *focus on the etiological or related factors.* If the probable cause can be influenced, the problematic health pattern should change.

Consider first a basic example: E (etiological factor) is the probable reason the P (problem) exists. If E is removed, the prediction is that P will be resolved. Intervention is directed primarily at E.

This abstract reasoning is applicable to clinical situations. Recall the 65-year-old woman whose diagnosis was social isolation/altered body image. After leg amputation she learned to use an artificial limb but continued to stay in her apartment and allowed no friends to visit. Before the amputation she went shopping, had friends in for coffee, and was socially active in her church. The outcome desired by the client and nurse was *resumes previous level of social relationships.* What shall be the focus of intervention for the visiting nurse?

Just recommending that the client socialize has a low probability of success. The problem alone does not offer a focus for generating interventions. If body image alteration is a major contributing factor, *influencing body image* may increase socialization. *Etiological factors identified in the diagnosis are the focus of intervention.* If these can be changed, the problem should begin to resolve.

Another example should help clarify the need to *focus on etiological factors in generating alternative interventions.* A second client also had alteration in socialization but the etiological factor was impaired mobility. This 65-year-old woman had been, as she described it, "a social butterfly," staying in the house was "confining"; she was becoming despondent. Visiting friends and going to holiday celebrations and the theater were important to her, yet the permanent peripheral vascular changes caused by diabetes impaired her mobility for stair climbing and walking distances.

The intervention for this client was entirely different, *although the problem specified in the nursing diagnosis was the same.* The focus for thinking about a solution was the etiological factor, impaired mobility. The nurse generated alternative interventions. Keeping these in the back of her mind, she encouraged the client to think of ways to circumvent the mobility impairment. The choice was to rent a wheelchair for steps (ramps) and distances; friends gladly helped. The visiting nurse arranged for the chair, and the client was delighted that they had found a way for her to resume social activities.

In these examples the alternatives for intervention were rather clear-cut. When more complex situations are encountered, the nurse must stop and think through the situation. The first step in deciding on an intervention is to answer the question, What is the therapeutic problem?

A *therapeutic problem* exists if interventions to attain outcomes either have a low degree of success; are unknown; or, while known, have been unsuccessful in the client's particular kind of situation. Aptly named, this is the *wicked decision problem.*

The nurse must define the therapeutic problem: Is it a behavioral change that is needed? Is it conflict resolution? Are there other ways of looking at the therapeutic problem? Keep etiological factor(s) and outcome in mind and then think of offbeat or "far-out" ideas; Osbourne (1963) and Gordon (1961) suggest methods such as this to increase creative thinking. Logical analysis is applied only *after* the ideas are generated.

Individualizing Interventions   During the process of generating alternative interventions, the nurse thinks about the contributing factors and the particular client and situation. Consideration of these factors individualizes interventions. *Individualizing interventions increases treatment success rate.*

The areas of information in which data are needed to individualize care are:

1 *Personal client factors* The client, whether an individual, family, or community, has unique characteristics. These influence intervention. If interventions are being considered for an individual, then age, developmental stage, gender, culture, religion, family structure, and other personal characteristics are considered. Some of these are equally applicable in family or community intervention. In some instances further data collection may be necessary.

2 *Client's perception* The client may associate various causal factors with his or her problem even though objectively they are unrelated. Unless correction of misperceptions and faulty associations about the cause of a problem is built into the intervention plan, intervention may fail because the client considers it unrelated and therefore meaningless.

3 *Current level of compensation* The client may have mobilized some strengths, defenses, or resources to compensate for the problem. Data about compensation help the nurse decide about the degree of nursing assistance required and also allow recognition of the client's strengths. Diagnoses can be classified as compensated (only monitoring is necessary), partially compensated (some nursing assistance is needed), or uncompensated (the client requires full nursing assistance).

4 *Problem magnitude and urgency* The acuity or severity of a problem influence the type and timing of intervention. Certain conditions are urgent and intervention must be immediate. These are health problems that can result in harm to the client or others.

As an example, a client who is having surgery in 24 hours and who is near panic and not coping effectively requires immediate intervention. Either the surgery has to be cancelled or the anxiety has to be reduced quickly. With diagnoses such as potential for injury or potential for violence, immediate reduction of risk factors is needed.

5 *Extended effects* Interventions have the potential for extended effects. Indirectly or directly they can influence members of the client's family, work group, or social circle. For example, what effects will a major diet change have on the other household members? Forethought is needed when interventions are planned, so that no additional problems will be created by their extended effects.

Interactions among nursing diagnoses should also be considered in planning intervention. If treatment for one problem is planned in isolation, there can be extended effects on coexisting problems. As an example, the usual treatment for one diagnosis may be contraindicated when another nursing diagnosis is present. Similarly the treatment for a nursing diagnosis may negatively or positively influence a disease or a medical treatment; the reverse can also occur. *Interactions among all diagnoses and all treatments have to be taken into account in decision making.*

6 *Cost-benefit factors* Consequences of treatments are a consideration in decision making. Each intervention has a "price." The costs can be financial, social, or psychological. *Benefits* are the advantages that accompany (or are expected to result from) the outcomes of treatment in terms of (1) optimum health and well-being or (2) an immediate or long-term life goal of the client. Possible benefits of the results of various interventions being considered are weighed against possible costs.

One dimension of cost-benefit considerations is psychological or social cost related to functional benefit. Before recommending or guiding clients to change their behavior patterns, consider the payoff. Be knowledgeable about the predicted benefits of change so that clients can weigh alternatives and make informed choices. Changing behavioral patterns is one of the most difficult things for people to do, especially during adulthood.

A client may value the expected outcome as a benefit but feel the cost (e.g., stopping smoking or giving up desired foods) is too high. In this situation the nurse and client should try to find a way to reduce the cost of the intervention. Perhaps a less valued outcome (e.g., switching to low-tar cigarettes) is all that can be accomplished at present. It may also be possible to increase the client's value rating of the beneficial outcome enough that the price will be paid.

A second dimension of the cost-benefit factor is financial cost related to the functional benefit of the expected outcome. Given today's soaring health care costs, if two alternative interventions for a diagnosis result in the same beneficial effect, choose the less expensive. *Before ordering consultations, equipment, or services for the treatment of the problem, consider whether the benefit is worth the cost.* Consumers are currently demanding that cost-benefit ratios be considered in treatment planning.

Predicting Effectiveness of Interventions   Consideration of the six factors just discussed should narrow down the treatment alternatives for a particular client's nursing diagnosis. The remaining alternatives have to be subjected to final scrutiny. The one that has the greatest probability of being effective is chosen.

The *predicted effectiveness* of an intervention is the probability that it will lead to the projected outcome. For example, suppose the probability that intervention A will lead to outcome C is 60 percent, whereas the probability that intervention B will produce outcome C is 90 percent. If A and B "cost" the same, B will be chosen.

Predicted effectiveness takes into account all of the six previously mentioned factors that are relevant to the diagnosis. Thus the predicted effectiveness is a prediction about individualized interventions for a particular client and situation. Obviously, the intervention with the highest probability of being effective is chosen and implemented.

Priority Setting   A client may have multiple diagnoses, not all of which can or should be treated at the time they are identified. Priorities for treatment depend on (1) the urgency of the problem, (2) the nature of the treatment indicated, and (3) the interactions among diagnoses.

Nursing diagnoses that if untreated could result in harm to the client or others have the highest priority for treatment. Examples include potential for violence, potential for trauma, and ineffective airway clearance. In these examples the priority is clear. In many other instances thorough knowledge of the client and situation is necessary before the nurse can be sure what patient conditions *are* urgent.

The type of treatment that is indicated also helps determine priorities in particular cases. If a client is physiologically unstable, as might commonly be the situation in an intensive care unit, treatment of diagnoses requiring learning of behavioral changes would not be given a high priority. Intensive care units are not designed for treating knowledge deficits about postdischarge health management; nor is an emergency room designed for treatment of noncompliance with a weight reduction program. *Consideration has to be given to the cost of keeping a client in an expensive nursing care setting for a problem that can be treated in a less expensive setting.*

Another factor that influences priority setting is the possibility of interactions among diagnoses. Suppose a 10-year-old client has the following diagnoses: chronic exogenous obesity/caloric intake-activity imbalance; dysfunctional grieving/loss of parent; and compromised family coping. Should priorities be set, and if so, how?

Although the coping and grieving problems are not judged to be probable causes of obesity, they are two problems that potentially can interact. Improved family coping may provide greater support to the child and assist in resolving the grief process. When these problems begin to improve, the child can be helped to lose weight, ideally with family support. Priority setting enhances treatment when the client has multiple problems. *Yet priority setting would be impossible without clearly identifying the nursing diagnoses.*

Implementation and Evaluation   After decisions about interventions and priorities are made, the treatment plan is begun. During implementation of the plan, continued assessment provides feedback that is used to evaluate prior diagnostic judgments and treatment decisions. Assessing the client's progress toward the projected outcomes enables the nurse to evaluate the effectiveness of the interventions. Progress toward outcomes is evaluated during the course of nursing intervention by *problem-focused assessment* as described in Chapter 6. Data collected about the status of the problem are the basis for evaluative judgments. If the intervention is effective, the signs and symptoms used to diagnose the problem should be changing.

At this point we may summarize the use of diagnoses in problem identification and problem solving. The nurse's first concern is to identify the client's health problems and apply diagnostic labels. Then use of a systematic problem-solving process takes precedence. During this problem-solving phase of the nursing process, diagnoses are the bases for projecting desired outcomes, deciding on interventions by which to attain the outcomes, implementing interventions, and evaluating the attainment of diagnosis-specific outcomes.

After one has completed this process of problem identification and problem solving, it appears in retrospect to have been a *sequence* of steps. In actuality, the entire set of activities is always in mind. *Each decision influences other decisions.* It is a matter of greatest importance to maintain open-mindedness about observations and new data that are collected during all phases of nursing process. Never be hesitant to consider new data and revise judgments; this open-mindedness is the key to handling uncertainties in clinical information.

NURSING PROCESS IN DISEASE-RELATED CARE

Nursing process is a problem-identification–problem-solving process. As such, it is adaptable to domains of problems other than nursing diagnoses; one domain is that described by medical disease. Although the subject of this book is nursing diagnoses, some consideration should be given to nurses' disease-related care activities and the clinical judgments upon which care is based.

The first judgment when a client is admitted is based on the quick-scan emergency assessment described in Chapter 6. This assessment differentiates between emergency and nonemergency situations. For example:

> Mr. F. was brought to the emergency room by ambulance after a fall. Head injury was obvious from his bleeding laceration, minimal spontaneous activity, and sluggish response to verbal communications. The situation was judged to be a medical emergency and a physician was immediately summoned.

Judgments about emergencies and the need for a particular health professional are continuously made in nursing. Although the need for medical evaluation was quite obvious in this case, frequently judgments are uncertain when clinical signs are ambiguous.

> Further physical assessment of Mr. F., a 45-year-old man in previous good health, involved the search for cues to his neurological status. The most likely possibility was intracranial bleeding from trauma. Signs observed signified moderate head injury (concussion).

A client from the emergency room with a history such as Mr. F.'s would require immediate assessment upon admission to an acute care unit and continued close observation. Judgments about the level of nursing care required are based on a nurse's medical knowledge. Irrespective of whether or not physician's orders were written, Mr. F. would be observed for increased intracranial pressure, intracranial bleeding, associated spinal cord injury, other undetected injuries, and infection of his head laceration. These hypotheses would be generated from the cues present on admission and the medical diagnosis. Hypothesis testing would involve a search for cues defining these conditions.

> Two hours after admission Mr. F. had changes from baseline data collected at admission (decreased level of consciousness, no spontaneous motor activity, reaction only to strong stimuli, increased dilation and fixation of right pupil, and changes in vital signs).

The observed physical signs suggested the hypothesis of further intracranial bleeding and a subdural hematoma. Having generated this hypothesis, the nurse caring for Mr. F immediately called the physician and anticipated surgical intervention. Mr. F.'s physiological problems and the nurse's responses demonstrate similarities and differences between nursing diagnoses and disease-related nursing judgments:

1 *Similarities* Assessment or information collection, hypothesis generation, and hypothesis testing. (Only one set of cognitive behaviors need to be learned.)

2 *Differences* The kind of information collected and processed and the actions taken. (A body of knowledge in medical science and experience in its application is required.) The problem is referred.

When a hypothesis about disease progression or complications is supported, judgments are made to verbally inform the physician, note the information in the client's record, carry out or withhold treatments designated by existing physician's orders or nursing protocols, carry out palliative treatments based on nursing judgment, or execute a combination of these actions. In contrast, the main responsibility after *nursing diagnosis* is to plan and execute treatment and to facilitate treatment coordination by communication with other health care professionals.

Treatment Coordination

When a client has both nursing and medical diagnoses, treatment has to be coordinated. Otherwise interventions could conflict and outcomes might not be attained. Having regularly scheduled time for mutual sharing of information among the professionals involved in client care is ideal. Regular communication promotes understanding of each care provider's diagnostic judgments and treatment decisions. It increases the probability of integrated care and also promotes working relationships.

It is easy to understand the need for coordination. Yet implementation in certain settings requires ingenuity and initiative. Who shall take the initiative? In acute care settings, such as hospitals, nurses have 24-hour responsibility for implementing client's medical and nursing treatments and for seeing their families. Accordingly, nurses need to be aware of the total care plan. To gain this overview, nursing staff may need to take the initiative to institute change in communication patterns. Care conferences between the client's primary nurse and physician could be scheduled.

Change takes time and is sometimes accomplished by small steps. Minimally, a front sheet on the client's chart could be used for the care providers from all professions to record their diagnoses. A perceived need for scheduled joint conferences might evolve from this beginning. If physicians and nurses have separate rounds on all clients, they could be combined. The methods employed to promote change have to be specific to a particular institution.

NURSING DIAGNOSIS AND COMMUNICATION

When more than one person is responsible for health care, communication is necessary. Actually, even in private practice, records of diagnoses and treatments have to be kept. In this section the relevance of nursing diagnoses to various types of written and verbal communication within and among professions will be examined. The problem oriented permanent record and the nursing care plan are important methods of communication and will be discussed in detail. It will be seen that nursing diagnoses provide a concise and organized means of communication.

Communicating one's diagnoses and interventions in writing has benefits, yet it is difficult to get health professionals to "do their charting." Perhaps an awareness of the benefits would increase the motivation to document:

1 Prevents memory strain and errors due to memory lapses
2 Encourages a person to organize their data, diagnostic judgments, and treatment decisions
3 Facilitates continuity and coordination of care when two or more people provide care
4 Provides a record in the event of alleged harm to a client
5 Permits research and reviews of care (quality assurance) that can lead to the improvement of care
6 Provides data for staffing, cost reimbursement, and health statistics

The costs in time and effort are minimal when compared with these benefits and the legal protection documentation provides.

Verbal Communication

Nurses use verbal communication in shift reports, informal discussions of client's health problems, formal case conferences, nursing rounds, and reports to supervisors. These are examples of nurses' communications with other nurses. During nurse-physician communication, a physician may inquire about a client's sleep pattern or nutritional pattern during hospitalization, or the nurse may initiate a verbal communication about a nursing diagnosis that will have an impact on medical treatment.

In all these kinds of communications, nursing diagnosis provides a succinct and clear mode of communication. Consider the following examples:

1 *Shift report* "Ms. K is ineffectively coping with the threat of impending surgery. I have . . ." [night nurse lists interventions and outcomes].
2 *Coffee break* "I'm really having trouble coming up with a way of dealing with Mr. G. He has a potential for fluid volume deficit and I can't get him to drink anything. I hate to see him have an I.V. [intravenous infusion]. Can you think of anything?"
3 *Case conference* "I've picked Mr. L because of his major problem that is common to so many of our clients. His diagnosis is self-care deficit due to left-sided neglect. We aren't treating this effectively and so I have done a review of the literature that may suggest some additional possibilities."
4 *Nursing rounds* "Mr. F. is a 45-year old construction worker; his medical problem is myocardial infarct, uncomplicated. Currently he has an independence-dependence conflict. The probable cause is the restriction of his activity and self-care. I am . . ." [states intervention].
5 *Report to supervisor (service director)* "I have one client with impaired home maintenance management/decreased activity tolerance. I taught her energy conservation techniques but I've decided she also needs a homemaker 2 days a week. Tomorrow I'll orient the homemaker. I also have two clients for

whom the referral states alterations in parenting. I'll see them tomorrow. The home health aide is implementing my plan for Ms. S. Her mobility has decreased and . . ."

6 *Nurse-physician* "I finally found out that Jamie's passive dependence is not due to fear but to parental overprotection. I'm helping his parents develop a plan for allowing independence. When you talk to the parents . . ."

The preceding communications are concise and to the point. Hesitation and confusion over a multiplicity of signs and symptoms are avoided. Data have been organized by use of nursing diagnoses.

Written Communication

In contrast to verbal communication, which relies on human recall and human interaction, written information takes on a quality of permanence. In the developed nations, important observations and decisions are nearly always recorded. One hour, one day, or years later others can read how an event was seen and interpreted.

In health care situations written communications provide a sequential record of the client's health status as well as care provider's diagnostic judgments, treatment plans, and actions. These records provide the means for continuity and coordination of plans across settings, care providers, and time. Written records not only preserve data; certain methods of recording also provide a means for checking thought processes.

Nurses and other care providers use various modes of written communication. Some are permanent records of the client's progress and others are working records that are summarized and discarded at intervals.

A permanent record, commonly referred to as the medical record or client's chart, is used in private, institutional, and community practice. Its main purpose is to provide continuity of care, but it also is used for research and teaching purposes. In addition, this record is used as evidence in legal proceedings. State laws require that a record of care provided to an individual or family be kept for a number of years.

Different chart formats are in use, particularly for nursing recordings. Some institutions separate medical and nursing notes within a chart. Others use one section for all health care providers' histories, examinations, progress notes, and treatment orders.

Historically nurses communicated important observations and actions in long paragraphs. Adding to the record occurred at least three times a day, once on each work shift. Communications of certain observations were required: sleeping, eating, comfort, and a doctor's visit. Sometimes long dissertations were critically important and sometimes not. Little evidence existed that physicians or supervisors read nurses' notes, and after the client's discharge they were discarded. Understandably, this type of nurse's note has become nearly extinct. In addition, the nurse's judgments were to be carefully worded in the written record. Every student learned the cautious, conservative phrase "appears to be" in the first nursing course. These words were modestly applied to nurses' judgments—"appears to be bleeding," "appears to be uncomfortable," or even "appears to have expired."

In recent years judgment has been emphasized in nursing. Most importantly, *nurses* are beginning to believe their observations, diagnostic judgments, and treatment decisions are important. They diagnose and treat health problems within their scope of practice and communicate these in the permanent record.

Computer-Based Communication

It is predicted that most health care agencies will use computer-based clinical records by the mid-1990s. Currently a number of hospitals and community agencies have discarded paper records and all charting is entered into the computerized system. Printouts provide the nursing care and medical care plans for daily care; laboratory and other data are also entered into the computerized record. The computer provides a readily accessible system of information to guide daily care activities. When an entire hospital uses computerized records, the term hospital information system is used. The nursing portion of the system is called the nursing information system. More will be said about computerized systems in the next chapter. For now it will suffice to say this type of clinical record permits documentation and access to

1 Current nursing diagnoses and supporting data
2 Projected outcomes
3 Treatment orders and progress notes
4 Personal data about the client (age, next of kin, etc.)
5 Current medical diagnoses, treatment orders, lab tests, progress notes, and other health care professionals' treatment plans and notes
6 History of dysfunctional patterns and illnesses
7 Name of primary nurse and physician

A computerized system of clinical data recording produces a printout of the current nursing and medical plan of care to guide daily activities. Appendix I lists suggested components of a practice-based computerized system for nursing care delivery.

FORMATS FOR DOCUMENTATION

Each health care agency develops a specific format for documentation that is useful for their client population and setting. This section will review general formats that are in wide use; these include problem-oriented recording (POR) and the Kardex. The sections of the POR and Kardexes organized by nursing diagnosis-outcome-intervention contain similar elements to those used in a computerized system. Also, consideration will be given to the documentation of disease-related care.

Problem-Oriented Recording

In 1969, Lawrence Weed, a physician concerned about the poor quality of records, designed a format that organizes information around client problems. This format has been implemented in many care delivery settings. Interestingly, it was about the same time that many nurses began to think about their practice in terms of nursing diagnoses. Merging the two ideas permitted nurses to move easily into the new charting system.

Realizing that the content of records was usually inadequate and information difficult to find, Weed introduced the idea of a problem-oriented charting and indexing system. It is designed to facilitate care, teaching, and research. The structure has four parts:

1 *A problem list* This is a cumulative listing of client problems and potential problems providing a continually updated indexing system. All health care professionals list their diagnoses with a number, date of diagnosis, and date when resolved, on the master problem list. This list is found at the front of the chart. Nursing diagnoses (problem/etiological factors) are recorded on the master problem list and assigned the next consecutive number. (If other professionals do not wish to use this listing, only nursing diagnoses may appear on the list or it may be agreed that nurses copy the medical diagnosis from the progress sheets so that they may index their charting.) Problems that are of a very transitory nature should not be listed on the master problem list. An example of a problem list from a chart is contained in Table 9-4.

2 *A defined data base* The term *data base* refers to all the information about the client's health. The nursing component would include the nursing history and examination, including supporting data for nursing diagnoses.

TABLE 9-4
ADMISSION PROBLEM LIST FOR ONE CLIENT

Problem no.	Active problems	Date entered	Date problem inactive
1.	Diabetes mellitus	5/20	
2.	Hyperglycemia; acidosis	5/20	
3.	Exogenous obesity/activity-caloric intake imbalance	5/20	
4.	Potential for injury	5/20	
5.	Four-day history of not taking insulin	5/20	

3 *Initial and revised plans* This component includes all professionals' treatment plans, revisions in plans, and discharge plans.

4 *Progress notes* All professionals caring for the client chart their observations about the client's progress or lack of progress on sheets called progress notes. Each entry is labeled with the number of the diagnosis being addressed. Thus, to review the progress of problem resolution, one can go through the notes and read about the particular numbered problem.

Documentation: Admission Assessment The nursing history and examination are documented on progress sheets in the form illustrated in Appendix D. The process of recording data in this manner helps the clinician to think through the problems that have been identified. The objective is to be clear, concise, and complete. The documentation of an admission assessment has two purposes: (1) it provides a baseline to which changes can be compared and (2) it is a record of the health status of the client when admitted to the nurse's caseload. The latter is important from a legal perspective in the event of a malpractice suit against the health care agency or the nurse.

Conciseness and clarity in documentation are important. First, others may want to review the nursing assessment and, second, a nurse's time should not be wasted with wordy descriptions. Note how extraneous words are deleted in the examples of admission assessments in this text and in Appendix D. For example:

1. *Not concise* The patient says he has a dull, aching pain in his right knee when he walks to the bathroom or around the house.

2. *Concise* Reports dull aching pain in right knee when ambulating.

To assure clarity in documentation use quotes to signify client's words. This will distinguish verbal reports from a nurse's observation or inference:

1. *Concise but not clear* Husband gets angry and beats the kids when he gets drunk. Has essential hypertension, diagnosed in 1982. Work is stressful for him.

2. *Concise and clear* States "husband gets angry and beats the kids when he gets drunk." Reports "essential hypertension diagnosed in 1982." States work is "stressful."

Documentation of the nursing history and examination has to be complete. First, data on each functional pattern should be documented even if there are no problems. *If assessment is deferred in a pattern area, the reason should be stated concisely.* Second, it is not advisable to only record conclusions about important data; rather, all data should be documented. For example:

1 *Incomplete* Seems anxious about surgery.

2 *Complete* Restless, in and out of bed 5 times this morning; eyes darting about; startled response to noises; reports feeling "anxious" about the outcome of surgery, whether he "will ever go back to work."

Documentation: Nursing Diagnoses/Treatment Plans The problem-oriented recording system has a particular format for documenting diagnoses and treatments. The format is concise and permits organization of the products of clinical reasoning. The components are:

1 *The health problem (P)* As defined in Chapter 5.
2 *Subjective clinical data (S)* Client reports, as described in Chapter 6.
3 *Objective clinical data (O)* Nurse observations, as described in Chapter 6.
4 *Assessment (A)* Analysis and interpretation of reasons for the problem (etiological or related factors, as described in Chapter 5) and any factors related to the prognosis of the problem. Also include strengths of the client situation that would influence treatment plans.
5 *Plan (P)* The desired outcomes and the treatments to be carried out. (Some authors suggest adding a sixth component *(O)* for outcomes to the list; it seems useful to include all elements of nursing process and adapt the format to *SOAOP.*)

The formulation of nursing diagnoses has been discussed in other chapters. An example of documentation of one of the problems listed in Table 9-4 would be:

#4. Potential for injury

S: Reports reduced touch sensation in legs; minimizes bruise and scratch on legs; can't recall trauma; "they're nothing"; uses scatter rugs without nonskid padding; "At times I hate to wear my glasses around the house"; does not put lights on to cross hall to bathroom during the night; hates to arouse her dog.
   O: 3-cm bruise on left leg; scratches on both lower legs; diabetic neuropathy (see physician's notes); decreased sensitivity to touch.

What outcome(s) would be projected?

What would be the treatment plan for this diagnosis?

While the reader is thinking about these questions, it is important to point out that a treatment plan is written for each diagnosis. Plans always include items 1 and 2 below; depending on the diagnosis, item 3 may be included. If the diagnosis is not completely formulated, item 4 would be expected on a care plan:

1 Projected outcomes
2 Treatment orders
3 Patient education orders when indicated by the diagnosis
4 Collection of further diagnostic information

Projected outcomes clarify the behavior that will indicate resolution of the risk state (or in the case of actual problems, the resolution of the problem). These outcomes will be the criterion for judging the quality of care delivered. Thus, it is important that outcomes are realistic, clear, concise, and emphasize critical indicators of problem-resolution. For the previous client with potential for injury, the outcomes and treatment plan stated at admission were:

O: Outcome: Absence of leg injuries; states plans for implementing measures in home to prevent injury.

P: P_{Dx}: Observe degree of caution exercised.

P_{Tx}: Room-check for jutting objects, slippery floors; eyeglasses worn during ambulation; adequate lighting at all times when ambulating.

P_{Ed}: Potential for injury with sensory deficit to be explained. Teach precautions regarding ambulation, adequate vision, lighting, scatter rugs, slippery floors, jutting objects, ill-fitting shoes or boots, nail cutting.

The diagnostic plan (Dx) at admission was to collect further information about the degree of caution exercised by the client when ambulating in the hospital. In addition, plans for further data collection should always be included when the problem list includes uncategorized but potentially important signs, for example, problem no. 5 in Table 9-4 (4-day history of not taking insulin). Admission data may not be sufficient to specify etiological factors; this situation would also necessitate a plan for data collection.

The treatment plan (Tx) was designed to ensure safety during ambulation in the hospital and attain the stated outcome, absence of leg injury. While these interventions were being implemented, incidental teaching could be done. Yet, to attain the outcome *states plans for implementing measures in home to prevent injury,* an *educational plan* (Ed) was needed.

The P-SOAP (or SOAOP) format provides immediate feedback on cognitive processes. Contradictions can be seen. For example, one can check to see whether the subjective (S) and objective (O) data are sufficient to support the problem and etiology recorded. First, a cross-check with a manual of diagnostic category definitions may help. Second, the nurse can check to be certain that the outcome (O) projected is consistent with the problem and that the treatment plan is consistent with the etiological factors identified (or the risk factors of a potential problem). The checkpoints in Table 9-5 from the *Manual of Nursing Diagnosis* (Gordon, 1987) may be useful. Consider some examples of errors that occurred as nurses were learning to use nursing diagnoses and problem-oriented recording. Try to pick out the inconsistencies found in these three charts:

EXAMPLE 1

#1 Self-bathing deficit (level II)/extreme obesity-fear (falling)

S: Fears falling in shower; bathes self at sink daily but has difficulty reaching all body parts due to extreme obesity.

A: Has plans to lose weight.

TABLE 9-5

PROBLEM-ORIENTED RECORDING: GUIDELINES AND CHECKPOINTS

#____: Problem number and label

State clear, concise diagnostic label for the problem.

1. Check below that S and O contain sufficient supporting data (diagnostic criteria) for the problem.
2. If insufficient information available to label the problem, record the possible diagnoses being considered or major signs/symptoms; continue assessment.

S: Subjective data*

List pertinent diagnostic indicators from verbal reports of individual or family.

1. Record quotes when applicable.
2. Check for consistency with objective data. Attempt to resolve incongruities or inconsistencies in data before recording.

O: Objective data*

List pertinent diagnostic indicators from direct observation and examination of individual or family, observations of context or milieu, and observational reports of other care providers, if pertinent.

1. Check for measurement error, observer bias, and for consistency with subjective data. Attempt to resolve incongruities or inconsistencies in data before recording.

A: Assessment

State etiological or related factors contributing to the problem in #____.

1. Use clear, concise terms.
2. Check that S and O data provide diagnostic criteria for etiological factor(s).
3. If insufficient information available to label etiological factors, record possible etiologies being considered; continue assessment.
4. Include functional strengths pertinent to resolution of the problem and any relevant prognostic statements.
5. Potential problems have risk factors recorded in S and O. These are the factors contributing to the high risk state.

P: Plan

State projected outcome(s) and interventions.

Projected Outcome(s) State concise, explicit, measurable, critical, attainable outcome(s) for the problem. State time of outcome attainment (e.g., discharge, 3 days, 4-week visit). If applicable, state a sequential set of outcomes and time frame.

1. Check that outcomes are specific to problem in #____.
2. Check that date of outcome attainment is realistic. Consider etiological factors that may influence time for outcome attainment.

Interventions State intervention goal (optional). List concise nursing treatment orders. Include specific actions (time and amount, if applicable).

1. Check that treatment orders are consistent with etiological factors stated in A and are specific to the individual client. If potential problem, check that treatment orders will reduce risk factors specified under S and O.
2. Check that treatment orders have a high possibility for attaining outcome(s).
3. If useful, classify plan by treatment orders (P_{RX}), diagnostic orders (P_{DX}), and teaching orders (P_{ED}).
4. Check that treatment plan includes strengths that can be mobilized by the client/family situation to help resolve the problem or risk state.

After the format is learned, errors in documentation are usually attributable to errors in clinical reasoning.

---

*S and O data must provide sufficient diagnostic criteria to support problem and etiology. Use a manual to check defining characteristics of a diagnostic category.

O: Personal hygiene poor; body odor and urine odor detected; hair unwashed; skin unclean on admission.

P: 1. Obtain long-handled sponge and tub chair.

    2. Arrange for equipment to be used in shower at home after practice in hospital.

    3. Teach 1000 calorie diet.

EXAMPLE 2

#1 Sleep pattern disturbance

    S: "I am unable to fall asleep at least three or four times a week; I awaken easily and have nightmares when I take Valium."

    A: Job stress; family stress.

    P_{Dx}: Observe and record sleep pattern in hospital.

    P_{Tx}: Back massage at bedtime; check comfort level.

EXAMPLE 3

#1 Impaired verbal communication

    S: States husband died 8 months ago; 4 days ago was told she has extensive cancer of abdominal organs.

    O: Weak, halting speech; uses short sentences; no apparent shortness of breath.

    A: Decreased strength.

    P: 1. Facilitate verbalization of feelings.

       2. Provide encouragement, support, and motivation.

       3. Work with family.

In Example 1 a question may be raised about plan number 3: Is "teach 1000 calorie diet" an intervention for self-bathing deficit/extreme obesity-fear of falling? Obesity, especially the exogenous type, due to a caloric intake–energy expenditure imbalance, is a second diagnosis. It should be recorded separately as problem number 2. Further, the plan is inadequate for the diagnosis of obesity.

Example 2 illustrates a common error of the novice. The data base is inadequate for the diagnosis. The recorded data do not support the etiological factors stated in A, work and family stress. Actually the nurse had data to support this diagnosis in the role-relationship pattern recorded in the history. In addition, the plan is inadequate for the diagnosis. Palliative treatment is prescribed but no interventions are directed toward the stress factors.

Obviously the nurse who recorded Example 3 did not appreciate how problem-oriented recording provides a check on clinical reasoning. The data do not support the diagnosis. It appears that objective data were heavily weighted in the nurse's diagnostic judgment. Look at the subjective data; do they support the diagnosis? Absolutely not. Furthermore there is no data base to support "decreased strength," the etiology recorded under A.

In Example 3, if the nurse had reread and examined the consistency among problem, etiology, and plan, the errors would have been obvious. Facilitating verbalization, providing support, and working with a family are not the treatments for impaired verbal communication. Second, the plan, even if appropriate, is too vague. What does support entail? Work with the family toward what objective?

Rather than having to cross-check judgments and decisions in memory, one can use the written SOAP format. Instructors or clinical specialists can provide feedback, but it is important to learn how to pick up contradictions oneself.

Now consider some reasonably good examples of problem-oriented recording in Table 9-6. Try to discover the one element of the POR format (or of nursing process) that is missing.

Did you find difficulty in evaluating the treatment plan? That is because no outcomes are stated. In Table 9-6, noncompliance with activity prescription was a problem of a 35-year-old construction worker in an intensive care unit for treatment of myocardial infarction (heart attack). In this case the nurse did not have sufficient data to determine etiological factors. Thus, tentative hypotheses and the etiological factor ruled out (knowledge deficit) were recorded under assessment. An assessment of activity tolerance was included. Potential skin breakdown was diagnosed for another client during a home visit by a community health nurse. The wife was taking care of her husband, who had had a transection of the spinal cord at level of the third lumbar vertebrae. The third example was written in a psychiatric setting; the diagnosis was impaired socialization/inability to trust. Probably the reader is raising some further questions at this point that could be answered by considering ongoing documentation during care delivery. Questions could include:

How do I document what I do?

How do I know when to stop treatment?

Documentation: Progress Notes   Progress toward outcomes is charted on each problem by number on sheets called progress notes. Theoretically, progress notes are written only when a change is observed in the status of the problem or when there is no response or an unexpected response to treatment. In actuality, if treatment is aggressive, daily changes (hospital settings) or at each visit in private practice settings, clinics, or community nursing home visits, changes should be observed and documented. Not all components of the P-SOAOP format need be included in each progress note. If initial plans have not changed, no entry is made under plan (P). A progress note on the client with potential for injury (page 326) would be:

TABLE 9-6
RECORDED NURSING DIAGNOSES

Intensive Care Unit

1 Noncompliance with activity prescription

S: States feels better: "heart OK now," and "able to do my own bath." Told M.D. that he understood need for rest and wanted to "do everything to get it healed."

O: Out of bed × 3; stays at bedside; heart rate increased 5 beats per minute with no arrhythmias when out of bed; restless when in bed; activity prescription is complete bed rest.

A: Possible post-myocardial infarction denial or independence-dependence conflict; no knowledge deficit regarding activity limits; heart rate response to being out of bed suggests tolerance.

P_{Dx}: Reasons for noncompliance: Assess denial or conflict over required dependence.

P_{Tx}: Anticipate needs; discuss activity orders and patient's tolerance limits with M.D.; may need activity tolerance evaluation.

P_{Ed}: Problem-solve with client regarding activity restriction if prescription is not changed.

Community: Home Care

2 Potential skin breakdown

S: States likes to lie on left side to look out bedroom window, has no discomfort at site of redness.

O: 3-cm reddened area over left greater trochanter; no ulceration; decreased pain perception below L3.

A: Wife competent and will be able to carry out plan with neighbor's help.

P_{Ed}: Discuss with wife: (1) relocation of bed, OOB as tolerated when assistance available; (2) $1^1/_2$-hour position change and functional positioning; (3) signs of impending skin breakdown; (4) care of potential pressure sites; (5) adequate nutritional intake, especially protein.

Psychiatric Unit

3 Impaired socialization

S: States he doesn't want to sit with or talk to others; they "frighten" him.

O: Single; no family in this part of country; no group involvement; at times appears to be listening to group conversations from a distance but does not interact.

A: Inability to trust.

P: **a** Milieu activities with staff person he relates to.
b Explore these difficulties with patient when he is observed to be listening to conversations.
c Assist patient to develop plans for joining activities.
d Provide support from trusted staff person when he agrees to join in activities.

#4. *Potential for injury*

S/O: No further trauma to extremities. Keeps eyeglasses on top of bedside stand; uses when ambulating. 20-minute teaching session on sensory deficit and potential for trauma; she suggested she use a night-light in the hall and dog would accommodate; plans to talk to daughter re scatter rugs and waxed floors.

P: Other risk factors to be discussed tomorrow.

Note that it was difficult to separate objective and subjective observations. In this author's opinion this may not be so crucial in nursing as in medicine.

Reading this note, one is able to see that treatment is leading to risk factor reduction. The most important cue for future health management is her suggestion of a night-light and plans to talk to her daughter. One senses that the nurse engaged the client in solving her problem, rather than "telling" her what to do.

To return to the second question posed: *When should treatment cease?* The answer is simply when the projected outcomes are reached. One outcome was *absence of leg injuries.* This is a discharge outcome; therefore "room-check" and observation for leg trauma should continue until discharge. As a method of teaching and evaluation the nurse could observe the client's assumption of responsibility for room-check and if any risk factors are identified. The second outcome was *states plans for implementing measures in home to prevent injury.* When the client and her daughter outline plans for correcting the risk factors in the home environment, treatment can be discontinued. If this was a client receiving home visits, the community nurse would have described the outcome as *implements measures in home to prevent injury* and would *observe* for corrective actions. When the client can identify a podiatrist that can cut her nails and check her shoes/boots, this outcome will be reached. To evaluate teaching, the client could be asked to write her plan for preventing injury to her legs. She would then have a written plan to take home. When outcomes are reached, the client can be discharged from the primary nurse's caseload. At that point a discharge summary is written.

Documentation: Discharge Summary/Referrals   Nursing discharge summaries are similar to medical summaries. A note is written about the progress, or lack of progress, toward outcomes for each nursing diagnosis. Other care-related information that should be summarized for future care providers is included. In some agencies the nursing diagnoses on the discharge summary are coded so that the client's record can be retrieved easily for purposes of research or health statistics. Consider the discharge summary for the nursing diagnosis potential for injury:

> **#4.** *Potential for injury*
> Stated plan for implementing measures in home to prevent injury to legs (sensory loss-diabetic neuropathy). Observed caution in hospital and demonstrated understanding by writing plan for a night-light, padding for scatter rugs, and nonskid wax on floors. Wore glasses when ambulating and stated name of podiatrist who would check shoes/boots, cut toenails and corns. No trauma to legs at discharge.

Documentation: Disease-Related Care   The emphasis in this chapter has been on nursing diagnosis and treatment. Yet, as pointed out in Chapter 1, nursing practice also includes carrying out aspects of medical therapy that clients cannot manage for themselves. These aspects of nursing care are determined by physicians' orders or established protocols for medical treatment.

Disease-related observations and treatments have to be recorded. Presumably, if a disease or symptom has been identified the physician has recorded it on the problem list. In the sample problem list in Table 9-3 the physician made two entries: (1) diabetes mellitus and hypoglycemia; and (2) acidosis. In charting observations or treatments related to the disease process, the nurse can use the SOAP format previously described. The differences from that format are

1. The plan (P) is not used unless supplementary *nursing* orders are required; these may include "observe for . . . ," "watch for . . . ," or other monitoring orders and any individualized adaptations of the physician's order that do not alter the intention of therapy, such as "give with orange juice," "notify M. D. if systolic above 170," or other orders relative to equipment used in treatment.

2. The medical diagnosis and its number (from the master problem list or medical notes) are the title for charting the nurse's observations and actions relative to the disease. For example, if symptoms of thirst or frequent urination were observed, the nurse would record them using the heading: #1 Diabetes Mellitus.

As with nursing diagnoses, one must be aware of contradictions in the charting of disease-related information. For example, recording "able to administer own insulin injection effectively" under diabetes mellitus is a contradiction. The client's ability has no *direct* relationship to the pathophysiology of diabetes. This observation may indicate that a nursing diagnosis of knowledge deficit (insulin administration) was present but not diagnosed. *Beware of placing observations related to nursing diagnoses under medical problems.*

There is no need to create new terms for diseases or pathophysiological processes in order to chart disease-related observations and treatments. The medical diagnoses provide terminology. Use of those terms does not constitute medical diagnosis, provided that the physician has already identified and recorded them as his or her diagnostic judgment. If the medical diagnoses have not been recorded, either the symptoms were overlooked or new problems have occurred. In either case notification of the physician is appropriate.

Kardex Care Plans: Nursing and Medical Diagnoses

In addition to recording diagnoses and plans on the client's chart, many nurses use a Kardex, a flip-card tool that has a section for keeping information about each client. Usually the following information is recorded: name; age; room number; religion; admission date; medical diagnoses; scheduled medical tests (e.g., cardiac catheterization) and medical treatments; nursing diagnoses; nursing treatments; and nursing outcomes.

The main advantage of the Kardex is that it provides rapid access to the client's overall plan of care. It is used in shift reports, in planning staff assignments, and as a quick reference about all the clients on the hospital unit. The alternative way to acquire information is to leaf through each client's chart or problem list. Proponents of the Kardex system extol its merits. Some nurses decry the Kardex's usefulness. They claim the Kardex duplicates information on the chart, is usually not up to date, and is rarely used by the professional staff.

If a Kardex is used, nursing diagnoses provide a method of organizing treatment plans. The diagnoses are stated in the problem/etiological factor format and the interventions and outcomes are then listed. The data base for a diagnosis is not included, as may be seen in the following example of one nursing diagnosis of a client who has pneumonia and chronic lung disease (the data for diagnoses is on the chart):

Problem: Fear (inability to breathe)/pain on inspiration and cough.
Intervention: 1. Discuss with M.D. need for a liquefying cough medicine and humidifier.
2. Repeatedly reassure (regarding breathing problem) that nurses are present; provide call system that does not require verbalization (client is concerned that he will not be able to speak into intercom if respiratory problems occur).
3. Monitor breathing difficulty every $\frac{1}{2}$ hr.
4. Teach relaxation techniques.
5. Ensure adequate fluid intake to assist in liquefying secretions.
Outcomes: 1. Verbalizes perception of ability to breathe adequately.
2. Verbalizes comfort on inspiration.

In some institutions a nurse's order sheet specifying interventions is used as a supplement to the client's chart. Orders, for example, "teach relaxation techniques" are transferred directly from the chart to the order book.

Disease-Related Interventions Nurses write nursing orders for treating nursing diagnoses. In addition, they write orders related to a client's disease, possible complications, or adaptations of medical treatments. For example, a client may require observation for heart failure, bleeding, or change in neurological signs. Or observations and adaptations (e.g., "give with orange juice") may be necessary while the nurse is carrying out medical orders for drugs and other aspects of medical treatment.

In ordering or recording nursing interventions related to diseases it is not necessary to label disease-related care with nursing diagnoses. One simply records on the Kardex or in the order book the interventions required. The same format can be used as when recording nursing diagnoses except that the medical diagnosis is listed as the problem. For example:

Problem: Diabetes mellitus.
Intervention: Observe for irritability as sign of impending ketoacidosis. See that daily
                 blood samples are drawn *before* breakfast.
Problem: Right hip fracture.
Intervention: Obtain fracture pan; maintain functional alignment of right leg.

It is not necessary to change a diagnosis of diabetes mellitus to alterations in glucose metabolism in order to write interventions or make observations. Nor is it necessary to change myocardial infarction or congestive heart failure to alterations in cardiac output in order to observe for arrhythmias or pulmonary edema. It is expected that *after* a medical diagnosis is made, nurses will make pertinent observations and carry out appropriate treatments. Communications about these conditions are organized under disease labels, not nursing diagnoses.

In summary, nursing diagnoses organize written and verbal communications. They provide a concise label for a health problem and thereby increase the speed and clarity of communication. Use of the problem-oriented clinical information system is facilitated by nursing diagnoses. In fact, without diagnostic labels the system is difficult to use. In addition, if a nursing Kardex or nursing order book is employed, diagnoses organize the recording of nursing care plans.

NURSING DIAGNOSIS AND DISCHARGE PLANNING

The high cost of health care requires that needs and resources be correctly matched. Clients should receive a level of care and the technology appropriate to the acuity of their health problems. To match needs and resources may require that clients be transferred through many levels of care within a few months. The following are two rather typical examples:

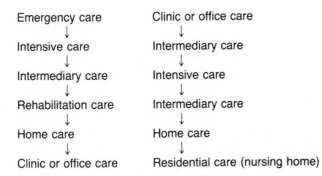

Emergency care	Clinic or office care
↓	↓
Intensive care	Intermediary care
↓	↓
Intermediary care	Intensive care
↓	↓
Rehabilitation care	Intermediary care
↓	↓
Home care	Home care
↓	↓
Clinic or office care	Residential care (nursing home)

These transfers offer the appropriate level of care for different phases of an illness; but from the client's perspective the repeated changes in care providers, routines, and the environment can be additional source of stress. By planning for continuity of care between levels, the nurse can decrease the impact of change.

Ensuring continuity of nursing care between acute care hospitals and the community has been problematic. In response to this difficulty many hospitals have established continuing care programs to assist in coordinating needs and available community resources. Even with these programs, continuity can be jeopardized. If needs are not clearly evaluated and communicated from one care setting to another, fragmented care results.

Requirements for continued medical care as the client moves from one setting to another can be clearly specified. Plans are organized and communicated from physician to physician by using the medical diagnosis. In contrast, nursing has not agreed upon the focus for predischarge evaluation or postdischarge communication of treatment plans. Additionally, many times medical and nursing plans for the client's continuing care have not been coordinated.

The set of decisions and activities involved in providing continuity and coordination of care after hospitalization is called *discharge planning.* In many instances it is required by federal or state law (McKeehan, 1979) or by hospital policy.

In the following sections it will be seen that nursing diagnoses provide an excellent focus for discharge planning. Communication of care requirements to nurses in community agencies and coordination of resources for continuing care are also facilitated. In fact, a nurse would not know that a client *needed* continued nursing care unless unresolved nursing diagnoses had been identified. A brief consideration of predischarge planning, referral decisions, and communication of nursing plans will illustrate how diagnoses facilitate these activities.

Predischarge Planning

Discharge planning begins when diagnoses are made. Outcomes that can and should be attained before discharge are projected. These discharge outcomes specify the level of problem resolution and probable time required before a client can (1) undertake independent health management at home or (2) manage with less than 24-hour acute hospital care.

Many currently identified nursing diagnoses can be treated with less expense to the consumer in nursing homes, rehabilitation centers, home care programs, or office and clinics than in hospitals. Thus a client's discharge is seldom delayed because of nursing diagnoses.

Time of discharge is a combined decision of all health professionals who treat the patient. Sometimes nurses and social workers leave this decision to the physician if it is assumed that the nursing and social work diagnoses (1) will be resolved before the physician is ready to discharge the client or (2) can and should be treated in another setting. In other instances coordinated discharge planning is necessary. No one professional should be expected to make decisions in isolation without information about the client's overall program of care. Too early discharge can result in harm, and delayed discharge adds to financial costs.

Most problems arise because of inadequate communications and delayed planning and intervention. The solution to these problems is (1) early discharge planning, (2) an established structure for multidisciplinary discharge planning, and (3) discharge nursing assessment.

Nursing Activities in Discharge Planning   The structure and implementation of multidisciplinary discharge planning has been described by McKeehan (1979, 1981). In order to participate in multidisciplinary planning, the nurse has to do the following:

1 Assess the level of problem resolution as discharge approaches. Review the status of each current nursing diagnosis. If there is doubt that all nursing problems have been diagnosed, a functional health pattern assessment is done.

2 By reviewing nursing treatment orders, decide what continuing care is needed.

3 Assess the client's capabilities as well as available family and community assistance. The client's (or responsible family member's or guardian's) understanding and plans for personal management of the medically prescribed treatment are also evaluated. (New nursing diagnoses may arise when medical discharge plans are formulated. These may include knowledge or planning deficits in management of symptoms, medication, diet or activity.)

Discrepancies between the nurse's and the client's (or family member's) assessments of capabilities for managing outside the hospital also need to be identified. For example, if a client does not feel capable of carrying out a health care recommendation, support services will have to be arranged until confidence is developed.

4 Assess the client's need for referral for continued care. When the nurse knows the current diagnoses, the posthospital nursing care that will be required, and the client's capabilities and environmental resources, the next questions are: What care will not be handled adequately by the client, family, or friends? What home or environmental adaptations that are necessary for optimal (or at least acceptable) health promotion cannot be handled by the client, family, or friends? The answers to these questions provide the basis for matching the client's needs for continued nursing care, the available community resources, and the client's preferences about continuing care.

Referral Decisions

The last step in planning for a client's discharge is to determine what type of referral to make. Some options for postacute nursing care are listed in Table 9-7. Clinics, nurses in private practice, health maintenance organizations, and

TABLE 9-7
POSTHOSPITAL RESOURCES AND FACILITIES FOR CONTINUED NURSING CARE

Hospital clinics
Private office practice
Health maintenance organizations
Neighborhood health centers
Rehabilitation centers
Hospital home care programs
Home health care agencies (visiting nurse or public health agencies)
Hospices
Residential centers (long-term care)
Nursing homes
Long-term care hospitals

---

neighborhood health centers provide periodic nursing care. The emphasis is on health maintenance and promotion. Clients with nursing diagnoses requiring follow-up care on an ambulatory basis would be referred to nursing services such as these.

With certain nursing diagnoses a long period of time and highly skilled nursing care are required to reach optimal outcomes. In these situations plans may be initiated to refer clients to rehabilitation centers or rehabilitation units within acute care hospitals. Specialized services may be considered with diagnoses such as impaired mobility, self-care deficit, perceptual deficit, or chronic pain self-management deficit. Referrals for rehabilitation are appropriate only for clients who have the potential for improvement of their functional pattern. Reliable predictions of potential are important.

Both hospital-managed home care programs and community nursing agencies provide family-centered care and help with adaptations from hospital to home. Clients with nursing diagnoses requiring continued home care or supervision are referred to visiting nurses in these agencies. Examples of such diagnoses are potential noncompliance (disease management), self-care deficit due to short-term memory loss, potential for injury, and unresolved grieving. Actual or potential family problems in coping, interaction, or home maintenance may also require home visits for evaluation and treatment. The availability of professional visiting nurses, homemakers, and home health aides varies from 24 hours a day in some communities to 8 or fewer in others; thus client and family capabilities have to be carefully determined.

Residential and hospice centers provide living environments for clients who cannot manage in their homes. Conditions such as profound mental retardation or severe cerebral palsy may require long-term residential care in a sheltered environment. A hospice is both a living environment and a philosophy of care for terminally ill clients. Residential care and hospice centers, respectively, are options for clients with nursing diagnoses related to permanent cognitive or motor impairments and terminal illness.

Depending on the resources available, a diagnosis such as severe chronic mobility impairment may be treated in the home or may require long-term institutional care. If continuous 24-hour nursing care is required over a period of time, nursing homes or long-term care hospitals may be chosen. The period of care may be weeks, months, or years, depending on the client's progress toward independence in decision making, mobility, and self-care.

The nurse discusses with clients and their families the type of care required and the options available, or clients and their families may attend multidisciplinary planning conferences. These conferences include all health team members involved in the client's care and discharge planning.

Two or more clients may have the same nursing diagnosis but different discharge plans. This is to be expected because interventions are always individualized. Consider the example of two clients with total self-care deficit (level III) due to sensorimotor loss (spinal cord transection). After rehabilitation, both were able to manage self-care with the assistance of one person and assistive devices. One client was referred to the visiting nurse service for home care. The other was discharged to a long-term care facility. Why the difference? The first client's spouse and neighbors valued home care and were able to adapt the home setting and provide care with the assistance of the visiting nurse. The second client had no family and lived alone although he liked social contact. Twenty-four hour home services were not available; even if they had been they would probably have been too costly and would not have provided sufficient social interaction. A nursing home was chosen where he could be near his friends.

Before discussing the writing of referrals, it is important to examine why discharge planning begins when nursing diagnoses are made and outcomes projected. If referral for continuing care will be necessary, information will be needed for making decisions about the referral. A great deal of information can be collected and charted while daily care is being given. Without this ongoing information gathering, discharge planning appears very time consuming—it is rushed and ineffectively done.

Discharge planning judgments are critically important both for the client's safety and for the quality of the person's life. Diagnoses have to be made accurately. If the capabilities of the client or situation are overestimated, further problems can arise; if they are underestimated, the client is subjected to unwarranted financial expense. The best data available have to be obtained.

Communication of Plans

The communication of plans is as important as planning. Clear and concise treatment orders and the bases for orders have to be communicated to the next care providers. Good communication increases the probability that nursing care will proceed without interruption.

Nursing diagnoses organize communications and clarify the rationale for nursing orders. Problem oriented recording of the diagnoses (SOAP format) further facilitates concise communication of critical information.

Standardized forms are used in most hospitals for client referrals to frequently used community agencies; visiting nurse referral forms are an example. Discharge summaries can also be used by nurses to refer clients with unresolved diagnoses. A discharge summary referral would be sent to nurses in clinics, private practice, and other ambulatory care settings. When particular attention needs to be called to some problem or aspect of follow-up care, a telephone call may be used.

The following two examples of the use of nursing diagnoses in writing referrals demonstrate the clarity and conciseness of communication which results. The first client was a 12-year-old intelligent, sports-loving boy referred for periodic nursing care at a hematology (blood) clinic. His medical diagnosis was hemophilia. The following two nursing diagnoses and SOAP notes were recorded on the nursing section of a referral:

ND_x:[1]   **1** Potential for injury

    S: Likes sports, especially football; active child; states thinks he can still play on team if plays a different position.

    O: Factor VIII deficiency, 1% plasma factor activity; recent football injury.

    A: Moderately severe risk for hemorrhage; knows about bleeding problem and that he will not be able to play football but can attend games; overheard telling mother he could play.

    P_{Dx}:   Assess whether he has resigned from Little League team.

    P_{Ed}:   Repeat instructions regarding caution in avoiding trauma. If trauma occurs mother is to bring child to emergency room.

ND_x: **2** Potential parental overprotection

    S: Mother states, "I feel so guilty, but I'll be sure he doesn't get hurt"; father says he will buy books and child can come home and read after school; asking if they should get rid of dog.

    O: Both parents express concern and nervousness whenever child's activity discussed.

    A: Parents understand tendency for overprotection and say they will try to avoid it; plan to contact National Hemophilia Foundation and join parent support group.

    P_{Dx}:   Assess for restrictions placed on child by parents; check to see whether they have joined parent support group.

    P_{Tx}:   Continue to reassure parents that guilt is normal reaction; assist them in identifying their strengths as parents; to hospital for plasma factor VIII if trauma and bleeding occur.

A second example is that of a referral to a visiting nurse. The client's medical diagnosis was adult onset diabetes mellitus. She was a 65-year-old retired

---

[1]Abbreviation for nursing diagnosis.

secretary. In the nursing section of the visiting nurse referral the following appeared:

ND$_x$: **1**   Dysfunctional grieving

    S: States lost her father 1 year ago; cared for him at home before he died of cancer; verbal expression of distress, sadness; states she has no one now and doesn't know what to do.

    O: Altered sleeping, eating, and dream pattern in hospital; mild inability to concentrate; crying spells.

    A: Loss; possible fear of newly acquired independence. States will try to become involved in community activities after discharge.

  P$_{Dx}$:   Evaluate state of grieving after return home.

  P$_{Tx}$:   Encourage contact with son and his family for support. Encourage joining voluntary community group; client expressed interest in this.

ND$_x$: **2**   Disease management deficit (insulin administration)[2]

    S: "I don't know if I can do this injection adequately. I could never give my father injections." States knows importance of insulin administration.

    O: Has successfully administered morning insulin twice. Hand shakes; dexterity is fair. Client has asked to practice on an orange. Able to draw up dose accurately.

    A: Fear (perceived incompetency and error). Motivated but still needs supervision. Supervision and experience increase confidence.

    P: Supervise insulin administration in home $\times 2$ (likes to eat breakfast at 9 a.m.) Reevaluate competency.

ND$_x$: **3**   Disease management deficit (compensated)

    S: Reassured by plans for nurse's home visit.

    O: Verbalizes correct dietary and activity plans. States principles of skin care, urine testing, and signs of complications to be reported; skills demonstrated.

    P: Review management during home visit. To be seen in doctor's office in one month.

Nursing referrals about unresolved diagnoses help community agencies to provide continuity of care. Referrals should also be sent from these agencies when their clients are treated in hospitals.

In summary, nursing diagnoses facilitate continuity of care among care settings. Diagnoses provide focus for early evaluation of continuing care needs, and suggested plans can be communicated in a concise, organized manner. Most importantly, individualized interventions can be written and communicated for each problem. Good communication between care providers decreases the client's stress in adjusting to different health care providers, routines, and environments.

NURSING DIAGNOSIS AND THE LAW

From the perspective of many nurses, nursing diagnosis merely recognizes what nurses have always done. This may not be the view of hospital admin-

---

[2]Note: The problem label heads the referral. Etiological factors are under assessment (A).

istrators, lawyers, or physicians, for many of whom the term *nursing diagnosis,* when heard for the first time, sets red lights flashing. The lights usually change to green when the concept is explained.

Even nursing colleagues are heard to say, "Legally, you can't do that" or "You'll put your license in jeopardy." Another often-heard comment by nurses is, "Our hospital hasn't accepted nursing diagnosis." The purpose of the discussion in this section is to explore whether the first statements are true or false and to see whether the latter has any relevance. The concepts of duty, cause, and harm, as they relate to negligence, will first be examined in order to provide a basis for judging the truth of the above statements or similar ones encountered in practice. It will be seen that *formulating and documenting nursing diagnosis can help nurses and institutions avoid negligence claims.*

Negligent conduct on the part of a nurse is a basis for malpractice litigation. The client, relative, or other has to provide evidence about four issues: (1) duty, (2) breach of duty, (3) cause and effect, and (4) personal or economic harm (Mancini, 1979, p. 337).

An example will clarify. A nurse, hospital, and physician were sued by the wife of a client. Her husband fell in the hospital and fractured his femur. She maintained that his care was negligent. The facts of the situation were as follows:

> On December 1 the patient, an athletic appearing, sociable, 30-year-old male was admitted to a hospital because of slight muscle weakness. The chart stated that tests for multiple sclerosis were to be done. According to the wife, she told the admitting nurse that her husband had fallen twice at home. The physician's ambulation order was "out of bed as desired." On the morning of December 2, the nurse told the client he could wash in the bathroom and left to care for others. The client fell going to the bathroom. X-rays revealed a fractured femur. The client was unable to reach the call light; the private room door was shut, and it was maintained he lay in pain for one-half hour before the nurse returned.

Element of Duty

The first element to be established when the possibility of negligence is being assessed is *duty* to the client. Basically, the nurse must protect the client against unreasonable risks by adhering to a certain standard of conduct. How is a nurse to know what the standard of conduct is?

In response to this question, the ANA standards of practice may come to mind, or the ANA code of nursing ethics. These nationally accepted, professional guidelines for the *conduct* of nursing practice can be used by a trial lawyer. The situation would be similar to obtaining a nurse expert witness. A lawyer would ask, "Would this [citing alleged negligence] be common practice by a nurse?"

As previously discussed, the *Standards of Nursing Practice* state that nurses assess and that nursing diagnoses are derived from health status data. There was no indication in the chart that the nurse had assessed mobility or gross muscle strength even though they were the reason for admission.

A nurse expert witness would probably testify that it was reasonable to expect that the risk factors (history of falls, muscle weakness, and possible multiple sclerosis) would suggest the diagnostic judgment of potential for injury. Recognition of potential for injury would be followed by supervision while ambulating and other preventive measures. Although this diagnosis was within the domain of nursing practice (Appendix A), there was no evidence that the diagnosis was made and supervision instituted.

Before resorting to the standards or nursing textbooks, the client's attorney would check the state nurse practice act. The incident occurred in one of the states whose nurse practice law includes the term *diagnosis.*

Lawyers also examine rules and regulations promulgated by state boards of nursing; some states specify the nursing process components as functions of the registered nurse. State practice acts and board of nursing rules and regulations are the legal basis for nursing; standards are professional, not legal, guidelines.

Breach of Duty

The second element that must be present in negligence is breach of duty to a client. The chart, in this man's case, was evidence that the nurse did not conform to the state practice act: No diagnostic judgment was on record about the potential for injury. Most importantly, there was no indication that ambulation was being supervised by nurses.

Cause and Effect

A relationship between the nurse's conduct and an alleged injury is the third element necessary for demonstrating negligence. In the case cited, a reasonably close relationship had to be demonstrated between the fracture and the nurse's lack of client supervision. *Why* the nurse did not supervise the client's ambulation is irrelevant from the legal perspective. The court is interested only in the fact that there was negligent supervision. Nurses and hospital administrators ask why in order to prevent future occurrences; for example, why was a nursing history and examination not done at admission?

Nursing diagnosis represents a synthesis of clinical data and a judgment about whether or not a health problem is present. Once this synthesis and problem identification take place, it is difficult to ignore the state of the client. The nurse becomes motivated to act. This is how diagnosis helps prevent a breach of duty that results in harm to the client.

Harm or Injury

The fourth element to be proven in a negligence case is actual injury (physical, psychological, or both) and loss, including economic loss. In the case illustrated, x-ray reports demonstrated a fractured femur. Because of the long period required for healing, economic loss as well as injury was claimed.

The main point to be understood from this discussion is that the law is concerned with diagnosis in only one respect. That is, the court wishes to establish what the state of the client is. Once this is established, the law is primarily concerned with nursing actions appropriate to the client's state. An act that is *committed* or *omitted* in regard to that state *and* results in harm is a basis for a malpractice determination. As Fortin and Rabinow state, "the law is primarily concerned with diagnosis-related action" (1979, p. 553).

Legal Decisions

No cases have been found in which the court cited nursing diagnosis, although "judgment" increasingly appears to be something nurses are expected to exercise.

Can nurses make medical diagnoses? This is not the most fruitful way of framing the question. Rather, ask: What judgments are nurses expected to make? Two cases cited by Fortin and Rabinow (1979) may clarify that judgment is expected beyond the domain of nursing diagnoses.

In the first case, a company nurse was considered negligent for not recognizing a basal cell carcinoma and referring the employee who had developed it. As cited, the court said "a nurse . . . should be able to diagnose . . . sufficiently to know whether it is a condition within her authority to treat as a first aid case or whether it bears danger signs that should warn her to send the patient to a physician" (Fortin and Rabinow, 1979, p. 560). In the second case, nurses judged that a child's fever was not serious. No physician was called. The child died of congestive heart failure after an attack of rheumatic fever (Fortin and Rabinow, 1979, p. 560). In both cases, the courts required tentative medical diagnosis to some degree. In many states the extent of a nurse's responsibility for making medical diagnoses is unclear.

Interpreting signs and symptoms and judging how to treat them (nursing diagnoses) or making referrals (tentative medical diagnoses) are nursing responsibilities. In both instances the nurse has legal responsibility to use the diagnostic process skillfully. Otherwise, diagnostic judgments may lead to injury and risk of malpractice.

One additional point should be made. There are reasons why some physicians pale when encountering nursing diagnosis. They may believe they are legally responsible for *all* care. What needs to be clarified to such physicians is that a nurse practices under his or her own license, not the physician's. Second, one should clarify that the law requires nurses to make diagnostic judgments; it may be useful to cite the previously mentioned court cases. Third, the nurse can find out whether the state practice acts or rules and regulations specify diagnosis, diagnostic judgments, or merely judgment. If diagnosis is called for, copies of those documents can be obtained for physicians. They may not have had the opportunity to learn the legal scope of nursing. In many medical schools little is taught about nursing practice.

DIAGNOSTIC RESPONSIBILITY

Who should diagnose? The answer sought is usually a classification, such as clinical specialist or professional, technical, or practical nurse. At times the question is abstract; at other times it is highly pragmatic and is asked for legal, administrative, or educational purposes. It also can be reworded: Who *can* diagnose? This wording introduces the idea of ability.

The answer is important when staffing and nursing care delivery are being examined. It is also important in decisions about delegating care to nonprofessionals when the nurse assumes managerial responsibility for groups of clients.

The answer depends on multiple factors. Exploration of these factors and the "state of art" of nursing diagnosis suggests that diagnosing is a professional activity influenced by the situation in which the professional is practicing. Bruce and Snyder provide an excellent review of rights and responsibilities in diagnosis (1982).

Legal Considerations

Laws regulating nursing practice are not worded consistently from one state to another. In some states, practice acts specify diagnosis as a function of the registered nurse (baccalaureate, associate degree, and diploma graduates). The question is sometimes asked whether initial assessment and diagnosis can be delegated to practical nurses. Practice acts controlling practical nursing usually state that the practical nurse must have the *direction and supervision* of a registered nurse, physician, or dentist. Diagnostic judgment cannot be directed; thus it cannot be delegated. Moreover, supervision during assessment would require presence of the registered nurse as data are being collected; thus there is no point in delegating assessment.

Direction and supervision usually refers to the activities of observation and treatment. These can be clearly directed *after* diagnoses are made. Noncomplex judgments related to observation and treatment are within practical nurses' scope of practice, but the complex diagnostic judgment is not.

The delegation of nursing diagnosis to practical nurses places a burden on them. If harm occurs, it can easily be established that they are not educated to diagnose and should not have accepted this responsibility. A comparable situation would exist if a physician delegated a liver biopsy to a registered nurse. Both risk malpractice if harm occurs.

This argument does not negate the fact that practical nurses contribute observations of importance to nursing diagnosis. Neither does it detract from their contribution to treatment, once the treatment plan has been specified.

Professional Considerations

Registered nurses consider assessment, diagnosis, care planning, and evaluation to be professional—as well as legal—duties to their clients. Standards of practice, nursing textbooks, and journal articles specify diagnosis as a professional function. In addition, standards of the Joint Commission on Accreditation of Hospitals state that a registered nurse assesses clients and plans their care (Joint Commission on Accreditation of Hospitals, 1981). Clearly, consumers deserve professional nursing care.

NANDA supports the concept that only registered professional nurses are responsible and accountable for identifying nursing diagnoses for their patient population (McLane, 1987). One argument for this statement rests within the educational curricula of nursing programs as will be seen in the next section.

Educational Considerations

Another way of answering the question of who should diagnose is to examine the curricula of nursing programs. Examination reveals that diagnostic judgment is seldom if ever taught in practical nursing programs. In baccalaureate and master's degree programs, nursing diagnoses and the judgment skills used in making diagnoses are usually integrated into nursing courses (McLane, 1981). In diploma and associate degree programs it may be expected that at least an introduction to nursing diagnosis is given when nursing process is taught. Currently diploma and associate degree graduates are prepared for registered nurse functions.

When competency statements for professional and technical practice (and thus, education) are discussed, professional competency includes formulating nursing diagnoses. Technical nurses' competencies are usually viewed as contributing observations to the formulation of diagnoses and understanding relationships between diagnoses and care planning.

Process Considerations

From previous chapters it should be clear that the diagnostic process is not a task to be undertaken by nonprofessional nurses. Diagnosing requires a good clinical knowledge base, training in inferential and analytical skills, and the ability to conceptualize a client's condition for purposes of intervention. Nevertheless it is not uncommon to hear that initial assessment or diagnosis can be delegated to nonprofessionals.

A distinct problem arises if one person collects clinical data, for example, takes the health history, and another tries to formulate diagnoses. A critical step is missed: branching on the basis of clinical knowledge and hypotheses. Discussion in previous chapters pointed out that assessment and diagnosis are not separate activities. The diagnostic process begins after the first few pieces of information signifying a possible problem are collected.

Further, a diagnosis dictates care. It is impossible to separate the components of nursing process into an assembly line activity. The nursing process is just that—a process—not independent steps.

A second major argument for diagnosis as a professional activity is the clinical knowledge base required. If all nurses had equally good diagnostic process *skills,* the successful and unsuccessful diagnosticians could probably be separated on the basis of their theoretical knowledge. This suggests that the best diagnosticians will probably be at the clinical specialist level. These are the nurses who should be used as consultants to the less knowledgeable and experienced.

An example may illustrate. Let us consider what many think is an "easy" diagnosis to make: potential skin breakdown. Anyone can recognize reddened skin if motivated to do so. Yet to make an early diagnosis and institute preventive care, one must weigh a multiplicity of factors in judgment. It is not just that a client is on bed rest; age, nutrition, current pathophysiology, motivation, and emotional state are also factors that determine the risk state. The weight of each factor has to be considered in making the judgment that the client is at risk for skin breakdown.

The current diagnoses (Appendix A) may appear very basic. In fact, from a cognitive perspective, they require more complex judgments than many medical diagnoses.

A third major argument for restricting diagnostic responsibility to professional nurses is the state of the art in nursing diagnosis. Professional nurses at this time are just learning how to formulate clients' actual and potential problems in diagnostic terms. Equally true, the diagnostic nomenclature still needs clinical testing and more explicit definition. When ambiguity exists in diagnosis, professionals are required. This is exemplified in the levels of certainty discussed in Chapter 2, page 53.

In other professions, it takes many years of training to be considered a good diagnostician by one's colleagues. Perhaps in the future, new nursing graduates, like medical interns, will routinely have an opportunity for a year of supervision. The value of postgraduate supervision of diagnosis and treatment is already recognized in psychiatric–mental-health nursing. Most people presumably would agree that clients with other conditions also deserve this quality control.

Situational Considerations

Not all clients who need nursing care have access to professional nurses. This is a reality. In some settings, such as primary care, the shortage of professional nurses can be related to insufficient reimbursement for nursing, a topic to be considered later. The lack of sufficient professional staff in hospital and nursing home settings is very widely recognized.

Why is there a shortage of *professional* staff? Conditions of employment have been implicated (Wandelt, Pierce, and Widdowson, 1981). Nursing as a profession has not articulated the client problems requiring professional care; in the absence of this information, staffing has been based on the only available data, the medical diagnosis and its acuity. Yet no administrator would be able to refute the need for staff if it is documented that nursing diagnoses are going untreated. Data about staffing needs in relation to the problems nurses treat take time to collect but may prove exceedingly useful in the long run to justify whether professional or nonprofessional staff are needed.

In response to shortages, busy nurses too often delegate the history, examination, diagnosis, or care planning at admission to a nonprofessional person. In actuality, it would be safer to turn over technical or administrative duties. Professional care planning makes a difference. More specifically, diagnosis-based treatment makes a difference. Many will attest to this.

Experiential Considerations

Among professional nurses there are both experienced and inexperienced diagnosticians. Some nurses may not have had the opportunity to learn diagnostic skills in basic or continuing education programs. Inservice programs or self-study groups can remedy this.

As competency is being attained, whether one is a student or graduate, it is important to recognize the need for consultation. No one is an expert on everything. Legal and ethical considerations suggest that assistance should be sought from colleagues or specialists in the problem area. As in medicine, general practitioners in nursing seek specialist consultation for complex diagnostic problems. The practitioner learns and the client receives quality care.

In summary, *registered nurses* have responsibility for diagnosis. Within this category may be varying levels of expertise. This variety is a result of the nature of educational programs as well as of continuing education opportunities.

Projections about the future indicate that clinical specialists will be the expert diagnosticians of the profession. Baccalaureate graduates will be competent in diagnosis and through experience will build on these competencies. The shorter programs cannot be expected to develop more than an introduction to the concept of diagnosis and diagnostic skills used in nurse-referrals. Practical nurses will be aware of diagnosis and of the relevant data to be documented. Projections are always tentative, especially when a profession is in the process of change; this is the current state in nursing. Furthermore, projections are not based on research in diagnostic competencies but rather on opinion derived from the legal, educational, and process considerations just discussed.

SUMMARY

The subject of this chapter was how to use nursing diagnoses in direct client care. Nursing process was described as the method nurses use to deliver care and to implement the concepts, values, and standards of nursing.

Two phases of the nursing process were delineated: problem identification and the *focus* of problem solving.

Nursing process involves an interrelated set of decisions. The chapter showed how, in the problem-solving phase, a nursing diagnosis, describing the client's present state, is used as a focus for projecting health outcomes. In combination the diagnosis and desired outcomes are used as a basis for decisions about nursing intervention.

One of the values held by the profession and expressed in its *Standards of Nursing Practice* (ANA, 1973) is individualized nursing care. Accordingly, although clients may have the same diagnosis and desired outcomes, their *individuality is considered in care planning. Personal factors, the client's perceptions about the problem, level of compensation, acuity, situational effects, and cost-benefit factors were discussed as considerations in care planning decisions that individualize care.*

To ensure *coordination of care,* and for legal reasons, communication of nursing process decisions is necessary. Both *written records and verbal communications* are enhanced by using nursing diagnoses to organize clinical data. The problem-oriented method of recording provides clarity of communication as well as an important cross-check on cognitive processes.

Using nursing diagnoses increases the clarity and conciseness of verbal and written communications. One result is improved coordination of care. Examples of communication in discharge planning demonstrated how diagnoses could be used to facilitate continuity of care.

In an examination of *nursing diagnosis and the law,* negligence was defined. In malpractice suits involving negligence, one criterion to be demonstrated is duty to the client. According to the professional standards of practice, duty includes diagnostic judgments. Some state nurse practice acts or board of nursing rules and regulations for practice also specify nursing diagnosis as within the scope of generic (general) registered-nurse practice. From a legal perspective, must the nurse diagnose? The law is concerned with whether harm and injury could have been prevented if a diagnostic judgment had been made and whether standards, acts, or rules and regulations were violated. Nursing diagnosis is a cognitive tool that directs conscious attention to the meaning of a set of cues. Attention to a client's need for care usually results in nursing action. This is how nursing diagnosis, as opposed to isolated and sometimes meaningless cues, protects a nurse against negligence litigation and a client against harm.

Who should diagnose? Standards and laws clearly dictate that this is a professional activity. Nonprofessionals contribute data after initial diagnoses are made. Can diagnosis be delegated to nonprofessionals? Certainly, just as cardiac surgery can be delegated to a registered nurse. No nurse would accept this delegation because none is prepared and licensed to practice medicine. The situation is similar where nursing diagnosis is involved. *Delegation is associated with legal risk,* both for the person delegating and for the one accepting. Nonprofessional activities, not assessment and diagnosis, are appropriately assigned to nonprofessional personnel. Professional authority cannot be used to subject others to situations they are unprepared to handle.

BIBLIOGRAPHY

American Nurses' Association (1985). *Code for nurses with interpretive statements.* Kansas City, MO.

American Nurses' Association (1980). *Nursing: A social policy statement.* Kansas City, MO.

American Nurses' Association (1973). *Standards of nursing practice.* Kansas City, MO.

Bloch, D. (1977). Criteria, standards, norms: Crucial terms in quality assurance. *Journal of Nursing Administration,* 7:20–29.

Bruce, J. A., & Snyder, M. E. (1982). Right and responsibility to diagnose. *American Journal of Nursing,* 82:645–646.

Combs, A. W., Avila, D. L., & Purkey, W. W., (1971). *Helping relationships.* Boston: Allyn and Bacon.

Crosley, J. (1986). Computerized nursing care planning using nursing diagnosis. In M. Hurley. (Ed.). *Classification of nursing diagnoses: Proceedings of the sixth conference.* St. Louis: Mosby.

Fortin, J. D., & Rabinow, J. (1979). Legal implications of nursing diagnosis. *Nursing Clinics of North America,* 14:553–561.

Gordon, M. (1987). *Manual of nursing diagnosis.* New York: McGraw-Hill.

Gordon, W. J. (1961). *Synectics: The development of creative capacity.* New York: Collier.

Joint Commission on Accreditation of Hospitals (1981). *Accreditation manual for hospitals.* Chicago.

Mancini, M. (1979). Proving negligence in nursing practice. *American Journal of Nursing,* 79:337–338.

McKeehan, K. M. (1979). Nursing diagnosis in a discharge planning program. *Nursing Clinics of North America,* 14:517–524.

McKeehan, K. M. (Ed.) (1981). *Continuing care.* St. Louis: Mosby.

McLane, A. (Ed.). (1987). *Classification of nursing diagnosis: Proceedings of the seventh conference.* St. Louis, MO: Mosby.

McLane, A. (1981). Nursing diagnosis in baccalaureate and graduate education. In M. J. Kim & D. A. Moritz (Eds.), *Classification of nursing diagnoses: Proceedings of the third and fourth national conferences.* New York: McGraw-Hill.

Orem, D. E. (1980). *Nursing: Concepts of practice.* New York: McGraw-Hill.

Osborne, A. F. (1963). *Applied imagination.* New York: Scribner.

Walter, J. B., Pardee, G. P., & Molbo, D. M. (1976). *Dynamics of problem-oriented approaches: Patient care and documentation.* Philadelphia: Lippincott.

Wandelt, M. A., Pierce, P. M., & Widdowson, R. R. (1981). Why nurses leave nursing and what can be done about it. *American Journal of Nursing,* 81:72–77.

Weed, L. L. (1971). *Medical records, medical education, and patient care.* Cleveland; Case Western Reserve University Press.

350

CHAPTER 10

RELEVANCE OF NURSING DIAGNOSIS TO PRACTICE ISSUES

In this chapter the relevance of nursing diagnosis to issues slightly removed from direct care will be considered. The *assurance of quality care* for populations of clients is one issue. This area will be examined in order to understand how diagnoses can be the focus for nursing quality assurance programs. Ideas in this section will be familiar because quality care review is a review of nursing process components discussed previously. It will be evident that nursing diagnoses have to be recorded during direct care in order for the required review to take place.

One factor that can influence quality care is the client's access to professional nurses. The section on *staffing patterns* demonstrates that current methods of allocating staff leave much to be desired, in the opinion of institutional administrators. Staffing patterns are unsatisfactory partly because nursing has not sufficiently described client needs from a nursing perspective. Studies are in progress to design staffing patterns that are based on clients' nursing diagnoses. The essential understanding to be gained from the discussion is that each nurse has to record clients' diagnoses and related interventions in order to help institutions plan professional staff allocations.

Access to professional nursing in the community is also problematic. The issue has some similarities to staffing problems in institutional care. In both settings, the rationale for reimbursement for nursing care is either vague or lacking. An understanding of *third party payment* for the treatment of nursing diagnoses may lead to clearer articulation of what should be reimbursed.

Nursing diagnoses, it will be seen, are relevant to determining the *scope of nursing practice.* Nurses need to communicate rather specifically to consumers, legislators, and administrators what health conditions they treat. In this chapter it is argued that the scope of practice will become much clearer when nursing diagnoses are identified.

Issues such as how to describe the domain of nursing practice will lead us to consider the development of nursing science. Nursing diagnosis is particularly relevant to this subject. It will be seen that diagnoses may offer a focus for the development of *nursing practice theory,* which will eventually provide scientific knowledge to be used in direct care activities.

Identifying health conditions that concern practicing nurses will have an impact on the previously discussed issues. Thus, we will come full circle: As nursing diagnoses are identified a focus will be provided for measuring quality client care, for allocation of professional staff, and for third party reimbursement.

NURSING DIAGNOSIS AND QUALITY CARE REVIEW

As costs rise, consumers demand quality goods and services. People have long been concerned about cost and quality of toasters, automobiles, and plumbers' services. Since more public funds have been funneled into government sponsored health programs, demands for assurance of quality care have been heard.

In 1972, the Congress of the United States mandated professional review of health care services, particularly emphasizing medical services. Since that time, care delivered to recipients of Medicare (people over 65 years of age), Medicaid (low-income populations), and maternal and child health programs must be reviewed. A national and statewide system of professional review organizations (PROs) was created. They are responsible for ensuring that all health care reimbursed from federal funds is *necessary.* In addition, care must (1) meet professional standards and (2) be provided economically in an appropriate setting (Public Law 92-603).

The legislation just described was based on the concept of *peer review.* This concept means that members of a profession that delivers a specific type of health care develop the bases for evaluation of that care. They also carry out the evaluation process. Care may be reviewed (evaluated) while it is being given or retrospectively. In the latter case charts are examined after the clients are discharged. The purpose of peer review is to identify less than acceptable care delivery. Once problems are identified, remedial action can be taken. Through educational programs, administrators and practitioners can be helped to bring care to an accepted level.

In addition to the required PRO review of hospital and long-term care, many institutions voluntarily submit to another type of care review carried out periodically by the national Joint Commission on Accreditation of Hospitals (JCAH). One of their requirements is a well-defined program for identification and correction of problems. The standard to be met in this area is:

As part of the hospital's quality assurance program the quality and appropriateness of patient care provided by the nursing department are monitored and evaluated and identified problems are resolved. (JCAH, 1982)

In the following sections, concepts of quality assurance will be reviewed. This review will provide a basis for understanding how nursing diagnosis can be used in care review, problem identification, and remedial actions. It will also be important to understand the concept of accountability to consumers that underlies quality assurance.

Terms will be introduced that are commonly used in quality assurance literature. Some will seem familiar because quality assurance deals with nursing process components previously discussed. Large populations of clients will be considered, not individual clients.

Assuring quality care for large groups of clients is sometimes thought of as a responsibility only of administrators. Actually, *concepts of quality assurance have to be integrated into every nurse's practice.* Irrespective of whether they are directly or indirectly involved in quality assurance, nurses should clearly understand issues, such as this, that affect their professional practice. Understanding is facilitated when each nurse becomes involved in developing standards, reviewing care, or in planning for care improvement. As professionals, all nurses are responsible and accountable for the standards that are set for their practice and the level of care delivered to consumers.

What are measures of quality nursing care?

This is the first question to be answered when a department of nursing begins quality care review. Various options exist. The competency of nurses certainly influences quality care, as do the resources they have available. Also, what nurses do for clients has an impact on care and can be measured. Finally, it is argued that the outcome of care, that is, the health state of the client, is one of the best measures of quality care delivery.

Overview of Care Review Concepts

The assessment areas just named represent the three components of care delivery that can be evaluated: structural, process, and outcome components. In each component, standards are developed from research literature and expert opinion. The three types of standards are defined as follows:

Structural standards are statements describing valued characteristics of the care delivery setting that indirectly influence care. Examples would be number and preparation of nurses, physical facilities, equipment, in-service education, policies, and procedures.

Process standards are statements describing valued characteristics of care delivery. They describe what nurses should do for their clients. The American Nurses' Association (ANA) standards of practice are process standards for assessment, diagnosis, planning, and so forth.

Outcome standards are statements describing health characteristics, behavior, or states of the client. Descriptions of clients' mobility and of clients' knowledge about their medications are examples of the focus of these standards. Outcomes are presumed to result from nursing intervention (although cause and effect relationships are hard to establish).

Theoretically, structural, process, and outcome standards are interrelated as are links in a chain. Structural resources are needed to carry out the processes of care delivery; in turn, processes (interventions) influence client health outcomes. Yet it is recognized that many other factors operating in either the client or the environment can influence outcomes.

Structural, process, and outcome standards are set for populations of clients. A *population* is a classification or grouping of clients that have some characteristic in common. A diagnosis may be a basis for grouping.

The setting of standards of care for client populations is an activity of great importance. Once standards are set, they cannot be ignored. In a sense they are a commitment to certain health care values. Suppose, for example, a standard of care is set in a hospital for clients with potential fluid volume deficit; ethically, the standard should then be met for every patient with that diagnosis. Standards should be based on the best scientific and clinical knowledge available. They have to be realistic and attainable in all situations unless extenuating circumstances can be demonstrated.

When quality assurance was mandated by legislation and accrediting agencies, the health professions had neither relevant research data nor standards with which to proceed. In the last 10 years many debates have occurred on how to measure quality. The major issue involves formulating reliable and valid standards and criteria for measurement. In essence the debate is whether the care (processes), the outcomes of care, or both have to be measured. Bloch (1975, 1980) in nursing and McAuliffe (1979) in medicine present reviews of the debate.

To experience the issue, imagine for a moment that your colleagues are going to use a set of standards to grade (evaluate) your nursing care or your clients' health outcomes. Imagine further that outsiders are going to know what grade you receive. Are you concerned about *what* is evaluated and *how* the evaluation is done? For example, do you want them to measure *what patient education you provided?* Or, instead, should they evaluate *your clients' health knowledge and skills?* Suppose you taught a client how to take his medications, but when your care was evaluated the client stated incorrect information. Does that mean you gave poor quality care?

There is a second important issue with which nurses must be concerned. Full accountability can be assumed only for health problems nurses diagnose and treat. This statement may seem so logical that it need not be said. As quality assurance began, however, clients were classified according to medical conditions such as myocardial infarction and appendectomy. This gave the impression that nurses were assuming accountability for quality of care not within their control. Actually, mislabeling of the populations occurred; many of the standards were nevertheless processes and outcomes of unlabeled *nursing* diagnoses.

Nursing diagnoses describe the independent domain of nursing practice. Thus nurses assume accountability for health problems described by these diagnostic labels. It follows logically that nursing diagnoses should be used to define client populations for care review (Gordon, 1980; McCourt, 1986; West-fall, 1984) and that diagnoses provide the ideal tool for writing nursing-specific process and outcome standards, identifying care delivery problems, and planning remedial actions.

Use of nursing diagnoses as a framework for care review brings some uniformity to quality assurance activities in different health care settings. Standards based on diagnoses rather than on unique features of one setting or another can be shared and consequently decrease the cost of implementing review programs. Also, multiple testing of standards in different institutions leads to the improvement of the standards.

Selecting Populations   In a health care setting a small, representative group of nurses usually undertakes the task of developing standards. This task requires a set of decisions. Because of time and costs, it is seldom possible to review all care given to all patients; therefore the first decision is to designate a few diagnostic populations. Later the number of populations can be increased. To decide which patient populations will be studied, high-incidence nursing diagnoses have to be identified by staff familiar with the setting. A listing such as that in Appendix A can facilitate the process.

Tracer methodology is a systematic way of making final decisions about populations. The common nursing diagnoses identified by staff can be narrowed by use of this technique. A tracer is a nursing diagnosis that can reflect the quality of care being delivered. For example, potential skin breakdown may be one good tracer for long-term institutional care. A tracer such as noncompliance may reflect an aspect of ambulatory care quality.

The questions in Table 10-1 can be applied to a list of diagnoses that are common in the particular setting. Those nursing diagnoses having most of the characteristics are probably good tracers, and the clients who have those diagnoses become the tracer populations.

Standards Writing   Sufficient nursing literature exists to enable nurses to begin to delineate processes and outcomes for currently approved nursing diagnoses. As clinical research on these conditions increases, standards will

---

TABLE 10-1
USEFUL QUESTIONS FOR IDENTIFYING TRACERS OF QUALITY NURSING CARE

---

1. Does the tracer diagnosis have a definite functional impact on clients?
2. Is the tracer diagnosis relatively well defined and easy to diagnose?
3. Is the incidence of the tracer diagnosis sufficiently high that adequate data can be collected?
4. Does the quality of nursing care influence progression of the tracer diagnosis?
5. Is the prevention or treatment of the tracer diagnosis sufficiently well defined?
6. Are the effects of nonnursing (environmental) factors on the tracer diagnosis sufficiently understood?

Source: Adapted from Kessner, Kalk, and Singer (1973).

TABLE 10-2
MODEL FOR WRITING STANDARDS/CRITERIA FOR NURSING DIAGNOSES

MODEL FOR WRITING STANDARDS/CRITERIA FOR NURSING DIAGNOSIS

---

1. Diagnostic category (taken from NANDA approved list).
2. Specific nursing diagnosis (related to category).
3. Assessment criteria (defining characteristics of nursing diagnosis).
4. Etiologies or risk factors (major cause of health problems).
5. Process criteria (interventions)(statements to guide nursing care of groups of patients).
6. Outcome criteria (projected goals)(changes in health status resutling from nursing interventions).
7. Review of literature (significant references).
8. Standards Committee, New England Sinai Hospital (date)

Source: Reprinted with permission. A. McCourt (1986). Nursing diagnoses: Key to quality assurance. In M. Hurley (Ed.), *Classification of nursing diagnoses: Proceedings of the seventh national conference.* St. Louis: Mosby.

have a more substantial scientific base. Until then theory, the available research, and expert opinion will prevail.

Table 10-2 illustrates a commonly used model for writing standards and criteria. When *process standards* are written both the problem and the etiological factors have to be considered. Look at differences in the standards in Table 10-3. Although the problem in the two diagnoses is the same, the standards are different because the etiological factor differs. The probable cause of a condition directly influences what is done to treat it; thus the acceptable standard for what is done changes with the etiological factors.

Outcome standards are characteristics of the client that describe a desired health state. They describe only the state of the client, not how it came about.

TABLE 10-3
DIAGNOSIS-SPECIFIC PROCESS STANDARDS

Diagnosis:	Impaired home maintenance management/decreased activity tolerance, level II
Process standards:	1. Energy conservation techniques for cleaning, cooking, lifting, pushing, etc., are taught.
	2. Assistance is given in planning home management activities and rest periods.
Diagnosis:	Impaired home maintenance management/knowledge deficit (hygiene practices)
Process standards:	1. Relationships between lack of hygienic home practices (cleanliness, food storage), spreading of harmful microorganisms, and human infections are explained.
	2. Assistance is given in planning home maintenance responsibilities with family.
	3. Information is given about methods and resources to prevent vermin.

If the health problem improves or disappears, the assumption is made that quality care was delivered. Outcome standards and their measurement were important when determinations were made about the appropriateness and effectiveness of care. As McCourt reports, they are extremely important today:

> Consideration is now being given to the feasibility of using outcomes as indicators for reimbursement, for determining level of nursing home placement, and even for licensure of long-term care facilities. This thinking reflects the rapidly changing climate of professional accountabilitity (McCourt, 1986).

When outcome standards are being written, the definition and defining characteristics of the problem statement are helpful; for accepted diagnoses these may be found in compilations of conferences on nursing diagnosis (McLane, 1987). When defining characteristics are converted to positive health behaviors, they provide the content for the outcome standards. For example, the standards indicating resolution of impaired home maintenance management could be those listed in Table 10-4. They are the opposite of the critical defining characteristics of the diagnosis. Similarly, converting the characteristics of a diagnosis such as ineffective coping to the signs of effective coping results in measurable outcome standards. In most instances, irrespective of the probable cause (etiology), with quality care the outcome standard should be attained. Therefore, etiological factors are not as influential when outcome standards for populations are written. Notice that in Table 10-3 the probable causes of the two diagnoses were decreased activity tolerance and knowledge deficit (hygienic practices). Clients with impaired home maintenance management from *either* cause should reach the same accepted outcome.

Although not influencing the *content* of outcome standards, etiological factors influence the *time* for reaching a standard. Standards must be realistic (attainable); hence the time frame may be different when etiological factors require complex, extended interventions.

In each standard the time by which the outcome has to be reached is specified. For a population with impaired home maintenance management, food stored safely (one week) would be an example. Some outcome standards also require consistency of client behavior across time, for example, food stored safely at three weekly visits (3 weeks). This would mean that the client's progress would be assessed, but outcome attainment would not be evaluated against the standards until after 3 weeks and three visits.

TABLE 10-4
DIAGNOSIS–SPECIFIC OUTCOME STANDARDS

Diagnosis:	Impaired home maintenance management
Outcome standards*:	1. Food stored safely
	2. Wastes disposed of safely
	3. Vermin absent
	4. Surroundings generally clean

*Time and methods of measurement are not specified.

Process standards also specify a time frame. It indicates the acceptable time(s) that a process of care (intervention) is performed. If the diagnosis is potential fluid volume deficit, for example, fluids offered every 2 hours might be the process standard. The diagnosis potential for violence might have a more frequent time frame, for example, agitation level checked every 10 minutes. One standard for noncompliance with medication therapy/regimen complexity might be: written list of medications, dosage, and time given before discharge. The above examples illustrate that time frames as well as content of the statements are standardized.

In addition to nursing diagnoses, nurses assume accountability for assisting clients in carrying out therapy ordered by physicians. Although no data exist, it may be estimated that nursing judgment is involved in nearly 50 percent of the disease-related acute care clients receive. This percentage includes making and reporting clinical observations and judgments about complications, administering "as necessary" medications, carrying out protocols, and taking other actions. How is this aspect of nursing care reviewed?

The quality assurance review of medical-diagnosis–specific nursing care requires only process standards. Nurses do not assume accountability for medical, or disease-related, outcomes.[1]

Process standards can be developed for complications, actions based on assessments, and actions based on physician orders or hospital protocols. Caution has to be exercised in writing these standards. Expectations cannot go beyond knowledge commonly acquired in professional education, and processes for the treatment of nursing diagnoses must not be mislabeled under medical diagnostic population groups.

Information Retrieval After standards are written, the quality of care is evaluated. The process is referred to as *monitoring standards.* Clients' permanent records are reviewed to see whether (1) admission was necessary (facility utilization review); (2) care being delivered is at an acceptable standard (concurrent review or retrospective review); and (3) outcome standards are reached (retrospective review). The time expenditures and other costs make it necessary for most monitoring to be done by reviewing clients' records. Thus it is extremely important that daily recordings be clear, concise, and complete.

There are difficulties, but not unsolvable ones, in grouping clients and writing standards according to nursing diagnoses. In most health care settings clients' records can be retrieved (selected for inclusion in the audit) only on the basis of medical diagnoses. This chart retrieval system exists because hospital statistical reports are based on medical diagnoses. Unless provision has been made also to record nursing diagnoses in the call-up system, record retrieval is difficult. For example, 100 charts of clients with ineffective coping patterns or impaired home maintenance management cannot be easily retrieved from among 10,000 records.

The mechanical problem of retrieval does not have to dictate the way stan-

---

[1]Nurses delivering primary care may have responsibility for treating some common diseases, but in most settings this treatment is given under physician supervision, orders, or protocols.

dards are written. Nurses are working toward the placement of nursing diagnoses on computerized or other information systems. Until this occurs other methods of record retrieval, such as depicted in Table 10-5, have to be used.

One method is to use medical diagnoses for retrieval and nursing diagnoses as a focus for writing standards (Gordon, 1980, pp. 85–86). This method requires

TABLE 10-5
MEDICAL DIAGNOSIS RETRIEVAL MODE AND NURSING DIAGNOSIS REVIEW

Retrieval Mode	Audit population	Process standards	Outcome standards
Right cerebrovascular accident*	Potential skin breakdown	1. Assisted to change position at least every 2 hours	1. Skin intact
		2. Special skin care (defined) every 2 hours	
		3. Protein intake monitored for deficits once daily	
		4. Elimination monitored for incontinence every 2 hours	
	Total self-care deficit (level III)/ uncompensated hemiparesis	1. Assistance required in bathing, dressing, grooming, feeding, and toileting assessed daily	1. Provides own self-care by using equipment or device in bathing, dressing, grooming, feeding, and toileting (level I)
		2. Use of adaptive equipment taught during bathing, dressing, grooming, feeding, and toileting	
		3. Compensation for deficit assessed daily	
	Ineffective family coping/role changes	1. Assisted in thinking through family management decisions until stated outcome obtained	1. Explains role readjustments made for family management
		2. Assisted in exploring role changes until stated outcome obtained	2. States no more than moderate concern about family role adjustments

*The population can be specified further (e.g., male, 45 to 65 years old, and married).

estimating what high-incidence nursing diagnoses occur with particular medical diagnoses. Table 10-5 presents an example: the medical diagnosis was cerebrovascular accident (stroke) and the predicted nursing diagnoses were potential skin breakdown, ineffective family coping/role changes, and total self-care deficit (level III)/uncompensated hemiparesis.

A second method of retrieval is to write discharge notes containing both resolved and current (unresolved) nursing diagnoses. This kind of discharge note facilitates record librarians' coding and retrieval of records by nursing diagnoses.

Interdisciplinary Reviews   Some institutions combine nursing, medical, and other health professionals' quality care reviews into one program (McCourt, 1986). Again, because of the retrieval process medical diagnosis is usually the main client classification. Nursing diagnoses can be a subset. The nursing standards could be similar to those in the example in Table 10-5.

Interpretation of Care Reviews   If standards are not reached by the specified time, two alternative interpretations are possible. One possibility is that quality care *was* delivered but client or situational factors interfered with the expected outcome. If clients with noncompliance/knowledge deficit become disoriented, it is understandable that they may not attain the knowledge level expected. This kind of situation would constitute an exception to the standard, but information about the disorientation would have to be found in the client's chart.

Not reaching an outcome can also mean that treatment of a particular nursing diagnosis was not at an acceptable level. This finding leads to the identification of care delivery problems.

Identifying Problems   The use of nursing diagnoses in population monitoring facilitates identification of care delivery problems. The group of clients receiving less than quality care is clearly specified and reasons for the inadequate care can be determined.

Problems in care delivery are identified by raising questions. For example, Why did 30 percent of the client population with the diagnosis of potential fluid volume deficit develop dehydration? Why did 10 percent of the population with potential skin breakdown develop decubitus ulcers (bedsores)?

Where do auditors find the answers to these questions?

The reader who thinks that possible answers lie in the processes of care (nursing interventions) or in the structural resources of the setting has grasped a major concept in quality care assessment. That is exactly where nurses look for the reasons why client outcomes are below standard. Charts that do not pass the outcome screening standard are examined. Process standards that have been developed for relevant diagnoses (for example, potential fluid volume deficit and potential skin breakdown) are compared to the actual care documented in the chart. It may be found that treatments for these diagnoses were not consistent with accepted standards of treatment. Why?

For answers, structural factors in the setting are examined. Was there sufficient staff competent in the treatment of these diagnoses? Did they have the necessary equipment and materials, such as special mattresses for prevention of pressure ulcerations? Does the method of nursing care delivery or philosophy of care promote individual accountability for treatment of diagnosed problems? These searching questions are asked by both practitioners and administrators.

It is advisable to begin a quality care assurance program with a concurrent audit of all (or a sample of) charts, using the ANA standards of practice. This preliminary audit can be done while committees are preparing diagnostic population standards. The major elements for this general audit are identified in Table 10-6. Included in the general process audit are assessment, diagnosis, outcomes, interventions, and evaluation of progress toward discharge outcomes. At this early point in the audit just the presence or absence of these elements is the objective of the audit.

An audit of this type will identify gross deficiencies. If nursing diagnoses, plans of care, progress notes, and discharge assessments of care outcomes are not recorded, monitoring of diagnostic populations cannot be done economically. Thus the first step is to determine whether broad standards are being met. If not, why not? After remedial actions are taken by nurses to correct these charting deficiencies, the previously described tracer population audits can be done from records.

When quality care assurance programs are built on nursing diagnoses, periodic review of the validity of diagnoses may be necessary. Nurses may not be making valid assessments or correct diagnostic judgments; these errors affect audits that are based on recorded diagnoses. Periodic review of items 1 and 2 in Table 10-6 would reveal these diagnostic errors. Actual reassessment of some clients could be done to check diagnostic accuracy, but this procedure

TABLE 10-6
GENERAL PROCESS AUDIT

---

1. Assessment contains information relevant to the 11 health pattern areas:

Health-perception–health-management	Self-perception–self-concept
Nutritional-metabolic	Role-relationship
Elimination	Sexuality-reproductive
Activity-exercise	Coping–stress-tolerance
Sleep-rest	Value-belief
Cognitive-perceptual	

2. Nursing diagnoses are supported by and consistent with history and assessment data.
3. Unstable or potentially unstable physical parameters are identified for observation, for example:
   Blood pressure
   Pulse
   Level of consciousness
4. Outcomes for diagnoses are stated.
5. Diagnosis-specific nursing activities are listed in the plan of care.
6. Progress notes are written about each diagnosis.
7. Information relevant to progress toward outomes is documented.

---

involves added time and expense. The same problem occurs in medicine. An elevated blood pressure may have been overlooked, but this lack of diagnosis and treatment would not be revealed in a process or outcome audit of a fractured femur population.

Taking Remedial Actions   Using nursing diagnoses for developing standards and identifying problems facilitates the next step in quality assurance. That step is the taking of remedial actions by nurses. Let us suppose that both the resources and the care provided are problematic for certain diagnostic populations. As an example, consider the situation in which the incidence of skin breakdown is too high. Nurses and administrators determine that the problem is twofold: inadequate professional staff and inadequate methods of prevention used by current staff.

The ultimate purpose of quality care review is to offer opportunities for institutional administrators and care providers to improve care. In the skin breakdown example, reasonable actions would include (1) obtaining more professional staff and (2) increasing staff education programs. The nursing diagnosis and management of potential skin breakdown would be an excellent topic for inservice education programs in this setting. Early diagnosis, judgments about risk factors, and prevention need emphasizing. If the problem was correctly identified and addressed, it should now be found that standards indicating quality care are being reached.

In summary, accountability to the consumer underlies quality assurance programs. Individual nurses of course evaluate the effectiveness of the care they give to individual clients; quality assurance evaluates the nursing care delivered to groups of clients. In essence, care review requires that nurses decide in what areas of health care their accountability lies. Clearly, nurses' accountability, first and foremost, is for the health problems described by nursing diagnoses. Just as physicians assume accountability for quality treatment of diseases described by medical diagnoses, nurses assume accountability for recognizing and intervening in the dysfunctional health patterns described by nursing diagnoses.

Writing standards, identifying problems that exist, and taking remedial actions are made easier when nursing diagnoses are used. Diagnoses impart clear direction to these activities. The result is that nursing assures quality of care within its own domain of practice. When each profession does this, overall health care quality is assured.

Future Directions

Two issues are clearly important as the future of quality assurance is contemplated. One is the need for a scientific base for nursing care evaluation. The second is the identification of care delivery problems and creative solutions that have immediate payoff in terms of quality.

Writing standards of care makes it clear to all involved that "mature knowledge" (replicated studies) in nursing is sparse. When a group of nurses try to state what nurses should do for a particular nursing diagnosis and what health results are expected, diversity of opinion exists. Even setting aside the matter of quality assurance, research is needed to determine effective treatments and related outcomes as a basis for everyday practice.

The second major issue for the next few years is the cost-benefit aspect of quality assurance. In simplest terms, activities have to pay off. This requires that problems in care delivery be prioritized. The highest priority must be given to those care delivery problems that have a significant impact on illness, death rates, and actual financial costs.

Inadequate preventive care is one example of a care delivery problem that when remedied can decrease health care costs. If potential problems were diagnosed and preventive care instituted, many dollars and days of disability could be saved. It is estimated that the treatment of a decubitus ulcer costs thousands of dollars but preventive nursing care of 2 hours daily costs less than $20 a day. As a second example imagine the reduction in cost, disability, and mortality if people were helped to improve their functional health patterns. Merely reducing the speed limit on highways has enormously diminished automobile accidents, one of the leading causes of death and disability.

One hospital, by focusing nurses' attention on the nursing diagnosis potential for injury, substantially reduced clients' falls (McCourt, 1979), Imagine the savings in money and days of disability and discomfort if even ten fractures of the hip were prevented. This is an example of identifying care delivery problems that have immediate payoff in monetary and human costs. Containing these costs will be the major emphasis in future quality assurance activities.

NURSING DIAGNOSES AND THIRD-PARTY PAYMENT

A large proportion of United States citizens pay for nursing care through a third party, commonly an insurance company. In fact, as will be discussed, a fourth party—the physician or hospital—enters into payment for nursing care. A brief overview of the current system of paying for care will demonstrate that some people have minimal access to nursing care and some have little choice. The historical development of the situation is interestingly portrayed by Welch (1975); change in the current situation, as will be described, can be facilitated by nursing diagnosis.

Rather than paying for health services at the time of care delivery, people pay monthly premiums to nonprofit (for example, Blue Cross and Blue Shield) or profit-making (Mutual of Omaha, Aetna, etc.) companies. Also, government funds are available for care of the elderly (Medicare) or medically indigent (Medicaid). Insurance companies and the government are referred to as *third-party payers,* and their process of payment is called *reimbursement.*

Treatment of a nursing diagnosis, except in a few instances, is not reimbursed. This means that consumers do not have direct access to nursing unless they are willing to pay the fees themselves. It means, further, that the poor and medically indigent have no choice in the type of care provider they can choose. Yet there are loopholes whereby payment for nursing occurs.

A client who wants nursing care can be admitted to a hospital or clinic; the nursing is included in the reimbursable bed and board charges or clinic fees. But to get into a hospital the client must have a disease or possible disease. Another route to take is to convince a physician that nursing care is needed. If a physician certifies the need, a client can obtain home nursing, private duty nursing, or community-based care by a nurse in private practice. As Jennings (1979) points out, although consumers are paying high premiums, in the current system a consumer is not entitled to receive any health care unless it is directed or executed by a physician.

Under the current system, many functional health problems are not diagnosed early or are not diagnosed until disease is present. Many cases could be cited: the untreated body image alteration that has to progress to a severe depression, the potential shoulder contracture that when fully developed a year after mastectomy requires surgery, and the ineffective coping pattern that is not diagnosed until child abuse results. As many have said, the current health care system is disease oriented rather than preventive care oriented.

What can be done?

Groups are currently working with legislators and insurance companies to determine reimbursement plans. This, of course, is a threat to the current system. Counteracting proposals, such as reimbursement for health education when ordered by the physician, continue to arise.

Consumers need to be informed about the controls the present system imposes on access to care. Public education requires clear communication about what is to be reimbursed. Communication should be focused on the actual and potential health problems nurses diagnose and treat rather than on tasks nurses do. Competency and quality care can be assured to consumers and third-party payers if the reasons (nursing diagnoses) for actions are specified.

In addition to these efforts to obtain reimbursement for community-based care, work is underway to study the use of nursing diagnoses to determine costs of hospital nursing. This work involves the concept of client classification for staff allocation, discussed later in this chapter.

Prospective Payment Programs

Prospective payment to hospitals for persons under the federal Medicare program was introduced in 1982. This means that hospitals know prior to care delivery what payment will be received for particular diseases. Previously, costs were established after services were delivered. This is similar to your employer (or school) telling your prior to a trip to Boston how much money you will receive to finance your trip, as opposed to submitting your actual costs after your return. Think for a minute how these two different situations could influence your behavior and you will appreciate the magnitude of change that has occurred in health care reimbursement. The reasons the federal government changed from retrospective to prospective payment are listed by Thompson and Diers (1985):

1 Spiraling health care costs
2 Increasing use of hospital services
3 Wide variation in care costs among hospitals

A method of payment based on a standard cost for specific disease groupings was instituted in the early 1980s. The method of payment is based on resources consumed. Payment remains the same regardless of the length of stay or the number of tests given. Clients with (1) similar conditions who supposedly use (2) similar resources which cost a (3) similar amount are grouped together. The 468 disease groupings are called diagnostic-related groups (DRGs). Hospitals classify individual clients into the DRG group that includes their disease/surgery/complications. There is a *standard payment for each DRG and a standard room and board for the length of stay* permitted under the DRG. Similar to the "prospective payment" for the trip to Boston, *hospitals keep the money if they can decrease costs and length of stay below the DRG. They absorb the cost if there are more services and a longer stay.* Hospitals, as well as the traveler to Boston, have to pay attention to cost control.

The DRG prospective payment system is saving money. For example, in 1985, a year when the system had been in full operation, these were the statistics:

1 The medical component of the Consumer Price Index increased 9 percent from 1983 to 1985 versus a 19-year-period of double-digit increases; there was a 6 percent increase in Medicare payments in 1985, the lowest in history.
2 The price of a hospital room in July 1985 dropped 0.4 percent for the first time in more than a decade. The average daily semiprivate rate was $212 compared to $79 in 1976.
3 Hospitals are getting fewer patients; admissions dropped 9 percent in first quarter in 1985.
4 The average length of stay of elderly patients was 8.8 days in 1985 versus 10.3 in 1982 (Social Issues, 1985).
5 There has been an increase in number of home health care visits (Taylor, 1985)

The results of these changes are: strain on home health care agencies; people going home earlier and sicker; people in hospitals more acutely ill; and many procedures and surgery, formerly done in the hospital, being done in clinics and health maintenance organizations. In 1985 this system of payment only applied to hospitals but is expected to expand to other health agencies and physicians. For example, Medicare paid hospitals $1200 to $1500 for placing an artificial lens in a patient's eye on an in-patient basis but paid hospitals or physicians up to $2800 for this procedure if done on an outpatient basis

(Social Issues, 1985); this will encourage extension of cost controls. After this introduction to prospective payment the question arises:

What is the relevance of nursing diagnosis?

In the next section it will be pointed out that nursing diagnosis accounts for a substantial portion of the costs of care and influences discharge from hospital settings.

DRGs and Nursing Diagnosis *The DRG only refer to medical diagnoses not nursing diagnoses.* This is because DRG (1) *only take into account therapeutic services* the client receives and (2) assume that *all care is disease-related* (Halloran and Halloran, 1985). Isn't that shocking? Traditionally, nursing has been part of the "bed and board" charges. It is covered under the per diem rate for a particular DRG along with housekeeping and meal services. A number of researchers have pointed out the problems [Halloran and Halloran, 1985; Halloran, Kiley, and Nadzam, 1986; Halloran, Nosek, and Kiley, in press; McKibbon, Brimmer, Galliher, Hartley, and Clinton, 1985]:

1 Not all clients within a DRG do require a similar intensity of nursing care; individual clients have different nursing diagnoses.
2 Nursing diagnoses are one reason that length of stay in a hospital varies.

This suggests that nursing diagnosis is extremely important to any cost containment program. Thus, it may be asked:

What increases resource consumption and costs?
What increases length of stay in the hospital?

Consumption of resources increases over the average for the DRG if complications result or the length of stay is exceeded. It is also important to keep in mind that too early discharge can result in readmission, complications, and death. Some points to remember in delivering care are

1 If potential for injury, potential skin breakdown, or potential for infection is not diagnosed and treated, costs can increase. In general, *risk factor control* is important both for cost containment and for preventing client discomfort.
2 Inattention to *early discharge planning,* especially with clients who have mobility impairments, pain management deficits, self-care deficits, or impaired home maintenance management can prolong the length of stay. Discharge planning should begin when the diagnosis is made and outcomes projected.
3 Delays in diagnosis and ineffective treatment plans can prolong hospitalization. In some instances lack of recognition of anxiety, ineffective coping, situational depression, or body image disturbances can influence the course of convalescence and produce complications. *Precision in diagnosis* and *effective and efficient treatment methods* are important.
4 *Quality care review and monitoring of outcomes attained* at discharge are necessary to prevent discharge before the client is ready and when community or family resources are absent.

Most nurses are employed by hospitals; if a hospital loses money the impact will be felt in salaries, reduced staffing, or layoffs. Nurses also appreciate the escalating costs of health care when they pay their own hospital insurance rates. They have always tried to prevent unnecessary hospital admissions and maintained that most clients do better at home. Thus, there is motivation to control costs, length of stay, and quality of care. A number of authors predict changes in the DRG system that will produce a more sensitive measure of the actual amount of resources consumed. It is likely that in the future DRG will be supplemented with an acuity of illness factor and nursing diagnoses.

Early in 1986, New York State began testing a model for prospective reimbursement in long-term care based on DRG. It is likely that ambulatory and community health settings will be next in doing this, followed by some method of controlling physician costs. As will be discussed in Chapter 11, prospective payment systems and other health care issues increase the need for clinical studies to refine nursing diagnoses and link diagnoses/outcomes/interventions to cost. Nursing is definitely a therapeutic service and nursing services have a definite impact on the cost and quality of care. It is important that this is demonstrated.

Halloran and his colleagues have utilized a nursing diagnosis classification system for determining staffing (Appendix F). For each client, nurses fill out a daily checklist of nursing diagnoses they are treating. Use of this classification method has revealed three things:

1 A greater percent of registered nurses on a unit decreased the cost of care delivery (Halloran, 1983).

2 Nursing diagnoses predict the client's nursing care requirements 50 percent better than medical diagnoses (Halloran, 1985; Halloran, et al., 1986).

3 Nursing diagnoses predict 20 percent more of the variation in the patient's length of stay in an acute care setting than the DRG (Halloran, et al., in press).

NURSING DIAGNOSIS AND STAFFING PATTERNS

Previously, number of professional staff was used as an example of a structural characteristic of a care delivery setting that influences quality of care. *Staffing pattern* refers to the allocation and utilization of nurses. An ideal pattern exists when the number and competency of the nurses who work in a setting match the nursing care requirements of the clients.

The degree of control a nurse has over the number of clients in his or her caseload varies with the institution. Whether or not involved in this determination, each nurse should have some understanding of how staffing is done and how daily assignments are made. If fewer staff are available than are needed, quality care or dedicated nurses suffer; if staffing is excessive, the cost to consumers and taxpayers rises.

This section includes a brief overview of how staffing patterns are determined. The influence of nursing care requirements and budgetary allocations on these decisions will be examined.

Current systems of classifying clients' care requirements receive much criticism. Equally true, the way hospitals are currently reimbursed for care does not allow for variability in nursing care requirements. This in turn has an effect on staffing. Two projects will be reported that involve studies of nursing diagnosis as a basis for determining clients' use of nursing services.

The following pages will emphasize that (1) both internal and external factors influence staffing on a unit, (2) nurses need to find ways of more accurately describing their practice so that staffing patterns support quality care, and (3) to study the potential uses of nursing diagnoses requires that every nurse incorporate diagnosis into practice.

Determination of Staffing Patterns

Nurses can set standards of quality care but standards will be difficult to realize if equal consideration is not given to staffing. Many factors influence the number of professional nurses you see on a hospital unit, clinic, or in a visiting nurse district. Two primary factors that we shall consider are client care requirements and budgetary allocations.

Classification of Care Requirements Client care requirements for a nursing unit can be determined by various means. The purpose is to predict the *nursing time* clients on a unit require. Quantifying care in terms of nursing time is the usual basis for allocating nurses.

Global approaches for determining nursing time, such as counting the number of clients, have been used. Such approaches are not too successful in predicting staffing needs because clients differ in their care requirements. Recognition of this has led to client classification as a basis for allocating nursing staff. *Classification* is the process of categorizing clients according to their nursing care requirements.

Classifications can be based on single or multiple indicators of care needs. For example, acuity of illness is one gross predictor of nursing time required. It is assumed that critically ill clients need more nursing care time than convalescent clients. If nurses did only physical care, the assumption might be true.

What if health counseling and teaching were used as indicators of nursing time required by clients? Then it might be found that convalescent clients need more or as much nursing time (and staff) as critically ill clients. Clearly, the indicator used for classifying clients ultimately influences decisions about staffing.

Most current systems of classification are based on task oriented, "doing for" views of nursing. Clients' needs for bathing, feeding, ambulation, and medication are not always valid predictors of professional nursing time required. These indicators do not take into account the scope of client problems and current standards of nursing care. By maintaining the status quo, classification systems of this type restrict developments in professional practice. In turn, clients are deprived of new developments in practice. A comparable situation would exist if a faculty-student ratio did not permit instructors to institute new methods of teaching or a physician-client ratio did not permit clients to benefit from new medical developments.

If professional staffing is based on poor predictor or poor use of predictors, shortages become the rule, not the exception. Understaffing readily limits the implementation of current practice standards including nursing diagnosis. Yet, if instituted, nursing diagnoses may provide a more valid measure of staffing needs.

Simmons (1980) has recognized the utility of diagnosis as a basis for staffing specifically in relation to community heath nursing. Her comments about the use of nursing diagnoses (nursing problems) apply to other levels of care also:

Problem labels and their signs and symptoms, stated clearly and concisely, can be useful in interpreting community health nursing services to others. A clear interpretation of services can be especially crucial when the agency must compete for funding and justify the need for existing or new programs.

Cost analysis and cost effectiveness can be enhanced by using the problem classification scheme. Nursing activities can be related to specific client problems resulting in cost centers for different client needs. Proficient use of the problem classification scheme will demand less time in recording and allow more nursing time for direct client care. (Simmons, 1980, p. 5)

Giovanetti (1978) notes that classifications are consistent with current ways of thinking about practice and with the nomenclature of the time. When nursing was conceptualized as tasks and procedures, the presently used classification systems developed. She states:

As the nomenclature changes, so will the basis for classification. Two relatively new nomenclatures to describe nursing process are now beginning to emerge: (1)patient problems and (2) nursing diagnoses. It seems reasonable to expect that as the validity of these descriptions becomes more evident, one or both may well lead to new patient classification systems, which, in turn, may be more responsive to the true nature of the patients' care requirements. (Giovanetti, 1978, p. 92)

Budgetary Allocations   A second important factor influences the number and competency of the nurses with which a unit is staffed. This factor is the budget for nurses' salaries in the institution. The nursing department budget for salaries is usually about one-third of a total hospital budget. To a great extent the hospital budget, and thus the salary budget, is controlled by outside forces.

Hospital income is based on direct client payments and reimbursement by insurance companies and public funds. The external control of reimbursement rates (by state agencies) directly influences nursing department budgets. State rate-setting commissions determine the reimbursement hospitals receive per client (excluding Medicare clients).

It must be recognized that in the majority of institutions the cost of nursing care *is included in the basic daily room charge.* This charge is a flat rate for all clients at particular levels of care (acute, intensive, long term). As an example, reimbursement is not provided for clinical specialist consultation. When nursing provided glorified maid service or apprenticeship training, inclusion in the "hotel rate" may have been appropriate.

Today many nurses argue that nursing should be a separate charge as are physical therapy, radiology, and other hospital services. Would this increase consumers' bills? Perhaps not; rather, there might be more equitable distribution. Those clients requiring minimal care would probably pay less than they now pay. Charging separately for nursing would also pressure the profession to determine the basis for fee-for-service charges. Actual and potential problems diagnosed and treated by nurses may be an answer.

In summary, hospital staffing patterns are controlled both from within an institution and by external forces. In institutions, clients are categorized (usually by medical diagnosis and acuity of illness) and their care requirements are estimated and translated into the nursing time that will be needed to give that care. This process is the basis for staffing patterns. More accurate predictions of nursing time requirements may result from using nursing diagnoses to estimate the care that will be needed.

Externally, the regulation of reimbursement rates by state agencies influences hospital budgets and, thereby, staffing patterns. Charges for nursing care are included in the daily room rate along with the cost of laundry, meals, and housekeeping. Other ways of establishing charges for nursing care are being studied; hospitalized clients of the future may pay a direct fee for nursing services.

As professionals, nurses have an obligation to clients to see that current standards of quality care are not compromised. The responsibility also exists to see that excess costs are not imposed by overstaffing. As employees, nurses seldom have much direct control over caseloads; as professionals, they are responsible for communicating clients' care requirements to enhance staffing pattern decisions.

NURSING DIAGNOSIS AND HEALTH STATISTICS

Florence Nightingale was the first to devise a system of gathering hospital and death statistics. This work was done in the middle of the nineteenth century. More recently the U.S. National Center for Health Statistics developed the Uniform Minimum Health Data Set. This data set is defined as "a minimum set of items of information with uniform definitions and categories, concerning a specific aspect or dimension of the health care system, which meets the essential needs of multiple data users." (Health Information Policy Council, 1983). Currently health statistics are mainly disease statistics; for example, the number of cases of morbidity and mortality caused by cardiovascular conditions or cancer are counted. Illnesses are classified using the World Health Organization's International Classification of Diseases (ICD) sanctioned by the World Health Organization. Every U.S. health care agency submits statistics to a national data bank for compilation of national statistics. In medicine, the Uniform Hospital Minimum Data Set (UHMDS) consists of the principal diagnosis, other diagnoses, and other relevant data.

A Nursing Minimum Data Set (NMDS) has been proposed for compiling health statistics at a national or international level (Werley and Lang, 1987; Werley, 1987). The data set contains 16 items, 11 of which are also included in other sets, such as date of birth, sex, and so forth. The items unique to the nursing minimum data set are

1 Nursing diagnosis
2 Nursing intervention
3 Nursing outcome
4 Intensity of nursing care
5 Unique identification number of principal registered nurse provider

The NMDS has been submitted to the U.S. Department of Health and Human Services. Before final acceptance the items will have to be field-tested to ensure that they can be retrieved from health care records in all settings. *If the NMDS is accepted nationally, it is important that nursing diagnoses be accurate and be recorded with the accompanying interventions and outcomes attained. Classification systems would provide measures of intensity of nursing care.* Clearly, computerized nursing information systems would facilitate collection of statistics at the agency level.

A second needed development in the collection of statistics regarding nursing diagnosis is a request to the World Health Organization to participate in the next revision of the ICD. One of the fields in this system or in a separate system could be devoted to nursing diagnoses, interventions, and outcome classifications. This would permit the collection of international statistics on nursing diagnoses. The development of the NMDS and an international classification system are important events in nursing. The reader will want to keep abreast of developments in these two areas.

NURSING DIAGNOSIS AND THE SCOPE OF PRACTICE

What is nursing practice? That question is asked by career-seeking high school students, by legislators who pass laws that regulate practice, and by hard-pressed financial vice presidents of agencies delivering nursing care. It is asked by educators designing curricula, by third-party payers, and by research funding agencies.

Nursing is caring for the whole person. Yet that statement is too vague for those who have to decide how many nurses to hire or what courses should be in a curriculum.

In recent years gigantic steps have been taken to define and describe the scope of nursing practice. Conceptual frameworks have been proposed to clarify the focus, and nurses now lament the proliferation of views. They forget that not long ago nursing was conceptualized only as being a handmaiden to other health care providers, who made all the decisions. The nursing process, requiring actions based on judgment, was "kept in the closet."

Theory and nursing process have led to even clearer articulation of the scope of nursing practice. In 1980 the Congress for Nursing Practice of the ANA defined 11 actual or potential health problem areas that exemplify the focus of nursing practice (ANA, 1980, p. 12). Within these areas, theoretical knowledge guides diagnosis and treatment.

Still clearer definition of the scope of practice will occur as nursing diagnoses are identified, standardized, and classified. Then nurses could point to a taxonomy of actual and potential problems and say nurses assume responsibility and accountability for the diagnosis and treatment of these. At a very specific, concrete level it can be said that nursing diagnoses are the focus of caring because they represent human health-related responses.

Both the ANA *Social Policy Statement* (1980) and the classification of problems in the domain of practice will increase nursing's future scope. If true responsibility is taken for a problem area such as knowledge deficit (health maintenance), imagine the opportunities for practice that will be open. Clinical research can be done about the quality and quantity of knowledge that correlates with health maintenance behavior. Nurses will be able to lobby for health education and learning centers; the media can be used to reach target populations, and third-party payers can be pressured to reimburse clients for preventive health education. These are only a few examples of what can occur as the domain of independent practice is clearly defined by nursing diagnoses.

NURSING DIAGNOSIS AND NURSING THEORY

The current effort to identify and classify nursing diagnoses has been described as theory development (Bircher, 1975; Henderson, 1978; Kritek, 1978, 1979). Interestingly, this position can produce various responses. One reaction is "If the work on diagnosis is theory development, then it's the *first* useful thing about theory I've seen." People with this point of view usually become involved in diagnostic category identification *even though* it could be theory development! The reaction that rarely leads to involvement is "Oh, another theory; probably too abstract for practice." Lacking appreciation of the use of theory in practice, nurses who hold this second view devalue diagnosis because it sounds theoretical.

Probably the most meaningful way for the learner to think about the issue is in the context of practice theory, as defined by Dickoff, James, and Wiedenbach (1968). They define four distinctive levels of theory. These levels will structure our discussion of the relationship between nursing diagnosis and theory. We shall see, as these authors propose, that theory begins and ends in practice.

Factor-Isolating Theory

Identifying and formally labeling phenomena is the first step in the development of theory in a science. This step is referred to as the factor-isolating level of theory development.

Phenomena of concern are isolated and categorized. Then the categories are given names. As previously described, categorization is a method humans use to deal with the otherwise overwhelming complexities of even their simplest environments. Things judged to be similar are given the same name. The names represent concepts or ideas that are the basic building blocks for other levels of theory.

Nursing practice has been commonly represented as a set of tasks related to clients' therapeutic needs. Categorization has been done in terms of needs for nursing such as "needs suctioning" or "needs emotional support." Grouping clients into a category like "needs emotional support" ignores the diverse health problems that may be present. These could be fear, anxiety, role conflict, and so forth. It also ignores the different interventions that may be required.

This type of categorization bears a striking resemblance to task-oriented categories in which *things are described by the actions performed in regard to them* (Bruner, Goodnow, and Austin, 1956, pp. 5–6). The formal categories of a science are established in quite a different way. Rather than describing phenomena by the response to them, *formal categories specify the intrinsic characteristics of phenomena.* In the case of nursing, intrinsic characteristics would be clusters of client characteristics such as the critical defining signs and symptoms. Formal categories such as nursing diagnoses provide a better cognitive focus for determining nursing intervention than do task-oriented categories with their prespecified interventions.

Currently, nursing diagnoses describing clients' actual or potential problems are being defined. Thinking of these as formal categories or concepts in a clinical science emphasizes the need for a scientific approach to their development. This approach will be discussed in Chapter 11 in a section on diagnostic classification systems. At that time, current identification and classification efforts will also be reviewed.

Having seen that the basic building blocks of nursing practice theories are diagnostic concepts, we can now consider other levels of theory. As will be seen, each level of theory presupposes development at lower levels (Dickoff, James, and Wiedenbach, 1968, pp. 415–435).

Higher Levels of Theory

The reader may have recognized that factor-isolating theories are the basis for concepts taught in courses such as physiology and chemistry. These disciplines isolate phenomena and create concepts such as chemical, atom, organ, and system. They then proceed to describe these and predict causal relations. This approach requires three levels of theory development: isolation, description, and prediction. As a practice discipline, concerned with intervention, nursing requires higher levels of theory development. As will be described, nursing extends beyond description and causal relations to the prescriptive theory level.

After actual and potential health problems are identified, their natural history can be described. This type of theory is called *descriptive theory*. It results in the depiction of relationships among factors in a client and situation. This description of relationships permits the study and development of third-level theories that are *predictive*. An example would be prediction of the effect A has on B. Situation A may be a nursing intervention and B a problematic health situation. Or A may be some causal factor in the development of B, a health problem.

Predictive theories are indispensable for the fourth level of theory. This is *prescriptive theory*, which assists in producing desired health outcomes.

> Prescriptive theories are situation-producing or goal-incorporating theories. They are not satisfied to conceptualize factors, factor relationships, or situation relationships, but go on to attempt conceptualization of desired situations as well as conceptualizing the prescription under which an agent or practitioner must act in order to bring about situations of the kind conceived as desired in the conception of goal (Dickoff, et al., 1968, p. 420).

In summary, identification and naming of health conditions described by nursing diagnoses is the first level of theory development. Building on these diagnostic concepts, higher levels of theory can be developed that will be a basis for treatment. In essence, the identification and classification of nursing diagnoses is the first step in developing a clinical science that can be used by all nursing clinicians. Theory development begins and ends in practice.

SUMMARY

Selected issues of practice have been examined to clarify the relevance of nursing diagnoses. It was argued that because the focus of nursing care is the client's diagnoses, it follows logically that diagnoses can provide a focus for programs designed to assure quality care.

Perhaps an even more basic issue is availability of and access to professional nursing care in institutions and communities. The suggestion was made that staffing of institutions may be improved if nursing diagnoses were considered in planning nursing staff allocations. In community practice as well as in institutions, financial reimbursement for care is an issue. As nursing moves toward third-party payment for services, nursing diagnoses will be a mechanism upon which to base reimbursement.

For many years it has been difficult to define the scope of nursing practice. Nursing diagnosis may make it possible to arrive at a clearer definition of nursing's domain of responsibility. Once the domain is defined, research and the development of practice theory can be focused on the health problems that are relevant to nursing.

Throughout this and the preceding chapter the reader may have thought that everything is being tied to nursing diagnosis! This observation is true. It suggests that perhaps clients' health problems are the basis for thinking about all nursing issues.

In essence, nursing's main social responsibility is to ensure that nursing services are available, accessible, and of a quality that promotes or maintains health. This is a huge undertaking unless the effort is narrowed to those conditions nurses are best able to prevent and treat. The next chapter deals with the ways those conditions can be identified.

BIBLIOGRAPHY

American Nurses' Association (1985). Personal communication.

American Nurses' Association Congress on Nursing Practice. (1980). *A social policy statement.* Kansas City, MO.

Bircher, A. V. (1975). On the development and classification of diagnoses. *Nursing Forum,* 14:20–29.

Bloch, D. (1975). Evaluation of nursing care in terms of process and outcome. *Nursing Research,* 24:256–263.

Bloch, D. (1980). Interrelated issues in evaluation and evaluation research. *Nursing Research,* 29:69–73.

Bruner, J. S., Goodnow, J. J. & Austin, G. A. (1956). *Study of thinking.* New York: Wiley.

Dickoff, J., James, P., & Wiedenbach, E. (1968). Theory in a practice discipline: Part I. Practice oriented theory. *Nursing Research,* 17:415–435.

Giovanetti, P. (1978). *Patient classification systems in nursing: A description and analysis.* (Publication No. HRA 78-22.) Washington, D.C.: U.S. Department of Health, Education and Welfare.

Gordon, M. (1980). Determining study topics. *Nursing Research,* 29:83–87.

Halloran, E. (1983). RN staffing: More care—less cost. *Nursing Management,* 14:18–22.

Halloran, E., & Halloran, D. (1985). Exploring the DRG nursing equation. *American Journal of Nursing,* 85:1093–1095.

Halloran, E., Nosek, L., & Kiley, M. (1987). Nursing complexity, the DRG, and length of stay. In A. McLane. (Ed.), *Classification of nursing diagnoses: Proceedings of the seventh conference.* St. Louis: Mosby.

Halloran, E., Kiley, M., & Nadzam, D. (1986). Nursing diagnosis for identification of severity of condition and resource use. In M. Hurley. (Ed.), *Classification of nursing diagnoses: Proceedings of the sixth conference.* St. Louis: Mosby.

Health Information Policy Council. (1983). *Background paper: Uniform minimum health data sets.* Unpublished. Washington, DC: U.S. Department of Health and Human Service.

Henderson, B. (1978). Nursing diagnosis: Theory and practice. *Advances in Nursing Science,* 1:75–83.

Jennings, C. P. (1979). Nursing's case for third party reimbursement. *American Journal of Nursing,* 79:110–114.

Joint Commission on the Accreditation of Hospitals. (1981). *Accreditation manual for hospitals,* Chicago.

Kessner, D. M., Kalk, C. E., & Singer, J. (1973). Assessing health quality: The case for tracers. *New England Journal of Medicine,* 288:189–194.

Kritek, P. B. (1979). Commentary: The development of nursing diagnosis and theory. *Advances in Nursing Science,* 2:73–79.

Kritek, P. B. (1978). Generation and classification of nursing diagnoses: Toward a theory of nursing. *Image,* 10:33–40.

McAuliffe, W. E. (1979). Measuring the quality of medical care: Process versus outcome. *Millbank Memorial Fund Quarterly, 37*:118–152.

McCourt, A. (1986). Nursing diagnosis: Key to quality assurance. In M. Hurley, (Ed.). *Classification of nursing diagnoses: Proceedings of the sixth conference.* St. Louis: Mosby.

McCourt, A. (1979). Personal communication.

McKibbin, R., Brimmer, P., Galliher, J., Hartley, S., & Clinton, J. (1985). Nursing costs and DRG payments. *American Journal of Nursing, 85:* 1353–1356.

Simmons, D. A. (1980). *A classification scheme for client problems in community health nursing.* (Publication No. HRA 80-16) Hyattsville, MD: U.S. Department of Health and Human Services.

Social Issues. (1985). Health care costs: The fever breaks, fierce competition—Will quality care suffer? *Business Week,* Oct. 21, 1985, pp. 86–88, 92–94.

Taylor, M. B. (1985). Effect of DRGs on home health care. *Nursing Outlook, 33*:288–291.

Thompson, J., & Diers, D. (1985). DRGs and nursing intensity. *Nursing and Health Care,* 6:435–439.

Thompson, J. D. (1981). Prediction of nurse resource use in treatment of diagnosis-related groups. In H. H. Werley & M. R. Grier (Eds.), *Nursing information systems.* New York: Springer, pp. 60–81.

Welch, C. A. (1975). Health care distribution and third-party payment for nurses' services. *American Journal of Nursing, 75*:1844–1848.

Werley, H., & Lang, N. (1987). *Nursing minimum data set.* New York: Springer.

Werley, H. (1987). Nursing diagnosis and the nursing minimum data set. In A. Mc Lane. (Ed.), *Classification of nursing diagnoses: Proceedings of the seventh conference.* St. Louis: Mosby.

Westfall, U. E. (1984). Nursing diagnosis: Its use in quality assurance. *Topics in Clinical Nursing,* 5:78–88.

CHAPTER 11

NURSING DIAGNOSIS: ACCEPTANCE, IMPLEMENTATION, CLASSIFICATION, AND RESEARCH

378

NURSING DIAGNOSIS: ACCEPTANCE, IMPLEMENTATION, CLASSIFICATION, AND RESEARCH

What is the status of nursing diagnosis in the profession, and what work is ahead? This chapter will attempt to answer these questions. Many of the realities have been saved until last in order to allow the reader to focus on the diagnostic process and its application. It will be evident in the first section of this final chapter that some nurses have difficulty with the term *diagnosis* but that the diagnostic process, or clinical judgment, are accepted as nursing functions.

The second section will review implementation in clinical units, including some suggestions for helping nurses acquire diagnostic skills. The novice in diagnosis may not have the responsibility of helping others learn to diagnose but when curiosity is expressed, suggestions can be offered.

A classification system for nursing diagnoses cannot be developed by armchair theorizing. Clinicians practicing nursing are the ones identifying client conditions and testing diagnoses in their daily care. For these reasons, even the beginner should appreciate how classification systems are developed, why they are developed, and how each nurse can contribute to the efforts of NANDA.

Progress in classification system development, including the identification of diagnostic categories and their taxonomic arrangement, will be discussed. Following this the research needed to facilitate classification system development will be described. The importance of clinical studies to validate and refine nursing diagnoses will be stressed in the last section of this chapter.

ACCEPTANCE IN THE PROFESSION

The idea of identifying a client's condition as a basis for planning nursing care is well accepted. That this condition should be conceptualized at a level beyond a set of observations is also accepted. What produces difficulty for some is the name applied to the process. The issue seems to be the word *diagnosis* and its association with medicine. Levine (1966) reacted to the term for reasons having to do with its legal implications and suggested *trophicognosis* as a substitute. Her concern was justified, since she conceived of nursing diagnosis as diagnosis of "disease and its manifestations . . . without using the formal language of medical diagnosis" (1966, p. 58). A few current diagnoses do fit her definition and increase the potential for harming clients if treated inadequately. These include fluid volume deficit, impaired gas exchange, alteration in tissue perfusion, and cardiac output (decreased). If placed in the position of consumer, this writer would request a physician rather than a nurse to treat these problems as they are currently defined. The secondary functional problems that occur because of these conditions certainly require nursing treatment.

A second reaction to nursing diagnosis is that it pigeonholes clients. This concept of nursing care has a negative emotional connotation. Humans are predisposed to categorize experiences in order to choose appropriate behavior in a situation. The need to categorize in order to understand is found in simple societies and even in cultures with a more holistic perception than ours. Nurses categorize clients' behavior; this act did not originate with nursing diagnosis. Among the categories sometimes used are "uncooperative," "turkey," "crock," and "vegetable." An article even exists with tongue-in-cheek specifications of etiological factors and treatment for one of these classifications (Whitney, 1981). Admittedly, pigeonholing and stereotyping happens. Inadequate knowledge of the person and too early closure on a diagnosis are errors that occur. Shall we blame the nurse or the concept of diagnosis? Perhaps sensitivity to these errors will prevent them.

Hagey and McDonough (1984) point out a number of legitimate concerns regarding the *social* use of nursing diagnoses in labeling clients. (Their comments are also reflected in the medical literature regarding physicians' use of medical diagnosis and reification.) The article should be studied in its entirety but the idea of ignoring the client's perspective, imposing erroneous meaning on a situation, and making decisions that implicate clients as the source of the problem which "absolves staff of their neglect" (1984, p. 153) deserves some reflection when using nursing diagnosis. Many comments center around the nurse in a bureaucratic environment where the purpose of using nursing diagnosis is to "save work" or "get the work done." In support of the author's criticisms, it is not unheard of to have nurses say they are not interested in nursing diagnosis unless it saves time. It is important to think about why some nurses feel this way; the authors suggest it is the work environment and working conditions "that interfere with in-depth problem solving and thoughtful nursing care" (1984, p. 157). It can also be asked why nurses committed to quality professional care tolerate a situation that does not permit time to listen to hidden meanings in clients' conversations and to think about them.

There was a time when nurses were not expected to think and thus were not given time for this; the "orders" for their work were written by others. As nurses change their perception of their role in the health care system, they may have to change the work situation to accommodate. Diagnosis requires time spent with clients and thinking through the meaning of situations to both the client and the nurse. It is not a simple stimulus-response activity.

IMPLEMENTATION

In this book, clinical judgment has been viewed as predominantly a logical process. Those who take this perspective believe that known components of the diagnostic process can be described in words, learned, and applied in practice to the extent one's intelligence allows. Some people, on the other hand, view judgment as an intuitive act; under this model, learning to make clinical judgments requires a description of the subjective, "aha" experiences of great nursing clinicians. This intuition model would seem to suggest imitation and apprenticeship training for the student of diagnosis.

By pulling together what is known about how humans reason, one can formulate a basis for clinical teaching and learning of diagnosis. Helping others to implement nursing diagnosis may be done informally in conversation or formally through conferences. In either case, being aware of current practice and steps in implementation will be useful.

Implementation in Practice

Not all professional developments in the health fields spread across the nation as fast as some people would desire. In medicine the application of new knowledge and techniques is sometimes delayed 5 or more years; the situation is no different in nursing.

One indicator of interest in a topic is the frequency of its appearance in journals and textbooks. Since the beginning of the national effort to identify nursing diagnoses in 1973, more than 100 articles have appeared in leading journals, and all recent textbooks in nursing process deal with the subject. Interest is high.

Interest does not help improve care, at least not until motivation leads to implementation. No data exist and thus no estimate can be made about how many nurses use nursing diagnosis to organize their clients' care.

The personal experience of the author suggests that many are implementing the concept in practice. Yet this impression is biased by association and contact mostly with those so motivated. In some regions the question of implementation has long passed. Nurses are discussing the application of diagnosis to quality assurance programs and the implications for clinical research. When a hospital requires that students know and use nursing diagnosis before affiliating for clinical experience, and when another advertises for a clinical specialist knowledgeable in nursing diagnosis, it is clear that diagnosis is established in those places.

Within the same or other regions situations are encountered in which even nursing process is not a familiar concept. Although different levels of competency are currently encountered, those interested in nursing practice are generally enthusiastic about learning nursing diagnosis. It is sometimes said that ideas arise from the academic ivory tower. This was not the case with nursing diagnosis. Clinicians seemed to appreciate its importance more than educators did in the early years.

Implementation in Education

Although interest has increased, diagnostic skills do not always appear "in bold type" in curricula of professional programs (McLane, 1982). Looking to the future, educators will have to assure that all students develop beginning competency in diagnosis and in treatment of common nursing diagnoses (Fredette and O'Connor, 1979). Otherwise, new graduates will not be prepared to practice at a level consistent with national standards of practice (see Table 9-1). State board examinations will begin to reflect this requirement as these standards are implemented. Competency in diagnosis is something graduates will use, as clinicians, the remainder of their professional lives. This usefulness criterion alone places nursing diagnosis into the category of essential content in educational programs.

Clinical experiences in disease-related judgment may not transfer to nursing diagnostic judgments. There are indications that beyond the general diagnostic process, knowledge is a significant factor in success as a diagnostician (Elstein, Schulman, and Sprafka, 1978). Clinical knowledge and nursing process have to be synthesized. Dealing with uncertainties and variability among clients requires repetitive experience in the diagnosis of common problems amenable to nursing care.

Clearly, the most economical way to acquire diagnostic skill is under the guidance of faculty. Feedback in early stages of training and guided clinical experiences offered in the educational setting are critical in developing this competency.

Currently, both remedial education and expertise in diagnosis have to be built into masters' degree and clinical doctoral programs. Graduation as a clinical specialist or teacher should guarantee to society that a nurse has the ability to diagnose and treat high-incidence nursing diagnoses in his or her speciality. Master's degree–prepared nurses are the ones who will act as consultants in differential diagnosis and provide feedback to generalists on the development of their competencies. They are also the more sophisticated clinical experts who have the responsibility for studying new or unlabeled conditions.

In-service educators continually remind us that they have to fill in the gaps that result not only from deficiencies in educational programs but also from new developments in practice or nurses' lack of continuing education. Orientation programs, workshops, and even classes in the identification and treatment of specific diagnoses are useful. Many in-service educators find, as Aspinall (1976) remarked, that nursing diagnosis and diagnostic judgment are the "weak link" in nursing process competencies. Clinicians are eager to learn. They find organizing their care around nursing diagnoses makes practice interesting and challenging and care planning more focused.

Assisting with Implementation

The usual roles of student and graduate may be reversed where nursing diagnosis is concerned. It is not uncommon to find students helping graduates learn about nursing diagnosis. This section will review the implementation process. It will be useful to be acquainted with methods and resources when opportunities to help are encountered. One should always use others' curiosity to advantage.

Nursing care settings will be encountered where the idea of nursing diagnosis is unheard of, controversial, seen as student activity, or considered interesting but unclear. In such settings it is appropriate for a student to present a brief description and examples of nursing diagnosis, if questioned. Follow this by suggesting some reading or a conference to discuss the idea. The staff may not be ready to think about diagnosis; a "back door" approach could include helping staff plan a conference on any of the following:

1 Are we implementing our institution's philosophy and objectives of nursing on this unit? (Each person at the meeting has a copy of the philosophy and objectives to examine.) Usually objectives specify identification of clients' health problems.

2 Is our practice on this unit consistent with national standards? (Each person has a copy of the generic or specialty American Nurses' Association (ANA) standards of practice to examine and perhaps also an article about legal aspects, such as the Fortin and Rabinow article listed in the Annotated Bibliography at the end of the text.) Standard 2 specifies nursing diagnosis.

3 Is our scope of practice consistent with the scope defined nationally? (Each person has a copy of the ANAs *Social Policy Statement* to examine.) Diagnosis is included within the scope of practice.

4 Is our practice consistent with the law? (Each person has copies of the state practice act and board of nursing rules and regulations; this approach is useful if diagnosis or judgment is specified in those documents.)

The topics provide a basis for thinking about current practice. The objective is to examine personal role concepts relative to outside criteria. This comparison, combined with one selected reading on the concept of nursing diagnosis, should lead nurses to consider the idea of using diagnoses, which is step one. Conversations and questions about diagnosis suggest readiness for step two.

The second step in implementation is to provide information. One or more of the following may be helpful:

1 Provide a small bibliography of two or three articles about nursing diagnosis, especially articles that are relevant to the type of clients the present staff serves.

2 Secure a speaker who is expert in nursing diagnosis, either a member of the staff or someone from elsewhere in the town or city.

3 Some staff members may be able to attend a continuing education offering about nursing diagnosis and report to the others.

Contact the local, state, or regional diagnosis association through the North American Nursing Diagnosis Association (NANDA). If interest in trying nursing diagnosis as a means of organizing nursing care is present, inform physicians before recording on charts. They may not understand the new way of recording. Think about (1) their level of knowledge and attitudes and (2) how nursing diagnosis may positively influence client care, and be ready with examples relevant to the particular physician's interest. Have the support within nursing before informing other professionals.

The group is ready for step three when even a few staff want to learn more. Step three begins the staff's educational process. The first learning objective is application of the definition of nursing diagnosis.

Diagnostic recognition exercises, such as those in Appendix G, are useful. These exercises require knowledge and application of the definition of a nursing diagnosis. Recognition of what is and what is not a diagnosis is present when discriminations can be made and reasons stated for choosing, and not choosing, items.

The group is then ready to move to *diagnostic selection exercises;* an example is provided in Appendix G. It is useful to prepare exercises at various levels of difficulty. For example, in vignettes the cues can range from obvious, critical defining signs and symptoms to cues which are ambiguous or conflicting. Also, a higher level of difficulty is attained if no diagnoses are provided at the end of the vignette and diagnostic hypotheses have to be generated during the reading of the vignette. A list of diagnoses and defining characteristics, such as those provided in a manual (Gordon, 1987) or book (McLane, 1987), are used to assist in problem-identification. An example of this second type of diagnostic selection exercise is contained in Appendix G. Early diagnostic concept learning is facilitated if (1) a language is provided (diagnostic labels) and (2) vignettes are constructed directly from defining characteristics of diagnoses. Ambiguities and uncertainties can be introduced *after* the basic concepts are acquired.

The next level of learning, problem formulation, utilizes total case data rather than vignettes. Learning can be facilitated by *diagnostic formulation exercises.* Examples are contained in Appendix H. This exercise is the most difficult but also the most meaningful. It stimulates the process used in actual client care. Answers to exercises in Appendix G and H are provided in Appendix O.

Repetition of diagnostic formulation exercises increases the group's skill in analyzing and integrating clinical data. When expertise is developed in formulating nursing diagnoses from simulated case data, each participant can be asked to bring to the group admission data and diagnoses from one of his or her own clients. Deficiencies in assessment, hypothesis generation, and testing, and in problem formulation can be discussed; this discussion can benefit both the individual and the group. After one or two experiences, diagnostic process (the hypothesis-testing model Chapters 7 and 8) should be discussed. This will focus attention on the *process* being used as well as on diagnostic labeling of health problems.

Step four involves using the diagnostic process with clients. One of the factors that facilitates formulating nursing diagnoses is collecting a *nursing* data base. Difficulties arise if the collected information is more appropriate to medical than nursing diagnoses. As implementation of the diagnostic process begins, nurses may become aware of needs to improve their interviewing and assessment skills. In addition, branching, hypothesis testing, and problem formulation usually need to be discussed. Some may wish not to record their first efforts in the client's chart. Provide opportunities for review by the group, a colleague, or whoever is guiding their learning. This helps alleviate anxiety about mistakes in labeling and charting.

Step five in implementation may last for a year. This is the questioning and doubting phase. Topics usually needing discussion include doctors' reactions, ways to treat diagnoses, the need for further work on terminology, and the creation of new terms to describe client conditions. The most common basis for discouragement in the novice is the time that diagnosis and care planning take.

One or more of the following approaches may help the staff get through the phase of feeling that "nursing diagnosis takes too much time":

1 Can I help? In what aspect are you having difficulty?

2 How many times have you gone through the diagnostic process (systematic health status assessments, problem identification, and care planning)? Oh, just once?

3 Do you remember how long it took you to give your first bath and make a client's bed?

4 Have you noticed how long it takes a medical student to do a history and exam? [Or] When you go to a physician for the *first* time, I imagine the history and examination take at least 30 minutes, and the doctor is probably experienced; I guess most of us would not refuse this much attention.

5 Oh, do you think there are areas in the functional patterns assessment that are not important? [This induces conflict.]

6 Could you be intervening as well as assessing? Oh, that's why it takes so long.

7 What nursing diagnoses did your client have? Oh, you wouldn't have wanted to miss *these*.

8 Yes, but now you have a base; daily assessments can be done from this base, and look how many problems you can prevent that would otherwise take nursing time to treat.

9 I promise that if you keep practicing, the *most complex* assessment, diagnosis, and care planning can be done in 30 minutes. For most clients this whole process may take 15 minutes.

10 Don't clients deserve the time functional health assessment takes? [This is the ethical-moral-legal appeal.]

Learning to systematically assess functional health patterns and identify and label problems, if there are any, takes time. This is why in other professions the skills are developed during the educational program. Those not having this opportunity to learn while in school will have to spend the time it takes, just as the others have had to do. There is nothing magical that will produce overnight the competency needed in current practice. The consolation is that diagnostic skills have lasting value, in contrast to learning how to use the latest machine that may be outdated in a year.

Resources Available The literature contains a number of articles useful in implementing nursing diagnosis in practice settings. Sharing even one of these may stimulate interest.

Feild's (1979) excellent description of her experience with the change process for implementing diagnosis is a good resource for staff, head nurses, and administrators. Dalton (1979) and Weber (1979) provide many insights about establishing diagnosis-based care in a community setting and private practice, respectively. Bruce (1979) describes a program of implementation stimulated by nursing administration and Rantz, Miller, and Jacobs (1985) discuss implementation in long-term care.

As implementation proceeds, resource information from articles listed in the bibliographies of chapters and the Annotated Bibliography at the end of the book may be helpful. NANDA, discussed in the next section, provides Nursing Diagnosis Newsletter containing national, regional, and local activities.

Clearly, the best way to exchange ideas about implementation is to hold local meetings, as is done in some regions. All participants in the monthly meetings comment on the learning that has occurred as a result of discussions with nursing colleagues. The local groups that have been formed in a few states can provide leadership through its members' practice and through conferences held in conjunction with state nurses' associations. Most importantly, having a local group offers a forum for nurses to extol or criticize the latest developments in nursing diagnosis.

In summary, one should not expect to find outstanding diagnostic competencies in all clinical settings. Change takes time. Yet the time can be reduced. Professional education can be designed to enable students to learn beginning diagnostic and therapeutic skills before graduation.

When students or staff begin to use nursing diagnoses in obvious places, such as care plans and charts, other nurses ask questions. In order to prepare the reader for these questions, a brief overview of stages of implementation and available resources has been provided. Introducing the staff to a professional role concept compatible with using nursing diagnosis is a basic step in implementing diagnosis; this leads them to examine the concept. The next steps in implementation center on the use of diagnostic nomenclature and process skills. No one has become an expert in diagnosis overnight, but once skills are developed they last a lifetime.

Diagnostic judgment is a process that requires a "language" for describing conclusions. In the next section, current developments in naming client conditions encountered in practice will be described.

CLASSIFICATION SYSTEM DEVELOPMENT

Diagnostic categories have been discussed throughout this book and at this point the reader needs to know where these categories originated and how they may change or evolve in the future. This brings us to the idea of classification systems in nursing. To understand the development of a diagnostic classification system, or taxonomy, it is necessary to review some terms and their definitions and the purposes of classification. Following this the Association that assumes responsibility for diagnostic classification, NANDA[1] will be described. The section will end with diagnostic category development, the elements of a classification system used most commonly in clinical practice.

Nursing Classification Systems

A diagnostic classification system is only one type of classification used in nursing practice. Classifications of interventions and outcomes need to be developed that interface with a diagnostic system. Clients have been classified in order to enhance staffing decisions. Except for the system using nursing diagnoses designed by Halloran (Appendix J), therapeutic needs or tasks requiring nursing time have been used. Clients are grouped according to acuity or intensity of illness. Classifications of nursing care providers have been attempted based on educational levels or roles and, of course, there is familiarity with the bureaucratic classifications of nurses along managerial lines, such as head nurse, clinical director, and director of nurses. None of the current classifications of nurses can be integrated with practice-based classifications because nurses have not been classified according to diagnostic and therapeutic expertise, other than that inferred by education. Similarly, no work exists on the diagnostic and therapeutic complexity of current diagnostic categories. The emphasis in this chapter will be on diagnostic classification.

Characteristics of a Classification System

A classification system is an arrangement of phenomena into groups or sets based on their relationships. For example, in a university students are classified by educational level: baccalaureate, master's, doctoral. Students working for a baccalaureate are further classified as freshmen, sophomores, juniors, and seniors. In the sciences and professions, classification is used to sort, code,

---

[1]NANDA, The North American Nursing Diagnosis Association, was formerly the National Conference Group for Classification of Nursing Diagnoses (1973–1982).

and order the phenomena of interest during first level-theory development, as discussed in Chapter 10. Biology is an example; it names and orders classes of living things. Chemistry classifies elements in a periodic table and medical science classifies diseases. *A class is a grouping of similar phenomena.* For example, apples are a class of fruit. In using the classification system, a piece of fruit that shares the same, or similar, characteristics as apples would be classified (named) *apple.* In nursing practice a diagnostic class is used to name a cluster of observed signs and symptoms when the observations correspond to the characteristics of the diagnostic class. (*The terms diagnostic category and diagnostic class are used synonomously.*)

Taxonomy is another term that will be heard in discussions of nursing diagnoses. It is used as a *synonym* for *classification* but also refers to the science of classification. A provisional diagnostic taxonomy of *human response patterns* will be discussed in this section.

Nomenclature is another term that will be encountered in discussions of classification. It refers to a *compilation of accepted terms for describing phenomena,* such as the names of nursing diagnoses. The diagnoses listed in Appendix A represent the currently developed diagnostic nomenclature in nursing.

Development of a classification system requires that (1) the purpose of the system is clear, (2) the conceptual focus and classes of phenomena are identified, (3) names are given to the phenomena, and (4) classes are systematically ordered according to an organizing principle. Hangartner (1975) in his discussion of classification systems uses the example of the common telephone book. The ideas of purpose, focus, naming, and ordering principle can be illustrated by enlarging his example of a simple classification system:

The *NYNEX Yellow Pages, Boston Area* includes a passage entitled "How to Use the Yellow Pages" that describes a system for classifying large and small businesses that provide a product or a service. Underlying the structure of this system is the everyday "theory" of classifying businesses according to their services. Purpose, focus, ordering principle, and description are evident. *Purpose:* "Telephone directories are provided as an aid to good telephone service." *Focus:* "Exclusively business related heading, 'Product or service.'" *Ordering principle:* "Headings are always alphabetical. Think of the heading most likely to carry what you want. Flip to it and you'll find names, addresses and phone numbers of business people ready to serve you. Forgotten the name? Again, turn to the heading best describing the firm's type of business. Glancing down the list [alphabetical] will usually bring the name back to mind" (*NYNEX* , 1986, p. 8). Under "employment" one finds employment agencies, employment contractors—temporary help, and employment training service. Under each is an alphabetical listing of names. This constitutes a three-level ordering hierarchy.

A classification system of nursing diagnoses might have a similar format: broad categories, diagnostic categories, and subcategories. This kind of system would provide a hierarchical reference to the health problems within the scope of nursing practice. Nursing diagnoses would be arranged at one horizontal level with similar problems separate from dissimilar ones.

Purpose of Classification

Why does nursing desire a classification system? What purpose will it serve other than filling the pages of a manual? These are critically important questions that have to be answered before beginning development. What is classified—that is, the focus of classification—and how the classes are ordered depend on the purpose of the system.

Classification systems designed for one purpose are more desirable than multipurpose schemes that have to accommodate to many types of operations. The initial purpose of developing a classification system in nursing was to facilitate practice. Diagnostic nomenclature did not exist; it was not a situation in which basic level diagnoses had been identified and standardized and were awaiting a system of classification that would be relevant to practice. It was necessary to start "from scratch." The task was to begin to develop a way of naming the client conditions that generated therapeutic concern. In essence, nurses had to sort and code their world of practice.

In their foresight, Gebbie and Lavin, coordinators of the First National Conference for Classification of Nursing Diagnosis, set the focus for classification system development: nursing diagnoses. A few articles had appeared in the literature but in the early 1970s most nurses still described their practice in terms of nursing objectives and tasks. The client conditions necessitating care were not articulated. In fact, the first classification system relevant to practice focused on therapeutic objectives as can be seen in the 21 problems listed in Table 2-1 (Abdellah, 1959, p. 26).

With a diagnostic classification system, or taxonomy, nurses in practice will be able to consult a manual that contains the entire diagnostic nomenclature. This will enable them to label client conditions consistently. When a diagnostic label is used, it will have a standard definition. This uniformity decreases the probability of communication errors.

A diagnostic classification system can be used to construct other systems with other purposes. There may be systems for computerizing nursing information; one such system of interest to nursing administrators would relate diagnoses to nursing care time. Classifying clients' diagnoses and the time required for intervention would assist in determining staffing patterns and hospital reimbursement. In addition, the development of a clinical science would be facilitated by classification of the client conditions amenable to nursing therapy.

In summary, current efforts in classification are directed toward establishing a system to facilitate practice. Yet this system can be used to design others. Let us now examine what progress has been made and the methodology used. Identification and ordering of diagnostic categories will organize the discussion.

Conceptual Focus for Classification

Since 1973, NANDA's efforts have been directed toward identification and naming health-related conditions of clients that nurses said they diagnosed and treated in their practice. Each nurse-participant's personal concept of nursing influenced the identification and development of diagnostic categories; no common conceptual focus was used. It is advantageous to represent the diversity in nursing but the disadvantage is that diagnoses are at various levels of abstraction and disparate in conceptual focus. In 1977 Sister Callista Roy, a member of the original task force concerned with diagnostic classification, convened a group of nurse theorists (Appendix K) to

1 Develop a framework for organizing diagnoses in a classification system
2 Make recommendations on the level of abstraction of the diagnostic labels
3 Correlate their work with the ongoing development of diagnostic categories
4 Clarify the relevance of the framework for nursing practice (Roy, 1984)

In their first and subsequent reports the Theorist Group presented a framework with the central concept, health of unitary man/human. Nine patterns of unitary man/human—environment interaction were identified:

1 *Exchanging* Mutual giving and receiving
2 *Communicating* Sending messages
3 *Relating* Establishing bonds
4 *Valuing* Assigning relative worth
5 *Choosing* Selection of alternatives
6 *Moving* Activity
7 *Perceiving* Reception of information
8 *Knowing* Meaning associated with information
9 *Feeling* Subjective awareness of information

Currently identified defining characteristics and diagnoses were grouped under these abstract pattern concepts representing unitary patterns of man/human—environment interaction. It was recognized that each pattern concept will require explicit definition. Basic assumptions underlying the framework are contained in the following narrative prepared by the Theorist Group in 1982 (Roy, 1982):

The first basic assumption about unitary man/human is the belief that unitary man/human is an open system, that is, a system in mutual interaction with the environment. Negentropy, a characteristic of open systems, is a process of continuous development toward increasing complexity and diversity. This process can be viewed from observations of individuals throughout the life process and observations from generation to generation.

The second basic assumption is that unitary man/human is a four dimensional energy field characterized by pattern and organization. Each human field has a unqiue pattern. The uniqueness of the pattern and organization of each field is manifest in nine man/human-environment interactional patterns.

The basic assumptions about health are that 1) it is a value, 2) it is a pattern of energy exchange, 3) this pattern enhances field integrity of unitary man/human (field integrity is denoted by completeness, efficiency, clarity, accuracy, and authenticity), and 4) it is manifested through nine man human/environment interactional patterns.

Nursing Diagnosis: Nursing is concerned with the health of unitary man/human. Nursing diagnosis is an integral component of the science and practice of nursing. It is a judgment about health based on data relevant to the conceptual framework of nine patterns. Diagnosis requires refinement of the patterns through identification of the characteristics.

The reader may note that this conceptual framework has assumptions similar to the work of Rogers reviewed in Chapter 3. The nine patterns were identified by the Theorist Group through analysis of the diagnostic list from 1977 to 1982. They are dynamically interrelated patterns and within their interaction is the unity of person interacting with the unity of the environment. In their 1982 report the theorists noted that the framework was incomplete and that a gap existed between the framework and the accepted nursing diagnoses (Roy, 1984). They recommended further refinement and research. Progress reports on the work of the Theorist Group (from 1978 to 1982) may be found in the proceedings of conferences (Roy, 1982; Roy, 1984).

Taxonomy Development

Further work on this framework by the NANDA Taxonomy Committee, chaired by Dr. Phyllis Kritek, continued between 1982 and 1986. The Committee's proposal to endorse the NANDA Nursing Diagnosis Taxonomy I (Appendix L) was accepted by the 1986 General Assembly of NANDA members. The following represent changes and additions from previous work (NANDA, 1986a):

1 The nine patterns listed above constitute the level 1 concepts, the most abstract level, and are called *human response patterns.* These patterns are the conceptual framework for organizing the taxonomy.

2 Level 2 concepts are less abstract and represent alterations in subcategories of human response patterns. Alterations are defined as "the process or state of becoming or being made different without changing into something else." Levels 2, 3, 4, and 5 contain current diagnoses.

3 Designations of actual or potential, acuity, and other qualifiers are defined in Appendix M.

The overall purpose of classifying human response patterns is to describe the structure and order of phenomena. The hierarchical arrangement of concepts identifies previously undiscovered properties of classes. Ordering also assists in the development of research hypotheses about relationships among concepts within the system (Sokal, 1974).

Classes are arranged in a hierarchy according to their level of abstraction. Each higher level class includes the classes at the lower levels. Consider a familiar example: *fruit* is at a higher level of abstraction than *apples* but *McIntosh apples* represent a lower level of abstraction than the general class, *apples.* In diagnosis, *alterations in nutrition* is at a higher level of abstraction than *protein deficit.* The reader may have figured out the reason one class, category, or concept is at a higher or lower level of abstraction than another. It is the distance from observable characteristics; the greater the distance from its observable characteristics, the more abstract (as opposed to concrete) the idea.

The levels within Taxonomy I represent a hierarchical ordering from abstract (level 1) to concrete (levels 4 and 5). The following example of a level 1 pattern concept, *feeling,* illustrates the idea of levels and order within the taxonomy; note that diagnostic categories from Appendix A are classified at various levels. This clearly points out that current diagnoses vary in level of abstraction:

Level 1	**9. FEELING**
Level 2	9.1 Alterations in Comfort
Level 3	9.1.1 Pain
	9.1.1.1. Chronic
	9.1.1.2. *Acute*
	9.1.2 *Discomfort*
Level 2	9.2 *Alterations in emotional integrity*
Level 3	9.2.1 Anxiety
	9.2.2 Grieving
Level 4	9.2.2.1. Dysfunctional
	9.2.2.2. Anticipatory
	9.2.2.3. ?
Level 3	9.2.3 Potential for Violence
	9.2.4 Fear
	9.2.5 Post Trauma Response
Level 4	9.2.5.1 Rape Trauma Syndrome
Level 5	9.2.5.1.1 Rape Trauma
	9.2.5.1.2 Compound Reaction
	9.2.5.1.3 Silent Reaction
	9.3?

The question marks represent possible diagnostic classes and sets yet to be identified. Italics signify classes created by the Taxonomy Committee. Examination of this pattern and the eight others in Appendix L makes it clear that (1) further development of diagnostic nomenclature is necessary and (2) the current difficulty in using some diagnostic categories in practice is because they are too general; further specification is necessary. This, of course, is the value of classification as opposed to alphabetical listing.

Examination of this evolving taxonomy raises a number of questions, some of which were raised by the NANDA General Assembly in 1986:

Where do functional health patterns fit into Taxonomy I?

At what level of the taxonomy are the diagnoses used in care planning?

Will some diagnoses not be acceptable if they don't fit into a higher level set or pattern concept?

The answers to these questions will in some cases require a crystal ball and it should be clear that the following "answers" represent speculations of the author and not the NANDA Taxonomy Committee.

Taxonomy I and Functional Health Patterns   Functional health patterns are frequently used as a format for organizing assessment data. The novice diagnostician also uses the functional pattern groupings of diagnostic categories (Appendix C) to facilitate the process of going from data to diagnosis. In addition, in some curricula nursing knowledge is organized within the patterns. Let us consider how the functional health patterns are related to the taxonomy.

Level 2 Concepts   In the author's opinion Taxonomy I is compatible with the functional health patterns and, although implicit, for the most part the dimensions of the patterns are included. For example, if the term *alterations* is removed from level 2 terms in Appendix L, the following listing of level 2 concepts is parallel to the functional patterns in most cases:

Level 2 concepts* (*N* = 27)	Functional Health Patterns
Physical Integrity (Suffocation, Trauma, etc.) *Participation* (Noncompliance) *Physical Regulation* (Infection)	Health-Perception–Health-Management Pattern
Nutrition *Physical Integrity* (Skin Tissue) *Physical Regulation* (Body Temperature)	Nutritional-Metabolic Pattern
Elimination	Elimination Pattern
Activity *Recreation* *Activities of Daily Living* Self-Care *Oxygenation* *Circulation* *Growth and Development*	Activity-Exercise Pattern
Rest	Sleep-Rest Pattern
Sensory-Perceptual Knowledge *Learning* Thought Processes Comfort	Cognitive-Perceptual Pattern
Self-Concept *Emotional Integrity* *Meaningfulnesss*	Self-Perception–Self-Concept Pattern

(continued)

Level 2 concepts* (N = 27)	Functional Health Patterns
Socialization *Communication* *Role* (Performance, Family Process) *Emotional Integrity* (Violence)	Role-Relationship Pattern
Sexuality *Role* (sexual)	Sexuality-Reproductive Pattern
Coping	Coping-Stress Tolerance Pattern
Spiritual State	Value-Belief Pattern

*Italics refer to the category sets created by the Taxonomy Committee to provide a level 2 concept for currently identified diagnoses in levels 3 and 4.

Although it would be possible to convert the functional patterns to the more specific level 2 concepts (e.g., coping pattern or role pattern), this would increase the memory requirements to twenty-seven areas of assessment. Note that *growth and development* is placed under moving in the taxonomy. Actually, this is a characteristic of *each* of the nine human response patterns and *each* of the eleven functional health patterns.

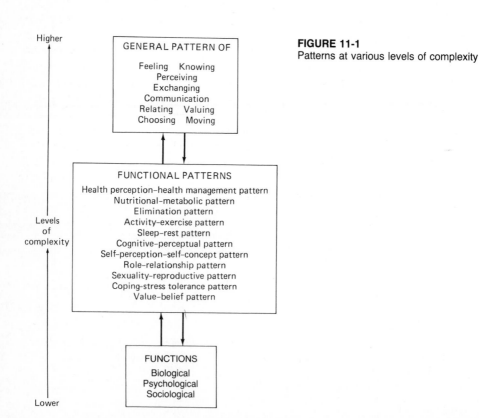

FIGURE 11-1
Patterns at various levels of complexity

Level 1 Concepts   Figure 11-1 represents the author's idea of how the functional patterns fit with superordinate level 1 pattern concepts. There is no one to one matching. The patterns of exchanging, relating, and so forth are a synthesis of functional patterns, just as functional patterns are a synthesis of lower-level biological, social, and psychological functioning. For example, as the reader has already learned, functional patterns are biopsychosocial patterns. It is the interaction of the parts that makes up the whole, that is, a pattern at a higher, more complex level of human functioning. Is this not the same case with the taxonomy pattern concepts? A higher level of synthesis of human behavior exists within the concept of exchanging, relating, and so forth. Now consider the health-perception–health-management pattern and the definitions of the taxonomy pattern concepts. Perception of one's health status and management of health (and disease, if present) is influenced by a person's pattern of knowing, perceiving, feeling, relating, valuing, choosing, moving, and exchanging. As Figure 11-1 illustrates, each functional pattern *contributes to and is influenced by* the person's general pattern of knowing, feeling, and so forth. This has implications for diagnosis.

Taxonomy I: Implications for Diagnosis   The implications of Taxonomy I for diagnosis are both obvious and not so obvious as one looks into the crystal ball. Consider first a prediction. When the nine pattern-concepts are more clearly defined they may represent a structure for the diagnosis of *life patterns.* These diagnoses would describe health problems at a higher level than currently identified. Instead of a cluster of signs and symptoms, this level of diagnosis would represent a cluster of "diagnoses," or problems and their etiological factors. A life pattern may be seen as a thread that seems to tie together and explain current health problems or risk states. As envisioned, this level of diagnosis may also explain particular sets of problems. To make this type of diagnosis it may be necessary to move from (1) assessment data to diagnoses, as currently conceived, and then (2) to a synthesis that results in problem identification (within a category of knowing, choosing, and so forth). The example in Figure 11-2 illustrates that discernible behavior may be described as self-concept dis-

FIGURE 11-2
Possible levels of diagnosis.

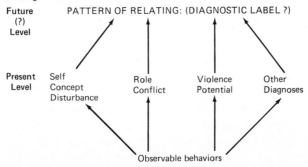

turbance, role conflicts, violence potential, and other problems. A synthesis of these problems may reveal a larger problem with relating in general, as yet unnamed. If intervention deals with the client's pattern of relating, then the more concrete diagnoses may all improve. Identification of general patterns has been discussed by others (Rossi and Krekeler, 1982; Field, 1982; Weber, 1982; Kirk, 1986). It is unlikely that this level of diagnosis will be resolved in a 2-day hospital stay. Although diagnosis is possible, it is likely that this level of diagnosis will need longer-term treatment. Perhaps the likely prediction is that nursing diagnosis and treatment will be at both the dysfunctional pattern level and the higher level of life pattern.

Congruence Between Taxonomy I and Diagnoses   The reader may be thinking: Will the taxonomy control acceptance of diagnoses or will new diagnoses possibly force changes in the taxonomy as needed? As Kritek (1986, p. 36) reports ". . . generation and classification should occur in tandem. Each process enhances, and challenges, the other. To continue to develop, test, and approve labels in a conceptual vacuum makes little sense." As the NANDA Taxonomy Committee report suggests, the answer lies in clinical studies to test both the taxonomy and the diagnostic categories. In order to identify diagnostic categories at the higher level of human response patterns, research will be needed to identify and label patterns of relating, exchanging, and so forth.

There is a deeper question that plagues taxonomy development. Are the human response patterns too abstract to guide identification of client conditions? What, exactly, is it that we are identifying and classifying—conditions resolved by nursing treatment or all health problems of concern in practice? The concepts, human response patterns, client-environment interactions, unitary man/human, and so forth, still do not provide an answer. Yet, there is a distinct feeling we are getting closer to an answer. The reader just entering the profession will be pleased that there still is intellectual work for the next generation of nurses.

The NANDA taxonomy is provisional in nature and will be further developed. Revisions will be presented at NANDA biennial conferences. This will give opportunities for further comments by the membership and the nursing community between conferences. It is predicted that the taxonomy will continuously evolve through theoretical work and research, as well as through interaction with the diagnostic nomenclature being developed.

Diagnostic Category Development

As seen in the previous discussion, a taxonomy consists of various levels. *The level that contains diagnostic categories is the one used most commonly.* This level contains the classes used in nursing practice to label diagnostic judgments about health-related conditions. Each class, or category, is defined by a cluster of observable characteristics. The characteristics are used in practice as diagnostic criteria for a judgment that a condition is present or absent.

Since 1973 NANDA has been classifying health-related conditions that nurses say they diagnose and treat in their daily practice. The state of development of diagnoses reflects the overall state of knowledge development in nursing. By no means are all the currently identified diagnostic categories based on a sound conceptual or theoretical base, a complete description of health conditions treated by nurses, or always precise enough to assure agreement among nurse-diagnosticians viewing the same client.

Current diagnostic categories share the same problems as some of the categories in medicine and psychiatry. Yet, with all their deficiencies, clinicians are reporting their usefulness in direct and indirect care activities. This is probably because (1) having language symbols (diagnostic terms) for recognizing and thinking about problems encountered in practice increases sensitivity to cues and awareness of clients' conditions and (2) provides a "resting point" for thinking about how to provide professional help and guidance. The widespread use in practice is why it is so important for nurses to recognize the need for refinement of categories used in clinical reasoning and to make a concerted effort to improve currently identified categories.

Conceptual and structural aspects of diagnostic categories will be examined in this section. The ideas may prove useful in developing and refining the categories used in clinical practice. The views represent the author's opinion and not, necessarily, that of the North American Nursing Diagnosis Association.

Conceptual Basis of a Diagnostic Category   A diagnostic category represents a conceptual view, or model, for thinking about a set of observations. Previously, the term *conceptual model* has been used to refer to a perspective, or way of thinking, about *all of nursing.* The difference in the use of the term here is that it is applied to *one phenomenon* in nursing, that is, one phenomenon described by one diagnostic concept.[2] *Each diagnostic category serves as a model to organize and account for empirical observations.* Think a moment about that statement.

As the reader has learned, concepts are created and the "creation" represents the perspective of the "creator." If a diagnostic concept survives in the "marketplace" of clinical practice and is used by others, it may be concluded that the concept of the health problem represents a useful and meaningful way of thinking about observed behaviors. As knowledge increases, models may change and categories will be changed or modified.

Knowing the conceptual meaning of a diagnostic category permits interpretation of clinical observations. *Meaning* refers to the conceptual basis of the diagnostic category, that is, the synthesis of theoretical and empirical knowledge about the health problem. There could be a discrepancy between your idea of the meaning of anxiety and another nurse's; therefore, the meaning needs to be specified to prevent miscommunication and errors in the use of the category. The conceptual basis of *each* diagnostic category needs to be specified. Norris (1982), and many of the manuscripts in Nicoll's compilation (1986), provide guidelines for developing the conceptual basis of each diagnostic category.

---

[2]It is more appropriate to use the term *diagnostic concept* in this discussion; recall that the terms *category* and *concept* refer to the same thing, but are used in different contexts.

Work in this area would lead to clear definitions and permit development of precise measurements. The questions and related activities that direct this work are

1 What is the current state of knowledge in each area described by a diagnostic category? Review the research literature related to each category; start with high incidence diagnoses.

2 Write up the conceptual basis citing references. Point out agreements, disagreements, gaps.

3 Does consistency exist between current concepts and each label, definition, characteristic, and etiological factor? Identify consistencies and inconsistencies.

4 Write up the conceptual analysis of elements in item 3. Identify further conceptual analysis, research, and development needed to improve the category. Is there a basis for any immediate improvements? Suggest these. Share findings.

5 Begin the analyses and research indicated.

The above plan needs to be implemented. Items 1 to 4 may provide sufficient basis for suggesting revisions in current categories to NANDA Diagnosis Review Committee (Appendix N). Item 5 will provide a program of theory development and research and can be the basis for further revisions. Revisions and reformulations will continue as long as the condition described by the category is of concern to nurses.

Some current categories could be improved by merely structural analysis and expert opinion. Even improvements in the structure of categories will begin to eliminate one source of diagnostic errors. Yet, it is important to be aware that tidiness is only a "minor virtue," in contrast to the underlying conceptual insights which are of major concern.

Structure of Diagnostic Categories Structure of diagnostic categories refers to the content and format of labels, definitions, major characteristics (diagnostic criteria), and minor characteristics (supporting data), and etiological factors. These are the elements of a category that are most frequently used in everyday practice. The level of theoretical development of a concept influences what is included in the structural elements. For purposes of discussion let us assume that this knowledge is not deficient and review some considerations in creating a diagnostic category suggested by Gordon (1985, 1986).

Level of Generality Recall that it was said that patterns, categories, classes, or concepts could be at various levels of abstraction. Abstract categories are more general descriptions (e.g., color) than concrete categories (e.g., red). A general term is inclusive, that is, it includes many things. Categories at a high level of generality, or inclusiveness, are not useful for planning treatment. For example, a *very* general category is *dysfunctional elimination pattern.* It is so inclusive that it includes all the diagnoses and certainly wouldn't be used to plan treatment. *Dysfunctional bowel pattern* includes less diagnostic categories and is less abstract but still not at a useful level. Proceeding toward the concrete:

Does *intermittent constipation pattern* provide a focus for recognizing a specific condition in clinical situations, clustering observations, and planning treatment? Probably so, because this category seems to be at a useful level of generality. In previous chapters categories, such as alteration in parenting or skin integrity, were used as examples of general and inclusive categories. When encountering this type of category, one is prompted to say: What kind of alteration? As may be seen in Appendix L, categories at a high level of abstraction or generality are at level 1 and 2, whereas the useful categories are probably at levels 3 and 4 (perhaps at level 5). *When refining or constructing categories, aim for the level of generality that is "appropriate for using, thinking about, or naming" the condition* (Rosch, 1978). This is the level needed for "thinking about" the condition and for "using" the diagnosis in treatment planning.

   Naming and Defining Categories   Consistency should exist between (1) the meaning of the diagnostic concept and (2) its structural elements which are the category name, definition, and major characteristics (diagnostic criteria for making the diagnosis). For a double-check see that internal consistency exists among the elements themselves. This applies to categories used to describe an actual or potential problem or to describe an etiological factor, as illustrated in Figure 11-3.

   Consistency is defined as agreement or harmony among (1) parts or features and (2) between parts and the whole. When internally consistent, there are no contradictions among the elements in Figure 11-3. For example, logical consistency and consistency in description would be: (1) Conceptual meaning is reflected in the descriptive label (name), (2) the label concisely summarizes the definition, and (3) the major characteristics permit discriminations between the presence or absence of the phenomena described by the definition and name.

FIGURE 11-3
Relationships among components of a diagnostic category.

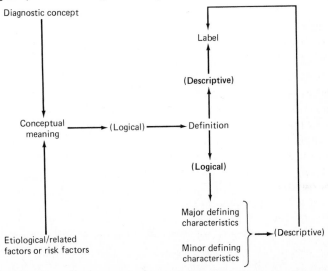

Naming a diagnostic category requires consideration of how the category is to be used in thinking and communicating. As discussed in Chapter 7, categories are used as diagnostic hypotheses. It is common in practice to hold a few hypotheses in memory while asking the client questions and while making observations. The limited memory capacity of human beings suggests that *names be concise and descriptive of the diagnostic criteria.* The category name should provide a *memory probe* for retrieval of knowledge about definition, major and supporting characteristics, and possible etiological factors. (Later, interventions, outcomes and other relationships will be retrieved in the same way.)

Consideration should also be given to the overall system of naming categories. For example, is there a difference in the attention paid to a problem when labeled as "Potential . . ." as opposed to "High Risk for . . ."? Levine has suggested that consultation with language experts is necessary to overcome some other labeling problems (1987). Communication is a second consideration in naming. The goal is to develop terms that describe the signs and symptoms clearly and concisely. There are advantages and disadvantages to selecting words that have meaning to nurses. An advantage is that the term(s) look familiar and are acceptable. The disadvantage is that old, familiar, personal meanings may be attached to the category which are inconsistent with its "scientific" meaning.

A clear, concise definition has to accompany each diagnostic category.[3] The words employed should be consistent with the conceptual meaning of the category and the list of major characteristics. *A definition differentiates a category from all others.* Current definitions are a base for revisions. As an example, let us revise a definition, step by step, according to: (1) conceptual meaning, (2) clarity and conciseness of label and definition, and (3) consistency with diagnostic and supporting criteria. To avoid any bias, look at the old alphabetical listing and pick the first diagnostic category: activity intolerance. The definition in 1986 was

A state in which an individual has *insufficient physiological or psychological energy* to *endure or complete* *required or desired* daily *activities.*

Taking the role of our old grammar school teachers, the major concepts have been italicized and spacing increased so they stand out from the rest of the sentence. Read the following slowly and think about the ideas.

The definition could be more concise with a deletion. Doesn't the following express the concept of activity intolerance?: *Insufficient physiological or psychological energy to endure or complete required or desired activities.* The thought expressed by the definition is highly complex. Complexity results from the two disjunctive concepts, energy and activities. Disjunctions are connected by an "or": (1) physiological *or* psychological energy and (2) endure *or* com-

---

[3]Definitions were introduced for diagnoses that lacked this component in 1986 by the NANDA Diagnosis Review Committee (McLane, 1987). The definitions were designed to be a base from which revisions could be submitted.

plete . . . activities. The latter disjunctive concept (endure or complete activities) may not be intended to be a disjunction. Commas inserted to indicate that *endure* is further explicated by the word *complete* would change the phrase to: *endure, or complete, . . . activities.* This is the likely meaning, as endurance is measured by the ability to complete an activity across time. When there is an inclination to write a disjunctive definition, consider whether two distinct entities are being considered under one category.

When the conceptual basis of this diagnostic category is considered, a question arises about the two types of energy: Are the definition and label consistent with the meaning of the concept being described? First, we will assume that the label is consistent with the concept it describes and then we will check the definition for consistency. The expectation would be to find the meaning of the two words *activity intolerance* and their connection. *Tolerance* is defined as "to endure or complete required or desired daily activities." Toleration of an activity is usually measured by the degree of completion and the deviation from resting levels both during and post activity. A person could very well *endure* an activity until it is completed but exhibit serious signs of activity intolerance during and after the activity. Should this be considered in defining the concept of activity intolerance?

The second concept in the diagnostic label is *activity*. Note that the definition is restrictive. It focuses on daily activities; daily are specified versus weekly, monthly, or yearly. Removing the restriction would result in: *insufficient endurance for completion of required or desired activities.* The definition of activities appears sufficiently inclusive; both required and desired activities are specified. The sentence may be clearer with some minor changes in wording: *insufficient endurance to complete required or desired activities.* The problem of using the same word, activity, in both the label and definition still exists. Also, should activities be specified as *energy consuming*? Perhaps not; the usual connotation is that activity is energy consuming and adding modifiers increases complexity. Thought should also be given to the restriction implied by *endurance.* Is endurance the only basis for not completing activities? Strength is another common factor. Whereas endurance is usually associated with cardiac and circulatory factors, strength is associated with muscle mass, tonus, and metabolism. Both strength and endurance interact in "completing activities" and the amounts needed vary with the activity. Another consideration is that defining characteristics will have to specify levels of "insufficient endurance." The levels could specify degrees of not completing required or desired activities within the time span dictated by the particular activity.

Let us now shift focus from label to the definition. We will assume that the definition captures the essence of the diagnostic concept and examine the label. Consider *physiological* or *psychological energy.* These are probably categories containing reasons for insufficient endurance (or tolerance). A lot of conceptual and format questions arise. Are these categories of etiological or contributing factors? Are we restricting the use of a diagnostic category if the etiological factors are built into a definition? (The author has been guilty of this in the past.) Yet, do these concepts, insufficient physiological energy or insufficient psychological energy, provide a clear focus for intervention? Isn't psychological energy an umbrella concept for a cluster of signs and symptoms indicating various conditions? Does psychological energy mean volition, which is as important in voluntary activity as is strength and endurance? It is necessary for both terms to be operationally defined before a decision can be made.

Notice that in analyzing a diagnostic category, we examined each idea, or concept, in the label and definition individually and in relation to each other. What we needed in this examination was the conceptual basis used by the author of the definition. Perhaps proceeding from the conceptual basis to a succinct definition and then to a label would be most profitable for clarity. It will be interesting in the following section to further examine the consistency among the defining characteristics, label, and definition of activity intolerance.

Defining Characteristics Structurally, a defining characteristic is *a value of an attribute of the client, environment, or both that serves as an indicator of the condition* described by the category.[4] Major characteristics are present in all clients with the condition; thus, these would be the *critical characteristics* or *criteria for making the diagnosis.* Major diagnostic criteria require attention because they discriminate between clients who have the condition and those who do not. They also permit the diagnostician to discriminate among conditions. The major characteristics, as previously stated, need to be clear, precise, express the essential nature of the category, and differentiate the category from all others. Each characteristic needs to be concrete and measurable through observation or client reports. If it is possible to quantify the characteristic, then consistency across clients and agreement among diagnosticians can be increased. The following are the major and minor characteristics listed for activity intolerance by NANDA in 1986 (Hurley, 1986):

1 Verbal report of fatigue or weakness[5]
2 Abnormal heart rate or blood pressure
3 Exertional discomfort or dyspnea
4 Electrocardiographic changes reflecting arrythmias or ischemia

In examination of the category *activity intolerance* we began with the definition: *A state in which an individual has insufficient physiological or psychological energy to endure or complete required or desired activities.* We ended with the definition: *Insufficient endurance to complete required or desired activities.* Using either definition, and examining the consistency of the characteristics with the definition, we find a critical characteristic is missing in the above list: noncompletion of activity (to some degree). Without this characteristic there is no consistency with the label *(activity)* or the definition.

This discussion could continue but there have been sufficient examples of

---

[4]Previously, when considering the clinical practice context, defining characteristics were called signs and symptoms. Two types of defining characteristics are identified by NANDA: (1) major characteristics are present in *all* clients with the condition and (2) minor are present in *most* clients with the condition (Kritek, 1986).

[5]Verbal report of fatigue or weakness has an asterisk because it is designated as the major critical defining characteristic, or diagnostic criterion.

questions to raise in the analysis of a new or current diagnostic category. It has to be kept in mind that this writer may have imposed meanings that were not compatible with the intended meaning (unspecified). For example, "to endure" may not have meant endurance in the physiological sense, but rather "to bear up under a burden" in the psychological sense. Specifying the conceptual basis and the definition of terms is very important when categories are to be used by thousands of nurses in clinical practice and research.

Etiological Factors   The discussion above pertaining to concepts also applies to what is commonly called *etiological factors*. These factors are explanatory concepts used to describe a probable cause of a problem. As stated previously, etiological factors and problem statements are related by theoretical knowledge derived from research, logical argument, or personal experience. This knowledge is used to support the judgment that a factor is contributing to the problem.

Identification of etiological concepts for each health problem by discovering the statistical relationship between problems and etiological factors is a major task. The first step in dealing with currently specified factors is concept analysis as discussed above. Once the proposed etiological factors are operationalized, research to determine the probability of relationships between a health-related condition and contributing factors can follow.

General Criteria for a Useful Category   Categories have to be valid representations of reality and must facilitate clinical reasoning and judgment. Otherwise they are not useful. The following criteria may be helpful in developing categories to be used in nursing diagnosis:

1 The category is within the conceptual focus of nursing and within the limits set by nurse practice acts. Nursing intervention can usually resolve the problem.

2 The level of generality, or inclusiveness, is appropriate for use in outcome projection (problem statement) and planning intervention (etiological factors).

3 The name given to the category is descriptive, concise, and clear. It conserves memory resources during hypothesis generation and testing.

4 A specific, concise definition is stated. The definition is consistent with the conceptual or theoretical basis of the concept and the diagnostic criteria that make the definition operational.

5 Valid diagnostic criteria (major characteristics) are designated. These characteristics permit discrimination among categories and are useful in hypothesis generation and testing.

6 Categories designated as etiological factors are valid, conceptually defined, have major characteristics that operationalize their definition, and facilitate therapeutic judgment.

Standardization of Diagnoses   Diagnostic labels will someday be standardized. This means there will be an established usage and meaning for each diagnostic label. All those who have been educated in the profession will know the proper usage and employ it. Yet standardization does not imply that the labels will be written in stone. As with dictionaries, periodic revisions will occur.

Why standardize? Before answering this question directly, let us try something important. Please turn to the back of this pamphlet.

If you are confused, that is expected. The *standard usage* of the word pamphlet was not employed; I described what you are reading as a pamphlet instead of a book. This resulted in poor communication between us. The situation is similar in nursing practice. Phenomena have to be called by the same name or communication suffers; different labels generate different meanings.

Whether or not to standardize is not the question. The issue is what word labels describe the clusters of signs and symptoms that are of concern to nursing. Are the to-be-named clusters human processes or patterns, or are they states?

Many of the labels in the current list of diagnoses (Appendix A) describe *states:* constipation, pain, fluid volume deficit, knowledge deficit. Others describe behavioral *processes* or *patterns:* impaired mobility, self-care deficit, sleep pattern disturbance. From a treatment perspective, one removes a state or at least modifies it. A state closely borders on an entity or static condition. Medicine also describes states; cancer, diabetes. Current nursing diagnoses are not as rigid; no *client* could be called a constipatic or a grievic, as in the use of diabetic, schizophrenic, cardiac, or asthmatic.

Standard average European (English), as our language is called, leads to defining client conditions as if they were concrete, material objects. The idea of change, which certainly we recognize, is not readily expressed in English (Warner, 1976).

Although diagnoses describe the state of the client at the time of encounter, is that the state of a pattern or process or a state-as-entity? For example, do we treat "pain" as an entity? Or do we treat "pain self-management deficit" as a subclass of comfort management and a human functional pattern? Do we treat constipation-as-entity or an intermittent constipation pattern?

Functional patterns or processes are close to the concept of "human responses" in the ANA statement on scope of practice (ANA, 1980). Patterns and processes also approach a more holistic (total person) philosophy, especially when the defining signs and symptoms are biopsychosocial. But can all therapeutic concerns be expressed in one naming format? Will this prove useful for treatment decisions? We do not know.

NORTH AMERICAN NURSING DIAGNOSIS ASSOCIATION

NANDA is an international organization of nurses (predominately, the United States and Canada) who have assumed responsibility for the classification of nursing diagnoses. Its history extends back to 1973 and the First National Conference in the United States. This conference was coordinated by two faculty members at St. Louis University, Kristine Gebbie and Mary Ann Lavin. At this conference, the Task Force for the Classification of Nursing Diagnosis was formed to continue work on the identification and classification of diagnoses. The Task Force held national conferences in 1975, 1978, 1980, and 1982. In

1982 the North American Nursing Diagnosis Association was formed. The name reflected the 9-year history of participation by nurses from Canada and the United States in development of diagnoses. Conferences have been held every 2 years since 1982 in conjunction with meetings of the General Assembly; in 1986 there was more than 600 participants.

Purposes of the Association

The purposes of NANDA are "to develop, refine, and promote a taxonomy of nursing diagnostic terminology of general use to professional nurses" (NANDA, 1982, 1986). These purposes are implemented through a set of standing committees chaired by members of the Board of Directors. The committees and their functions are as follows:

1 *Diagnosis Review Committee*   Reviews diagnoses and prepares diagnoses for membership voting

2 *Taxonomy Committee*   Develops and regularly reviews a taxonomic system for diagnoses, promotes the taxonomy, and promotes collaboration with groups supporting other established health-related taxonomies

3 *Research Committee*   Promotes research and reviews research papers for the publications of the Association

4 *Membership Committee*   Provides information to those interested in membership and reviews and accepts applications

5 *Program Committee*   Plans General Assembly meetings and provides consultation to regional or special interest groups desiring to conduct programs of interest to members.

6 *Publications Committee*   Oversees the publications of the Association and recommends editors of publications to the Board

7 *Public Relations Committee*   Promotes relationships with nursing and other health professionals, keeps the membership informed of trends/activities, and is advocate/spokesman for the Association

8 *Regional Affairs Committee*   Promotes the involvement of members of the Association and provides a mechanism for bringing issues of regional concern to the Board and Association.

Membership

Membership is open to registered nurses and associate membership includes professional nursing students and nonnurses. The association had approximately 1500 members in 1986.

Liaison Activities

Since 1974 there has been a formal liaison with the ANA through its Cabinet for Practice and its Task Force on Classification of Nursing Phenomena, as well as with the Nursing Organizations' Liaison Forum (NOLF). Communication has occurred with other nursing organizations and groups engaged in classification, or related work. It will be necessary to expand international communications as diagnoses have been (or are being) translated into Japanese, Chinese, Spanish, Italian, and French. Communications can occur through nursing associations of various countries, the International Council of Nurses, or the World Health Organization.

Implementation of Purposes

One purpose is classification system development. Diagnoses are submitted to the Diagnostic Review Committee from individuals or groups according to the guidelines and review cycle presented in Appendix N. The final acceptance of a diagnostic category depends upon a vote of the membership by mailed ballot. Taxonomy development is an ongoing activity. The Association has designated funds for supporting research and plans are underway for a review of research methodologies. Important issues in diagnosis have been addressed by invited speakers at biennial conferences; however, basic educational programs are viewed as a responsibility of regions or localities.

The *Nursing Diagnosis Newsletter*, is published quarterly by NANDA; it serves as a mechanism for members and others to obtain information, raise questions, react to issues, and report activities through letters to the editor. In addition, the Association has an office in St. Louis which acts as a clearinghouse for information on nursing diagnosis and related issues. The address is:

North American Nursing Diagnosis Association
St. Louis University School of Nursing
3525 Caroline Street
St. Louis, MO 63104

Groups have formed in many parts of the United States—regional, state, and local—and in some regions and provinces in Canada. These groups provide a mechanism for discussion of issues related to development, implementation, and research at the local level. Efforts are currently underway to increase networking among groups and between NANDA and the regions across Canada and the United States through the Committee on Regional Affairs. Some groups have begun their own newsletter in order to promote communication.

Nurses working on identification, development, and classification are an enthusiastic group who see the potential for nursing diagnosis in clinical practice, theory development, and organizing nursing knowledge. They are a group of nurses committed to the improvement of nursing care delivery through clarification of that area of nursing practice that involves diagnosis and treatment.

RESEARCH ON NURSING DIAGNOSIS

Clinical opportunities are plentiful for collecting data that could be used in clinical studies of nursing diagnoses. Students in professional education programs may have opportunities to do a clinical study as part of a research or senior elective course, or within a faculty's research project. After graduation there will be opportunities for collaboration or independent research; in some settings research is required for promotion to senior primary nurse.

The work associated with development and classification of diagnoses has gone through a period of identifying common conditions nurses said they diagnosed and treated in their practice. It was important to describe nurses' perceptions of these conditions and publish a listing that could be used to focus research on each diagnostic category. The problem of credibility arises if the acceptance and revision of categories continues to be based on opinion. As Fuller (1978, pp. 701–702) has suggested basing acceptance of diagnoses on nurses' recall and opinions "runs the risk of defining nursing practice by consensus rather than by inquiry. . . . If unity and order are to be identified in the practice of nursing, the identification will surely come from the quiet pursuit of knowledge using the scientific method." Most would agree that research and field testing are the necessary criteria to substantiate proposals of new diagnoses and revisions. Expert opinion can be used to evaluate the research base.

Research focused on diagnostic categories has increased considerably since 1980 but still falls below what is needed. There is nearly an equal distribution of nurse consensus studies and clinical data-based studies of categories. Epidemiological research has been reported; studies in the medical-surgical setting are most common. There also have been some studies in the area of nurse staffing, quality assurance, and other areas of application.

This section will provide a brief, introductory overview of the types of studies needed in nursing diagnosis and related areas. No attempt will be made to review particular studies. Consideration will be given to the identification of new diagnoses and testing and refinement of current diagnoses. Epidemiological surveys and studies in related areas will conclude the section.

Identification Studies

Most agree that the current listing of diagnostic categories is incomplete. When a clinician repeatedly observes a condition that cannot be labeled with a current diagnosis, attention should be paid to the manifestations observed in the client-environment pattern. Both conceptual analysis of the set of manifestations and studies to further describe the phenomenon are indicated at this point. Either qualitative, quantitative, or both types of methodologies can be employed to study the condition. It would be advisable after a few clients are observed to report the condition in the *Nursing Diagnosis Newsletter* mentioned above. This would alert others to the condition and simultaneous research can begin.

Some have suggested that diagnoses seem to cluster in a pattern, somewhat like a syndrome. Chronic pain, activity intolerance, and immobility each seem to be associated with a particular set of dysfunctional patterns (other diagnoses). Studies are needed to identify clusters of problems that are associated with a common etiological factor. Whether or not the cluster is more useful for care planning than each single problem is a second question for study that would determine if these clusters should be given a diagnostic label. The currently listed category, rape trauma syndrome, is an example of this type of category. Taxonomic pattern concepts (level 1) may also be a source of diagnoses at a higher level of synthesis than current categories. Research is needed to examine the potential of these patterns to generate new diagnoses that describe health-related life patterns.

Each category has to be examined for *reliability* and *validity*. These dimensions of a category specify its *dependability* and *applicability*. In one sense reliability and validity are a test of the conceptual clarity of the diagnostic concept; problems in attaining an acceptable level usually are solved by further concept development.Reliability and validity will be described in the next section when refinement studies are considered.

Refinement Studies

There is a critical need for refinement of categories that are widely used in practice. Many of the categories need the conceptual work outlined in the previous section and by Gordon and Sweeney (1979). After a category has been developed conceptually the next step toward refinement is to establish validity and reliability. Trying to attain absolute validity and reliability is an impossible goal for any research; what is expressed is the *degree* of validity and reliability attained. Users of the category can take these estimates under consideration and acceptable levels can be decided upon by the profession.

Reliability Whereas *credibility* of a category is determined by its validity, *dependability* is determined by its reliability, that is, during the diagnostic process, a category has to have defining characteristics that can be used by one or more nurses to arrive at the same judgment; this is referred to as *interdiagnostician* reliability. Also, it is important that an individual nurse be able to use a particular diagnosis consistently to describe the same condition in various clients; this is called *intradiagnostician* reliability. These will be recognized as the terms *intrarater* and *interrater* reliability. Reliability is important in preventing diagnostic errors.

To measure the degree to which the defining characteristics of a category can be used to arrive consistently at the same diagnosis, a group of experts skilled in the diagnostic process are used. The degree of reliability can be established by presenting a list of defining characteristics to experts and requesting a diagnostic judgment. Interdiagnostician agreement is a measure of the reliability of the characteristics. Another method is to use written or videotaped cases and determine the agreement among the diagnoses formulated. The problem with using clinical situations is that all the raters would have to be present during assessment if the possibility exists that the client's condition could change before all assessments are done. There also is the concern about exposing a client to repeated assessments that makes the simulated situation more attractive as a method. Reliability is a necessary but not sufficient condition for validity.

Validity Studies need to focus on the validity, or accuracy, with which a new or current diagnosis describes a condition occurring in practice. It should be noted that the label and definition are not the subject for research. These components are created by the category developer. *Validity* describes the degree to which a cluster of defining characteristics describes a reality that can be observed in client-environment interaction. Researchers need to be concerned with the extent to which observations (that are later formulated as the characteristics of a category) are authentic representations of what exists in clinical practice; this measure refers to the *internal validity* of a category. The degree to which the characteristics may be used, legitimately, to diagnose the condition across various groups of clients is the *external validity* of a diagnostic category. These two measures establish *construct validity*.

Clinton (1986) suggests that construct, predictive, and discriminant validity of a diagnostic category should be established. *Predictive validity* refers to the degree to which the cluster of defining characteristics (derived from descriptive studies and concept analysis) is associated with other theoretically related phenomena. The degree to which the cluster of characteristics can detect differences between groups of clients is a test of *discriminant validity*. The *known-groups technique* provides a measure to detect differences between a group of clients expected to have the condition and a group expected not to have the condition.

Fehring (1986) provides a model for establishing the *content validity index* (CVI) of diagnostic categories. He suggests each diagnostic category should have standardized validity measures, including *diagnostic content validity* (DCV), *clinical diagnostic validity* (CDV), and *etiological correlation rating* (ECR). The DCV is an index of content validity using experts' ratings of characteristics relative to the conceptual definition. Experts' observations of the characteristics in a clinical situation are the basis for a category's CDV index. From the DCV and CDV indices, the major characteristics (diagnostic criteria) of a category can be designated. Correlations describing the strength of association between problems and their etiological factors are represented by the ECR. Validity of categories has to be determined before correlations between, or among, categories; thus it would be important to know the DCV and CDV before attention is paid to the problem-etiological factor relationship.

Asking nurses or using the data of nursing assessments to establish validity requires some thought. Expert raters and astute clinical observers have to be used. It may also be important to establish the reliability of clinical data collectors' interviewing and examination skills and their sensitivity to cues. Other principles of validity testing also apply. Examples of studies using different methodologies may be found in the literature (Lackey, 1986; Lo and Kim, 1986; Vincent, 1986).

Validity provides a measure of the confidence that should be placed in the accuracy of a category to depict reality. Of course, conceptual reality is relative to the perceiver. It may be found that the characteristics are (1) present as a pattern in the client-environment interactions that are measured and (2) related to the conceptual definition of the diagnosis. Yet, nurses may not agree that the diagnosis is within the conceptual or legal focus of nursing practice. As Fehring (1986) suggests, a study of the consensual validity of the category from a random sampling of the population of nurses may be necessary. On the other hand, if the investigator has confidence in the conceptual and legal dimensions, survival in the "marketplace" of clinical practice will provide an indication of nurse consensus about the category.

Epidemiological Studies

Epidemiological studies are designed to document the base-rate occurrence of diagnoses in the population. A review of research from 1953 to 1983 revealed few studies and many methodological problems (Gordon, 1985b). Unless an acceptable level of reliability and validity is established for diagnostic categories, studies merely shed light on the diagnoses nurses use and record in their practice. This may be all that can be expected until categories are refined, but questions can be raised about the dependability of both the categories and the diagnostic skills of nurses who recorded the diagnoses. This assumption also has to be made in large epidemiological studies of medical diseases but it is clear that all physicians have training in diagnosis.

Various populations can be studied to determine the epidemiology of nursing diagnoses. Populations may be selected by medical groupings such as disease or diagnostic-related groups, by gender, ethnicity, culture, setting, phase of illness, and other variables. It would also be of interest to select a nursing diagnostic population, such as clients with immobility, and determine the co-occurring nursing diagnoses. Epidemiological studies add to the nursing knowledge base. The knowledge derived is used (1) in the diagnostic process to predict likely possibilities and increase sensitivity to cues, (2) to predict the nursing care requirement of specific populations, and (3) provide guidelines for essential content in education. Co-occurrence of medical and nursing diagnoses is of interest with the current prospective payment based on diagnostic-related groupings. Co-occurrence studies could help to establish the approximate cost of medical and nursing resources used by a population of clients (see Chapter 10). With the emphasis on cost containment and early discharge it would be interesting to study the nursing diagnoses at discharge and correlate these with the community nursing services available. Crosscultural epidemiological studies are also needed; these can contribute to further development of categories.

Diagnostic Process Studies

How nurses collect, interpret, cluster, and give names to their diagnostic judgments requires a great deal more investigation. Studies on aspects of the process, diagnostic errors, the effect of initial impressions and other potential biases, and the influence of various educational strategies on competency are needed. Task, personality, and setting variables also need to be the focus of research.

Diagnosis-Based Outcome and Process Studies

Studies to determine realistic outcomes for specified time periods would be a fruitful area of study. Research of this type would guide individual practitioners as well as quality assurance reviews. Experimental research on treatments for nursing diagnoses is a field of study that is critically needed to determine which interventions lead to desired outcomes in the most cost-efficient and humanistic manner. Retrospective studies of the treatment provided and outcomes attained would provide data on outcome-process linkages for each diagnosis. Also, the many variables that influence outcomes and treatments need to be identified. Some current diagnoses may have a sufficient level of reliability and validity for investigators to proceed with outcome and treatment studies. The increased use of computers in health care institutions will facilitate large-scale studies on each diagnosis, outcomes, and treatment. These studies will provide a research base for diagnosis-based outcome and process standards and provide data for cost-benefit analyses.

Studies in Ethics of Diagnosis and Treatment

Most studies in nursing ethics focus on the collaborative area of practice with physicians or with nurses' ethical responsibilities in personal-professional-bureaucratic conflicts. Research is needed on ethical issues in nursing diagnosis and treatment but this may have to await an increased consciousness of moral responsibilities in this area of practice. For example, many nurses state they do not have time for assessment beyond that required in their collaborative role. "No time for nursing assessment and diagnosis" is stated as a fact and does not appear to be viewed as a dilemma in allocation of resources. Respect for autonomy of clients, informed consent, and other issues is also relevant in the domain of practice described by nursing diagnoses.

Nursing diagnosis can help focus clinical research and provide a way of organizing knowledge gleaned from clinical studies of "problems," interventions, results of interventions, and the variables that influence any of these. Perhaps investigators will be sufficiently interested in one or more diagnoses to begin a program of research that will extend beyond the initial studies of a category to its use in nursing process.

SUMMARY

In this final chapter are four issues critical to future development of nursing diagnosis: acceptance of diagnosis, current status of implementation, problems and prospects in classification, and research. For various reasons not everyone accepts the term *diagnosis*. At this point the reader will have sufficient background in the subject to take a position. Should nurses use this term to describe the judgments they make? Or must we create a new word? That nurses make clinical judgments of the type described by nursing diagnoses is not the issue.

Implementation of nursing diagnosis and the diagnostic process is not seen in every clinical setting in North America. Yet when outside accreditors cite the organized approach to care resulting from diagnosis, nurses may consider the concept. When nurses become bored with a routine approach to every "gallbladder patient," they may consider using the diagnostic process. Diagnosis-based care planning may become so habitual during educational programs that new graduates will be unable to consider any other way of determining nursing interventions.

Classification of nursing diagnoses and related research has been reviewed. The problems and prospects are evident. The development of nomenclature and a classification system for nursing practice will not be done by an elitist group. Students, clinicians, and clinical specialists will have to be involved. It is hoped that this review will stimulate more nurses to become enthusiastic about contributing to the future direction of nursing diagnosis.

FUTURE DIRECTIONS

Many forces within and external to nursing will influence the future direction of nursing diagnosis in both North America and other areas. Nurses using diagnosis and those with whom they communicate in practice settings will encourage clearer definition of the concept. Shoemaker's (1984) report of a study on the "critical, defining characteristics" of a nursing diagnosis contributes to this. It may be expected that potential problems, requiring preventive nursing intervention, will continue to be defined as nursing diagnoses. As primary care specialists become more involved in identifying these high-risk health patterns, additional nomenclature will be added. Research will follow to identify methods of helping clients decrease health risks. When risk reduction can be demonstrated and related to cost and quality of life, the public may be persuaded to finance preventive care.

Financing of nursing care will be a major factor influencing development of a diagnostic classification system. Hidden within the costs of room and board or medical care, nursing is not clearly perceived by the public. What nurses do and why they do it will become obvious when direct reimbursement is a reality. At that point in time it will be important to articulate what actual or potential problems are treated, what outcomes result, and how these health outcomes contribute to goals society values.

In acute- and long-term care settings, nursing's concern with the quality of life will encourage assessment of functional patterns. Recognition of actual or potentially dysfunctional patterns will stimulate experimental studies of nursing intervention. Intervention-outcome links will be established which enhance decision making in care planning.

If current predictions are correct, the aged will comprise a high percentage of clients in health care settings. Ways will have to be found to sustain their optimal function. Otherwise, the dire predictions for the year 2000 made by some analysts of health care—financial collapse of the health care system and euthanasia—may come true. Nurses focus on optimal patterns of functioning; this focus is especially useful in health care of the elderly. If nursing's domain of practice is established as the detection of potential problems and restoration of integrated function after dysfunctional patterns occur, nurses may be the health care providers that assume major responsibilities for care of the elderly population. Beliefs and values traditionally held by nurses may influence society to recognize the aged for their wisdom, rather than their disabilities.

The validity of long-range prediction rests on attainment of short-term goals. One immediate goal is to assess the diagnostic reliability of currently identified signs and symptoms for each diagnostic category. If diagnostic category labels generally represent client problems encountered by nurses, reliability studies are worthwhile.

What would reliability studies accomplish? If a sign or symptom can be demonstrated to occur in 95 out of 100 clients, it is a reliable predictor of a condition. Nurses caring for clients need clusters of highly reliable cues to diagnose actual or potential problems, Without these predictors, diagnostic errors occur. Diagnostic errors lead to inadequate care plans and interventions. In turn, inadequate interventions rarely permit health outcomes to be attained and can result in harm and suffering.

Establishing the level of reliability of current lists of defining characteristics would greatly facilitate education. Students could learn the few critical cues that reliably predict the presence of a diagnosis. Other cues currently listed may be useful to support a judgment but are not critical. Noncritical cues can be learned later, as clinical experience in diagnosing a condition accumulates.

Future graduates of professional nursing programs will demonstrate competence in using diagnostic categories to organize client data and plan care. This will occur only if both diagnostic process and diagnostic categories are learned in educational programs.

Clinical studies of the diagnostic process used by health care providers will increase. The search for knowledge to increase diagnostic efficiency and validity of diagnosis will be influenced by a continued emphasis on cost and quality control. Expanding knowledge of the diagnostic process will facilitate teaching of the process in nursing. Studies will test the application of knowledge about cognitive processes to specific diagnostic situations in nursing. As faculty appreciate the need for training in uncertainty-based judgment, methods of controlling uncertainties will become part of the educational preparation of nursing practitioners.

Perhaps the future will reveal a unified perspective on what information is included in a nursing data base. A unified perspective on assessment would mean consensus had been reached regarding nursing's focus of concern. (It may be expected that multiple models of intervention and nursing goals will continue to be used.) Classification would be greatly influenced if a unified perspective was reached because diagnostic categories would have to be logically consistent with the agreed upon conceptual model. Some are concerned that professional nurses will divorce themselves from seriously ill clients, leaving this area of nursing to the technically prepared. This is unlikely. It is especially unlikely if studies demonstrate complex *nursing* diagnoses occur in intensive and acute care, as well as in primary care, settings.

A few of the issues that will influence the future direction of nursing diagnosis have been briefly reviewed. To those who have the sensitivity to see beyond the mere obvious, the curiosity to wonder why, and the intellect to reason how, is left the future of nursing and nursing diagnosis.

BIBLIOGRAPHY

Abdellah, F. G. (1959). Improving the teaching of nursing through research in patient care. In L. E. Heidgerken. (Ed.) *Improvement of nursing through research*. Washington, D.C.: Catholic University of America Press.

American Nurses Association. (1980). *Nursing: A social policy statement*. Kansas City, MO: Author.

Aspinall, M. J. (1976). Nursing diagnosis: The weak link. *Nursing Outlook, 24:* 433–437.

Bruce, J. (1979). Implementation of nursing diagnosis: An administrator's perspective. *Nursing Clinics of North America, 14:* 509–516.

Clinton, J. (1986). Nursing diagnoses research methodologies. In Hurley, M. (Ed.), *Classification of nursing diagnoses: Proceedings of the sixth national conference*. St. Louis: Mosby, pp. 159–167.

Dalton, J. M. (1979). Nursing diagnosis in a community health setting. *Nursing Clinics of North America, 14:* 525–532.

Douglas, J., & Murphy, E. K. (1985). Nursing process, nursing diagnosis, and emerging taxonomies. In J. C. Mc Closkey & H. K. Grace (Eds.), *Current issues in nursing*. (2d ed.). Boston: Blackwell Scientific.

Elstein, A., Schulman, L. S., & Sprafka, S. A. (1978). *Medical problem-solving: An analysis of clinical reasoning*. Cambridge, MA: Harvard University Press.

Fawcett, J. (1985). *Conceptual models of nursing, nursing diagnosis, and nursing theory development*. Paper presented at Annual Meeting of the Massachusetts Conference Group for Classification of Nursing Diagnoses, May 22, 1985. (Reprinted in *Newsletter, Massachusetts Conference Group*, Boston, May, 1985.)

Fehring, R. J. (1986). Validating diagnostic labels: Standardized methodology. In M. Hurley (Ed.), *Classification of nursing diagnoses: Proceedings of the sixth national conference*. St. Louis: Mosby, pp. 183–190.

Feild, L. M. (1982). Comments of clinical specialists on the unitary man framework. In M. J. Kim & D. A. Moritz. (Eds.). *Classification of nursing diagnoses: Proceedings of the third and fourth national conferences*. St. Louis, MO: Mosby, p. 265.

Feild, L. (1979). Implementation of nursing diagnosis in clinical practice. *Nursing Clinics of North America, 14:* 525–532.

Fredette, S., & O'Connor, K. (1979). Nursing diagnosis in teaching and curriculum planning. *Nursing Clinics of North America, 14:* 541–552.

Fuller, S. S. (1978). Holistic man and the science and practice of nursing. *Nursing Outlook, 26:* 700–704.

Gordon, M. (1987). *Manual of nursing diagnosis*. New York: McGraw-Hill.

Gordon, M. (1986). Structure of diagnostic categories. In M. Hurley. (Ed.). *Classification of nursing diagnoses: Proceedings of the sixth conference*. St. Louis, MO: Mosby.

Gordon, M. (1985a). Diagnostic category development. In J. McCloskey & H. Grace. (Ed.). *Current issues in nursing practice*. (2d ed.). Boston: Blackwell Scientific.

Gordon, M. (1985b). Nursing diagnosis. In H. H. Werley & J. J. Fitzpatrick (Eds.) *Annual Review of Nursing Research*. New York: Springer, vol. 3.

Gordon, M., & Sweeney, M. A. (1979). Methodological issues in nursing diagnosis research. *Advances in Nursing Science, 20:* 1–7.

Halloran, E. J. (1980). Analysis of variation in nurse workload by patient medical and nursing condition. Doctoral Dissertation, University of Illinois Medical Center. *Dissertation Abstracts International,* 41–09B.

Hangartner, C. (1975). Principles of classification. In K. Gebbie & M. Lavin (Eds.), *Classification of nursing diagnoses: Proceedings of the first national conference on classification of nursing diagnoses.* St. Louis: Mosby.

Hagey, R. S., & McDonough, P. (1984). The problem of professional labeling. *Nursing Outlook,* 32: 151–157.

Hurley, M. (Ed.) (1986). *Classification of nursing diagnoses: Proceedings of the sixth conference.* St. Louis: Mosby.

Kirk, L. W. (1986). The design for relevance revisted: An elaboration of the conceptual framework for nursing diagnosis. In M. Hurley. (Ed.). *Classification of nursing diagnoses: Proceedings of the sixth conference.* St. Louis, MO: Mosby.

Kritek, P. (1987). NANDA Taxonomy I. In A. McLane (Ed.), *Classification of nursing diagnoses: Proceedings of the seventh conference.* St. Louis: Mosby.

Kritek, P. (1985). NANDA procedures for diagnosis review. *NANDA Nursing Diagnosis Newsletter,* 12(3,4).

Lackey, N. R. (1986). Use of Q methodology in validation of defining characteristics of specified nursing diagnoses. In M. Hurley (Ed.), *Classification of nursing diagnoses: Proceedings of the sixth national conference.* St. Louis: Mosby, pp. 191–206.

Levine, M. E. (1987). Taxonomy development. In A. McLane (Ed.), *Classification of nursing diagnoses: Proceedings of the seventh conference.* St. Louis: Mosby.

Levine, M. (1966). Trophicognosis: An alternative to nursing diagnosis. In American Nurses Association. (Ed.). *Exploring progress in medical-surgical nursing.* Kansas City, MO: Author.

Lo, C. K., & Kim, M. J. (1986). Construct validity of sleep pattern disturbance: A methodological approach. In M. Hurley (Ed.), *Classification of nursing diagnoses: Proceedings of the sixth national conference.* St. Louis: Mosby, pp. 207–215.

McLane, A. (1987). (Ed.). *Classification of nursing diagnoses: Proceedings of the seventh conference.* St Louis, MO: Mosby.

McLane, A. (1982). Nursing diagnosis in baccalaureate and graduate education. In M. J. Kim & D. A. Moritz, *Classification of nursing diagnoses: Proceedings of the third and fourth conference.* New York: McGraw-Hill.

Nicoll, L. H. (1986). *Perspectives on nursing theory.* Boston: Little, Brown.

Norris, C. A. (1982). *Concept clarification in nursing.* Rockville, MD: Aspen Systems.

North American Nursing Diagnosis Association. (1986a). *NANDA Taxonomy I.* North American Nursing Diagnosis Association, St. Louis University School of Nursing, 3525 Caroline Ave., St. Louis, MO.

North American Nursing Diagnosis Association. (1986b). *NANDA Bylaws.* North American Nursing Diagnosis Association, St. Louis University School of Nursing, 3525 Caroline Ave., St. Louis, MO.

NYNEX Yellow Pages, Boston Area (1986). Boston: New England Telephone Co.

Rantz, M., Miller, T., & Jacobs, C. (1986). Nursing diagnosis in long-term care. *American Journal of Nursing.* 85: 916–917, 926.

Rogers, M. (1970). Introduction to the theoretical basis of nursing. Philadelphia: Davis.

Rosch, E. (1978). Basic level categories. In E. Rosch & B. Llloyd (Eds.), *Cognition and categorization.* Hillsdale, NJ: Erlbaum.

Rossi, L., & Krekeler, K. (1982). Small group reactions to the theoretical framework of unitary man. In M. J. Kim & D. A. Moritz. (Eds.). *Classification of nursing diagnoses:*

Proceedings of the third and fourth national conferences. St. Louis, MO: Mosby, p. 274.

Roy, C. (1982). Theoretical framework for classification of nursing diagnoses. M. J. Kim & D. A. Moritz (Eds.), *Classification of nursing diagnoses: Proceedings of the third and fourth national conferences.* New York: McGraw-Hill.

Roy, C. (1984). Framework for classification systems development: Progress and issues. In M. J. Kim, G. Mc Farland, & A. McLane (Eds.), *Classification of nursing diagnoses: Proceedings of the fifth national conference.* St. Louis: Mosby.

Shoemaker, J. (1984). Essential features of a nursing diagnosis. In M. J. Kim, G. Mc Farland, & A. McLane (Eds.), *Classification of nursing diagnoses: Proceedings of the fifth national conference.* St. Louis: Mosby.

Sokal, R. R. (1974). Classification: Purposes, principles, progress, prospects. *Science,* 185: 1115.

Vincent, K. G. (1986). Validation of a nursing diagnosis: A nurse consensus survey. In M. Hurley (Ed.), *Classification of nursing diagnoses: Proceedings of the sixth national conference.* St. Louis: Mosby, pp. 207–214.

Warner, R. (1976). Relationship between language and disease concepts. *International Journal of Psychiatry in Medicine,* 7: 57–68.

Weber, S. (1982) Comments of clinical specialists on the unitary man framework. In M. J. Kim & D. A. Moritz. (Eds.). *Classification of nursing diagnoses: Proceedings of the third and fourth national conferences.* St. Louis, MO: Mosby, p. 270.

Weber, S. (1979). Nursing diagnosis in private practice. *Nursing Clinics of North America,* 14: 533–540.

Whitney, F. W. (1981). How to work with a crock. *American Journal of Nursing,* 81: 86–91.

APPENDIXES

NORTH AMERICAN NURSING DIAGNOSIS ASSOCIATION APPROVED NURSING DIAGNOSES, APRIL 1986[1]

Activity Intolerance (Specify level)
Activity Intolerance, Potential
Adjustment, Impaired
Airway Clearance, Ineffective
Anxiety
Body Temperature, Potential Alteration in
Bowel Elimination, Alterations in: Constipation
Bowel Elimination, Alteration in: Diarrhea
Bowel Elimination, Alteration in: Incontinence
Breathing Pattern, Ineffective
Cardiac Output, Alteration in: Decreased
Comfort, Alteration in: Pain
Comfort, Alteration In: Chronic Pain
Communication, Impaired Verbal
Coping, Ineffective Individual
Coping, Ineffective Family: Compromised
Coping, Ineffective Family: Disabling
Coping, Family: Potential for Growth
Diversional Activity Deficit

Family Processes, Alteration in
Fear (Specify)
Fluid Volume Deficit, Actual
Fluid Volume Deficit, Potential
Fluid Volume, Alteration in: Excess
Gas Exchange, Impaired
Grieving, Anticipatory
Grieving, Dysfunctional
Growth and Development, Altered
Health Maintenance, Alteration in
Home Maintenance Management, Impaired
Hopelessness
Hyperthermia
Hypothermia
Incontinence, Functional
Incontinence, Reflex
Incontinence, Stress
Incontinence, Total
Incontinence, Urge
Infection, Potential for

---

[1]Definitions, defining characteristics, and related factors are included in McLane, A. (Ed.). (1987). *Classification of nursing diagnoses: Proceedings of the seventh conference.* St. Louis: Mosby.

Injury, Potential for (Poisoning, Potential for; Suffocation, Potential for; Trauma, Potential for)

Knowledge Deficit (Specify)

Mobility, Impaired Physical

Neglect, Unilateral

Noncompliance (Specify)

Nutrition, Alteration in: Less than Body Requirements

Nutrition, Alteration in: More than Body Requirements

Nutrition, Alteration in: Potential For More than Body Requirements

Oral Mucous Membrane, Alteration in

Parenting, Alteration in: Actual

Parenting, Alteration in: Potential

Post-trauma Response

Powerlessness

Rape Trauma Syndrome

Rape Trauma Syndrome: Compounded

Rape Trauma Syndrome: Silent Reaction

Self-Care Deficit (Bathing/Hygiene, Feeding, Dressing/Grooming, Toileting)

Self-Concept Disturbance (Disturbance in Body Image, Personal Identity, Self-Esteem, Role Performance)

Sensory Perceptual Alteration: Visual, Auditory, Kinesthetic, Gustatory, Tactile, Olfactory

Sexual Dysfunction

Sexuality Patterns, Altered

Skin Integrity, Impairment of: Actual

Skin Integrity, Impairment of: Potential

Sleep Pattern Disturbance

Social Interaction, Impaired

Social Isolation

Spiritual Distress (Distress of the Human Spirit)

Swallowing, Impaired

Thermoregulation, Ineffective

Thought Processes, Alteration in

Tissue Integrity, Impaired

Tissue Perfusion, Alteration in (Cerebral, Cardiopulmonary, Renal, Gastrointestinal, Peripheral)

Urinary Elimination, Alteration in Patterns

Urinary Retention

Violence, Potential for (self-directed or directed at others)

NOMENCLATURE DEVELOPMENT, 1973–1986

NOMENCLATURE DEVELOPMENT, 1973–1986*

The following table depicts diagnostic nomenclature development from 1973 to 1986. A horizontal reading provides information on how diagnoses (1) were added (blank spaces in previous years), (2) changed, or (3) deleted (blank spaces in subsequent year). A vertical reading of the columns for each year provides the list of accepted diagnoses in 1973 (first national conference), 1975 (second national conference), 1978 (third national conference), 1980 (fourth national conference), 1982 (fifth national conference), and 1986 (seventh conference; no changes in 1984).

1973	1975	1978	1980	1982 and 1984	1986
				Activity intolerance Activity intolerance, Potential	Activity intolerance Activity intolerance, Potential
Anxiety, mild Anxiety, moderate Anxiety, severe Panic	Anxiety, mild Anxiety, moderate Anxiety, severe Panic	Anxiety, mild Anxiety, moderate Anxiety, severe Panic		Anxiety	Anxiety
Body fluids, depletion of	Body fluids, depletion of Body fluids, excess Body fluid, excess	Fluid volume deficit Fluid volume deficit, potential Body fluids, excess	Fluid volume deficit Fluid volume deficit, potential	Fluid volume deficit, actual Fluid volume deficit, potential Fluid volume, alteration in: excess	Fluid volume deficit, actual Fluid volume deficit, potential Fluid volume, alteration in: excess
Bowel function, irregular: constipation Bowel function, irregular: diarrhea	Bowel elimination, alteration in: constipation Bowel elimination, alteration in: diarrhea Bowel elimination, alteration in: impaction Bowel elimination, alteration in: incontinence	Bowel elimination, alteration in: constipation Bowel elimination, alteration in: diarrhea Bowel elimination, alteration in: impaction Bowel elimination, alteration in: incontinence	Bowel elimination, alteration in: constipation Bowel elimination, alteration in: diarrhea Bowel elimination, alteration in: incontinence	Bowel elimination, alteration in: constipation Bowel elimination, alteration in: diarrhea Bowel elimination, alteration in: incontinence	Bowel elimination, alteration in: constipation Bowel elimination, alteration in: diarrhea Bowel elimination, alteration in: incontinence

1973	1975	1978	1980	1982 and 1984	1986
	Cardiac output, alteration in: decreased	Cardiac output, alteration in: decreased	Cardiac output, alteration in: decreased	Cardiac output, alteration in: decreased	Cardiac output, alteration in: decreased
	Circulation, interruption of	Circulation, interruption of Tissue perfusion, chronic abnormal	Tissue perfusion, alteration in subcategories (see Appendix A)	Tissue perfusion, alteration in subcategories (see Appendix A)	Tissue perfusion, alteration in subcategories (see Appendix A)
Cognitive functioning alteration in level of Distractibility Hypovigilance Hypervigilance					
		Consciousness, altered levels of			
Cognitive dissonance Inappropriate and unrealistic based thinking Decreased capacity for abstract conceptualization Inaccurate interpretation of environment Increased egocentricity					
Thought processes impaired Impaired perception Impaired retention Impaired reflection Impaired decision making Impaired judgment Confusion	Thought processes impaired Confusion	Thought processes impaired	Thought processes, alteration in	Thought processes, alteration in	Thought processes, alteration in

Comfort level, alterations in	Alterations in comfort: discomfort	Comfort, alterations in: pain	Comfort, alterations in: pain	Comfort, alterations in: pain	Comfort, alterations in: pain
Physiological comfort level, alterations in					Comfort, alterations in: chronic pain
Psychological comfort level, alterations in					
Environmental comfort level, alterations in					
Spiritual comfort level, alterations in					
Verbal communication, impairment of	Communication, impaired verbal	Communication, impaired verbal	Communication, impaired verbal	Communication, impaired verbal	Communication, impaired verbal
Nonverbal communication, impairment of					
Coping patterns, maladaptive (individual)	Coping, ineffective (individual)	Coping, ineffective (individual)	Coping, ineffective (individual)	Coping, ineffective (individual)	Coping, ineffective (individual)
Coping patterns, ineffective family	Coping, ineffective family: disabling	Coping, ineffective family: disabling	Coping, ineffective family: disabling	Coping, ineffective family: disabling	Coping, ineffective family: disabling
	Coping, ineffective family: compromised	Coping, ineffective family: compromised	Coping, ineffective family: compromised	Coping, ineffective family: compromised	Coping, ineffective family: compromised
	Coping, family: potential for growth	Coping, family: potential for growth	Coping, family: potential for growth	Coping, family: potential for growth	Coping, family: potential for growth
Adjustment to illness, impairment of significant others	Adjustment to illness, impairment of significant others	Adjustment to illness, impairment of significant others			
Adjustment to illness, impairment of all significant others					
Adjustment to illness, impairment of spouse's					
Adjustment to illness, impairment of child's					
Adjustment to illness, impairment of nonfamily's					Post-trauma response
					Adjustment, impaired

(continued)

1973	1975	1978	1980	1982 and 1984	1986
Digestion, impairment of (impaired digestion)					
			Diversional activity deficit	Diversional activity deficit	Diversional activity deficit
Faith, alterations in Faith in self, alterations in Faith in others, alterations in					
		Spirituality: spiritual concern			
		Spirituality: spiritual distress	Spiritual distress (distress of the human spirit)	Spiritual distress (distress of the human spirit)	Spiritual distress (distress of the human spirit)
		Spirituality: spiritual despair			
Fear Functional fear, mild Functional fear, moderate Functional fear, severe Functional fear, panic Nonfunctional fear, mild Nonfunctional fear, moderate Nonfunctional fear, severe Nonfunctional fear, panic			Fear (specify)	Fear (specify)	Fear (specify)
		Functional performance, variations in or Self-care activities, alterations in ability to perform			

		Home maintenanace management, impaired	Home maintenance management, impaired	Home maintenance management, impaired	Home maintenance management, impaired
Self-care activities, altered ability to perform	Self-care activities, alteration in ability to perform	Total self-care deficit	Self-care deficit (specify level)	Self-care deficit (specify level)	Self-care deficit (specify level)
Self-care in all spheres, altered ability to perform					
Impairment in performance of established hygiene activities	Self-care activities, alteration in ability to perform: hygiene		Self-bathing/hygiene deficit (specify level)	Self-bathing/hygiene deficit (specify level)	Self-bathing/hygiene deficit (specify level)
			Self-dressing/grooming deficit (specify level)	Self-dressing/grooming deficit (specify level)	Self-dressing/grooming deficit (specify level)
		Self-feeding deficit	Self-feeding deficit (specify level)	Self-feeding deficit (specify level)	Self-feeding deficit (specify level)
		Self-toileting deficit	Self-toileting deficit (specify level)	Self-toileting deficit (specify level)	Self-toileting deficit (specify level)
Grieving	Acute grieving	Grieving	Grieving, anticipatory	Grieving, anticipatory	Grieving, anticipatory
Normal grieving	Grieving, anticipatory		Grieving, dysfunctional	Grieving, dysfunctional	Grieving, dysfunctional
Normal grieving, potential	Delayed grieving				
Arrested grieving					
Arrested grieving, potential					
Delayed onset of grieving					
Delayed onset of grieving, potential					
					Growth and development, altered
					Health maintenance alteration
					Hopelessness

(continued)

1973	1975	1978	1980	1982 and 1984	1986
Injury, potential for Susceptibility to hazards		Injury, potential for Accidental falling, potential for	Injury, potential for (see subcategories Appendix A)	Injury, potential for (see subcategories Appendix A)	Injury, potential for (see subcategories Appendix A)
					Infection, potential for
		Knowledge, lack of (specify area)	Knowledge deficit (specify)	Knowledge deficit (specify)	Knowledge deficit (specify)
Understanding of state of health, lack of					
Understanding of etiology of state of health, lack of					
Understanding of preventive health measures, lack of					
Understanding of therapy, lack of					
Manipulation, verbal Manipulation, nonverbal	Manipulation				
Mobility, impaired Mobility, impaired physical Mobility, impaired social Mobility, impaired emotional Mobility, impaired intellectual Mobility, impaired developmental	Mobility, impairment of	Mobility, impairment of	Mobility, impaired physical	Mobility, impaired physical	Mobility, impaired physical
Motor incoordination Motor incoordination, gross Motor incoordination, fine					

Noncompliance	Noncompliance	Noncompliance	Noncompliance (specify)	Noncompliance (specify)	Noncompliance (specify)
Noncompliance with diet Noncompliance with drug therapy Noncompliance with environmental therapy Noncompliance with activity regimen	Noncompliance	Noncompliance	Noncompliance (specify)	Noncompliance (specify)	Noncompliance (specify)
Nutrition, alterations in: undernutrition	Nutritional alteration: less then required (MDR)	Nutritional alteration: less than body requirements	Nutrition, alteration in: less than body requirements	Nutrition, alteration in: less than body requirements	Nutrition, alteration in: less than body requirements
Nutrition, alterations in: obesity	Nutritional alteration: more than required	Nutritional alteration: more than body requirements	Nutrition, alteration in: more than body requirements Nutrition, alteration in: potential for more than body requirements	Nutrition, alteration in: more than body requirements Nutrition, alteration in: potential for more than body requirements	Nutrition, alteration in: more than body requirements Nutrition, alteration in: potential for more than body requirements
	Nutritional alteration: potential	Nutritional alteration: related to changes in body requirements			
		Parenting, alterations in: actual Parenting, alterations in: potential	Parenting, alterations in: actual Parenting, alterations in: potential	Parenting, alterations in: actual Parenting, alterations in: potential	Parenting, alterations in: actual Parenting, alterations in: potential
				Oral mucous membranes, alteration in	Oral mucous membranes, alteration in
Respiration, impairment of	Respiratory dysfunction	Respiratory dysfunction	Airway clearance, ineffective Breathing pattern, ineffective Gas exchange, impaired	Airway clearance, ineffective Breathing pattern, ineffective Gas exchange, impaired	
Respiratory distress					

(continued)

1973	1975	1978	1980	1982 and 1984	1986
Family process, inadequate Group relations, noneffective				Family process, alteration in	Airway clearance, ineffective Breathing pattern, ineffective Gas exchange, impaired Family process, alteration in
Social isolation				Social isolation	Social interaction, impaired Social isolation
Self-esteem or self-actualization, impairment of Self-concept, altered		Self-concept, alterations in: (self-esteem, role performance personal identity, body image)	Self-concept, disturbance in (see subcategories Appendix A)	Self-concept, disturbance in (see subcategories Appendix A)	Self-concept, disturbance in (see subcategories Appendix A)
Altered body image Depersonalization Identity conflict	Self-concept: alterations in body image				
Role disturbance					Body temperature, potential alteration in Hyperthermia Hypothermia Thermoregulation, ineffective

(continued)

		Rape trauma syndrome Rape trauma, compound reaction Rape trauma, silent reaction	Rape trauma syndrome Rape trauma, compound reaction Rape trauma, silent reaction	Rape trauma syndrome Rape trauma, compound reaction Rape trauma, silent reaction	Rape trauma syndrome Rape trauma, compound reaction Rape trauma, silent reaction
Sensory disturbance Sensory deprivation Sensory overload Sensory impairment	Sensory-perceptual alterations	Sensory-perceptual alterations	Sensory-perceptual alterations (see subcategories Appendix A)	Sensory-perceptual alterations (see subcategories Appendix A)	Sensory-perceptual alterations (see subcategories Appendix A)
Disturbances in visual perception Disturbances in auditory perception Disturbances in gustatory perceptions Disturbances in tactile perception					Unilateral neglect
Sexuality, alterations in patterns of	Sexual dysfunction	Sexual dysfunction	Sexual dysfunction	Sexual dysfunction	Sexual dysfunction Sexuality patterns, altered
Skin integrity, impairment of	Skin integrity, impairment of: actual Skin integrity, impairment of: potential	Skin integrity, impairment of: actual Skin integrity, impairment of: potential	Skin integrity, impairment of: actual Skin integrity, impairment of: potential	Skin integrity, impairment of: actual Skin integrity, impairment of: potential	Skin integrity, impairment of: actual Skin integrity, impairment of: potential
Skin, impairment of regulatory function of Altered internal regulatory function					Tissue integrity, impaired
Altered relationships with self and others				Powerlessness	Powerlessness

1973	1975	1978	1980	1982 and 1984	1986
Altered relationships with self and others				Powerlessness	Powerlessness
Altered external regulatory functions					
Sleep-rest patterns, ineffective	Sleep-rest activity, dys-rhythm of	Sleep-rest activity, dys-rhythm of	Sleep pattern disturbance	Sleep pattern disturbance	Sleep pattern disturbance
					Swallowing, impaired
Urinary elimination, impairment of	Urinary elimination, impairment of: alterations in patterns	Urinary elimination, impairment of: alterations in patterns	Urinary elimination, alteration in patterns	Urinary elimination, alteration in patterns	Urinary elimination, alteration in patterns
					Incontinence, functional
					Incontinence, reflex
					Incontinence, stress
					Incontinence, total
					Incontinence, urge
Inability to control initiation of urine flow	Urinary elimination, impairment of: incontinence	Urinary elimination, impairment of: incontinence			
Inability to control cessation of urine flow					
Inability to generate urine flow	Urinary elimination, impairment of: retention	Urinary elimination, impairment of: retention			Urinary retention
			Violence, potential for	Violence, potential for	Violence, potential for

*The books containing lists from which this was prepared are:
Gebbie, K. M., & Lavin, M. A. (Eds.). (1975). *Proceedings of the first national conference on classification of nursing diagnoses.* St. Louis: Mosby.
Gebbie, K. M. (Ed.). (1976). *Summary of the second national conference of classification of nursing diagnoses.* Clearinghouse for The National Group for Classification of Nursing Diagnoses, 1310 South Grand Blvd., St. Louis, Mo. 63104, 1976.
Kim, M. J., & Moritz, D. A. (Eds.). (1982). *Classification of nursing diagnoses: Proceedings of the third and fourth conferences.* New York: McGraw-Hill.
Kim, M. J., McFarland, G., & McLane, A. (Eds.). (1984). *Classification of nursing diagnoses: Proceedings of the fifth national conference.* St. Louis: Mosby.
Hurley, M. (Ed.). (1986). *Classification of nursing diagnoses: Proceedings of the sixth conference.* St. Louis: Mosby.
McLane, A. (Ed.). (1987). *Classification of nursing diagnoses: Proceedings of the seventh conference.* St. Louis: Mosby.

NURSING DIAGNOSES GROUPED BY FUNCTIONAL HEALTH PATTERNS[1]

An *asterisk* indicates diagnoses not currently accepted by NANDA; diagnoses in *italics* represent suggested changes in wording. The approved diagnosis Altered Growth and Development represents a condition that can occur in any functional pattern; the defining characteristics have been used to describe specific developmental delays.

HEALTH-PERCEPTION–HEALTH-MANAGEMENT PATTERN

Health Maintenance Alteration
*Health Management Deficit (Total)
*Health Management Deficit (Specify)
Noncompliance (Specify)
*Potential Noncompliance (Specify)
Potential for Infection
Potential for Injury (Trauma)
Potential for Poisoning
Potential for Suffocation

NUTRITIONAL-METABOLIC PATTERN

Alteration in Nutrition: Potential for More than Body Requirements or *Potential for Obesity*
Alteration in Nutrition: More than Body Requirements or *Exogenous Obesity*

[1]Definitions, defining characteristics, and etiological or related factors for diagnoses can be found in Gordon, M. (1987). *Manual of nursing diagnoses.* New York: McGraw-Hill. NANDA-approved diagnoses also can be found in McLane, A. (Ed.). (1987). *Classification of nursing diagnoses: Proceedings of the seventh conference.* St. Louis: Mosby.

Alteration in Nutrition: Less than Body Requirements or *Nutritional Deficit (Specify)*
Impaired Swallowing or *Uncompensated Swallowing Impairment*
Alteration in Oral Mucous Membrane
Potential Fluid Volume Deficit
Fluid Volume Deficit
Alteration in Fluid Volume: Excess or *Excess Fluid Volume*
Potential Impairment of Skin Integrity or *Potential Skin Breakdown*
*Decubitus Ulcer (Specify Stage)
Impaired Skin Integrity
Impaired Tissue Integrity
Potential Alteration in Body Temperature
Ineffective Thermoregulation
Hyperthermia
Hypothermia

ELIMINATION PATTERN

Alteration in Bowel Elimination: Constipation or *Intermittent Constipation Pattern*
Alteration in Bowel Elimination: Diarrhea or *Diarrhea*
Alteration in Bowel Elimination: Incontinence or *Bowel Incontinence*
Functional Incontinence
Reflex Incontinence
Stress Incontinence
Total Incontinence
Urge Incontinence
Urinary Retention
Alteration in Patterns of Urinary Elimination

ACTIVITY-EXERCISE PATTERN

Potential Activity Intolerance
Activity Intolerance (*Specify Level*)
Impaired Physical Mobility (*Specify Level*)
Total Self-Care Deficit (*Specify Level*)
Self-Bathing–Hygiene Deficit (*Specify Level*)
Self-Dressing–Grooming Deficit (*Specify Level*)
Self-Feeding Deficit (*Specify Level*)
Self-Toileting Deficit (*Specify Level*)
Diversional Activity Deficit
Impaired Home Maintenance Management (Mild, Moderate, Severe, Potential, Chronic)
*Potential Joint Contractures
Ineffective Airway Clearance
Ineffective Breathing Pattern
Impaired Gas Exchange
Alteration in Cardiac Output: Decreased or *Decreased Cardiac Output*
Alteration in Tissue Perfusion (Specify)
*Altered Growth and Development: *Self-Care Skills (Specify)*

SLEEP-REST PATTERN

Sleep-Pattern Disturbance

COGNITIVE-PERCEPTUAL PATTERN

Alteration in Comfort: Pain
Alteration in Comfort: Chronic Pain
*Pain Self-Management Deficit (Acute, Chronic)
*Uncompensated Sensory Deficit (Specify)
Sensory-Perceptual Alteration: Input Deficit or *Sensory Deprivation*
Sensory-Perceptual Alteration: Input Excess or *Sensory Overload*
Unilateral Neglect
Knowledge Deficit (Specify)
*Uncompensated Short Term Memory Deficit
*Potential Cognitive Impairment
Altered Thought Processes
*Decisional Conflict (Specify)

SELF-PERCEPTION–SELF-CONCEPT PATTERN

Fear (*Specify*)
*Anticipatory Anxiety (Mild, Moderate, Severe)
Anxiety
*Mild Anxiety
*Moderate Anxiety
*Severe Anxiety (Panic)
*Reactive Depression (Situational)
Hopelessness
Powerlessness (Severe, Low, Moderate)
Self-Esteem Disturbance
Body Image Disturbance
Personal Identity Confusion

ROLE-RELATIONSHIP PATTERN

Anticipatory Grieving
Dysfunctional Grieving
Disturbance in Role Performance
*Unresolved Independence-Dependence Conflict
*Social Isolation
Social Isolation (*Rejection*)
Impaired Social Interaction
*Translocation Syndrome
Alteration in Family Processes
*Weak Mother-Infant Attachment or Parent-Infant Attachment
Potential Alteration in Parenting
Alteration in Parenting

Impaired Verbal Communication
Potential for Violence
*Support System Deficit
*Altered Growth and Development: Communication Skills (Specify)
*Altered Growth and Development: Social Skills (Specify)

SEXUALITY-REPRODUCTIVE PATTERN

Sexual Dysfunction
Altered Sexuality Patterns
Rape Trauma Syndrome
Rape Trauma Syndrome: Compound Reaction
Rape Trauma Syndrome: Silent Reaction

COPING–STRESS-TOLERANCE PATTERN

Coping, Ineffective (Individual)
*Avoidance Coping
Impaired Adjustment
Post-trauma Response
Family Coping: Potential for Growth
Ineffective Family Coping: Compromised
Ineffective Family Coping: Disabling

VALUE-BELIEF PATTERN

*Spiritual Distress (Distress of Human Spirit)

NURSING HISTORY AND EXAMINATION

NURSING HISTORY

First visit of 50-year-old white male, industrial photographer who appears relaxed in chair. Diverticulosis diagnosed by x-ray 6 months ago. Purpose of visit: follow-up.

Health-Perception–Health-Management pattern States general health has been "good lately." While eating supper 6 months ago, had "severe stomach pains" with some diaphoresis, no nausea/vomiting; saw his physician the next day. Lower G.I. x-ray revealed diverticulosis. States he has gained weight; tried to take it off without success. No episodes of abdominal discomfort, constipation, or blood in stools in last 6 months. Reports that he has no problems in "watching his diet and fluid intake"; avoids getting constipated. Does not smoke; social drinking once or twice a month; takes no medications. One episode of "the flu," but "everyone had it."

Nutritional-Metabolic Pattern States typical daily food intake consists of toast and coffee in the morning, a sandwich, cake, and soda for lunch, and a large dinner meal consisting of meat, potatoes, vegetable, and cake or ice cream. Snacks during day: a candy bar or potato chips and sometimes cookies while watching T.V. at night. Takes no vitamin supplements. States drinks water throughout the day, one glass of fluid with each meal. Reports gained 20–30 pounds over the last 10 years due to "decreased activity"; usually hungry at meal-times, wife is a good cook. Intake of alcoholic beverages decreased in last few years to one–two drinks per month. No healing problems; no open lesions. Reports always has had "bad teeth" and had teeth replaced with both upper and lower dentures 5 years ago; states no problems with dentures fit; no gum problems visible.

Elimination Pattern   Usual bowel regimen is once a day in the a.m.; reports no constipation, narrow or loose stools, blood in stool, does not use cathartics. Voiding pattern: urinates three or four times during the day; no discomfort or changes in urination.

Activity-Exercise Pattern   States he has less energy than 30 years ago when he used to jog and play baseball. Exercises very little; usually only short walks once or twice a month; job requires little walking. Leisure: enjoys reading, T.V. and going to concerts. States "I guess I've gotten lazy." Full self-care in all areas.

Sleep Rest Pattern   Feels rested and ready for work in a.m. No problems in sleeping; no use of sleep medication; sleeps flat with one pillow.

Cognitive-Perceptual Pattern   States he must wear his glasses at all times for any activity; wearing glasses 35 years; last eye exam was 2 years ago. States no hearing difficulties. Attention span is good and converses easily, although somewhat reserved; often closes his eyes when talking about himself. Alert and oriented × 3 and states no changes in memory. Learns best "when I can understand and ask questions."

Self-Perception–Self-Concept Pattern   Describes self as "not really satisfied with the way life has turned out"; he always wanted to be a "big success" and make a large income. He regrets not ever getting a "formal education" (high school graduate), but that he has taught himself over the years and feels he is a "highly motivated" person, unlike "many of my friends." States he feels he is "too old" now to make major career/investment changes in his life, and that his focus in life now is his family's welfare.

Role-Relationship Pattern   States he has been married for 28 years; one daughter and three grandchildren. Lives with his wife; daughter, son-in-law, and grandchildren live in apartment upstairs; large house in suburbs. States living situation seems to work out well and that family members get along well with each other. Is oldest of seven siblings; helps support one financially. Took care of both parents when they were very ill (cardiac disease) 7 to 8 years before they died. States has always carried a large "responsibility role" in his family. States that marriage is "good"; he and his wife have things in common. Enjoys his work (industrial photographer), was in politics 20 years ago; was a band musician (trumpet player) in the Army in his early twenties.

Coping-Stress Tolerance   States life has been good to him; copes best by working when he has problems and talking things over with wife. He enjoys his grandchildren very much; tries to spend time with them. Finds that if he has information he can "cope" and "go on and do what I've got to do."

Value-Belief Pattern   Reports most important thing in his life at this point is helping his grandchildren "grow up right"; concerned about drugs in the schools. Used to be a devout Episcopalian; feels the church has changed over the years and he does not agree with many "things that church dictates these days"; attends every Sunday with his family and enjoys this but has "own faith in God" that he feels very strongly about.

EXAMINATION

General appearance, grooming, hygiene _Good_
Oral mucous membranes (color, moistness, lesions) _Within normal limits_
Teeth: Dentures _Yes_ Cavities _0_ Missing _0_
Hears whisper? _Yes_
Reads newsprint? _Yes_ Glasses? _Yes_
Pulse (rate) _84_ (rhythm) _Reg._
Respirations _20_ (depth) _wnl_ (rhythm) Breath sounds _Clear_
Blood pressure _130/82_
Hand grip _Strong_ Can pick up pencil? _Yes_
Range of motion (joints) _wnl_ Muscle firmness _firm_
Skin: Bony prominences _wnl_ Lesions _0_ Color changes _0_
Gait: _wnl_ Posture _wnl_ Absent body part _no_

Demonstrated ability for (code for level):
Feeding _0_
Bathing _0_
Toileting _0_
Bed mobility _0_
Dressing _0_

Grooming _0_
General mobility _0_
Cooking _0_
Home maintenance _0_
Shopping _0_

Intravenous, drainage, suction, etc. (specify) _NO_
Actual weight _200 LB_ Reported weight _195 LB_
Height _6' 0"_ Temperature _98.6°_

During history and examination:
Orientation _oriented × 3_ Grasp ideas and questions (abstract, concrete)? _Both_
Language spoken _Eng_ Voice and speech pattern _Clear_
Eye contact _Most of the time_ Attention span (distraction?) _No_
Nervous or relaxed _4_
1——5
(Rate from 1 to 5)
Assertive or passive _3_
(Rate from 1 to 5)
Interaction with family member/guardian/other (if present) _Not present_

(List nursing diagnoses, problem and etiological factors, and the data supporting diagnoses; list
interventions and outcomes.)

FUNCTIONAL HEALTH PATTERN ASSESSMENT: ADULTS

NURSING HISTORY AND EXAMINATION

1 Health perception-health management pattern
   a How has general health been?
   b Any colds in past year?
   c Most important things do to keep healthy?. Think these things make a difference to health? (Include family folk remedies, if appropriate.) Use of cigarettes, alcohol, drugs? Breast self-exam?
   d In past, been easy to find ways to follow things nurses or doctors suggest?
   e If appropriate: What do you think caused this illness? Actions taken when symptoms perceived? Results of actions?
   f If appropriate: Things important to you while you're here? How can we be most helpful?
2 Nutritional-metabolic pattern
   a Typical daily food intake? (Describe.) Supplements?
   b Typical daily fluid intake? (Describe.)
   c Weight loss/gain? (Amount)
   d Appetite?
   e Food or eating: Discomfort? Diet Restrictions?
   f Heal well or poorly?
   g Skin problems: Lesions, dryness?
   h Dental problems?
3 Elimination pattern
   a Bowel elimination pattern. Describe.) Frequency? Character? Discomfort?
   b Urinary elimination pattern. (Describe.) Frequency? Discomfort? Problem in control?
   c Excess perspiration? Odor problems?

4 Activity-exercise pattern
a Sufficient energy for completing desired/required activities?
b Exercise pattern? Type? Regularity?
c Spare time (leisure) activities? Child: Play activities?
d Perceived ability for: (code for level)

Feeding _____	Grooming _____
Bathing _____	General mobility _____
Toileting _____	Cooking _____
Bed mobility _____	Home maintenance _____
Dressing _____	Shopping _____

Functional levels code
Level O: Full self-care
Level I: Requires use of equipment or device
Level II: Requires assistance or supervision from another person
Level III: Requires assistance or supervision from another person or device
Level IV: Is dependent and does not participate

5 Sleep-rest pattern
a Generally rested and ready for daily activities after sleep?
b Sleep onset problems? Aids? Dreams (nightmares)? Early awakening?

6 Cognitive-perceptual pattern
a Hearing difficulty? Aid?
b Vision? Wear glasses? Last checked?
c Any change in memory lately?
d Easiest way for you to learn things? Any difficulty learning?
e Any discomfort? Pain? How do you manage it?

7 Self-perception–self-concept pattern
a How would you describe yourself? Most of the time, feel good (not so good) about yourself?
b Changes in your body or the things you can do? Problem to you?
c Changes in way you feel about yourself or your body (since illness started)?
d Find things frequently make you angry? Annoyed? Fearful? Anxious? Depressed? What helps?

8 Role-relationship pattern
a Live alone? Family? Family structure (diagram)?
b Any family problems you have difficulty handling? (nuclear/extended)
c How does family usually handle problems?
d Family depend on you for things? If appropriate: How managing?
e If appropriate: How family/others feel about your illness/hospitalization?
f If appropriate: Problems with children?. Difficulty handling?
g Belong to social groups? Close friends? Feel lonely? (frequency)
h Things generally go well for you at work (school/college)? If appropriate: Income sufficient for needs?
i Feel part of (or isolated in) neighborhood where living?

9 Sexuality-reproductive pattern
a If appropriate: Any changes or problems in sexual relations?
b If appropriate: Use of contraceptives? Problems?
c Female: When menstruation started? Last menstrual period? Menstrual problems? Para? Gravida?

10. Coping–stress tolerance pattern
    a Tense a lot of the time? What helps? Use any medicines, drugs, alcohol?
    b Who's most helpful in talking things over? Available to you now?
    c Any big changes in your life in the last year or two?
    d When (if) have big problems (any problems) in your life, how do you handle them?
    e Most of the time, is this (are these) way(s) successful?
11 Value-belief pattern
    a Generally get things you want out of life? Most important thing?
    b Religion important in your life? If appropriate: Does this help when difficulties arise?
    c If appropriate: Will being here interfere with any religious practices?
12 Other
    a Any other things that we haven't talked about that you'd like to mention?
    b Questions.

SCREENING EXAMINATION FORMAT

(May need to add other observable indicators to expand the examination depending on type of illness, age, and cues elicited in history.)
General appearance, grooming, hygiene_____
Oral mucous membranes (color, moistness, lesions)_____
Teeth: Dentures_____Cavities_____Missing_____
Hears whisper?_____
Reads newsprint?_____Glasses?_____
Pulse (rate)_____(rhythm)_____
Respirations_____(depth)_____(rhythm)_____Breath sounds_____
Blood pressure_____
Hand grip_____Can pick up pencil?_____
Range of motion (joints)_____Muscle firmness_____
Skin: Bony prominences_____Lesions_____Color changes_____
Gait_____Posture_____Absent body part_____

Demonstrated ability for: (Code for level)
Feeding_____
Bathing_____
Toileting_____
Bed mobility_____
Dressing_____
Grooming_____
General mobility_____
Cooking_____
Home maintenance_____
Shopping_____

Intravenous, drainage, suction, etc. (specify)_____
Actual weight_____Reported weight_____
Height_____Temperature_____

During history and examination:
Orientation_____Grasp ideas and questions (abstract, concrete)?_____

Language spoken_____Voice and speech pattern_____
Eye contact_____Attention span (distraction)_____
Nervous or relaxed (rate from 1 to 5)_____
1————————5
Assertive or passive (rate from 1 to 5)_____
1————————5
Interaction with family member, guardian, other (if present)_____

Grouping of Indicators, Demonstrating Relevance of Data to Pattern Description

Nutritional-metabolic pattern
Weight
Height
Temperature
(intravenous, drainage, suction)

Skin (bony prominences, lesions)
Oral mucous membranes
(color, moistness, lesions)
Teeth (dentures, cavities, missing)

Activity-exercise pattern
Gait
Posture
Absent body part
Hand grip
Coordination
Range of motion (joints)
Muscle firmness

Prostheses
Assistive equipment
Pulse rate, rhythm
Respiratory rate, depth, rhythm
Breath sounds
Blood pressure

Cognitive-perceptual pattern
Grasp of ideas, questions
Language spoken
Hearing
Orientation

Vocabulary
Attention span
Vision

Self-perception–self-concept pattern
Body posture
Attention span
Voice and speech pattern

Eye contact
Nervous or relaxed

Role-relationship pattern
Interactions with family member, guardian, other (if present) Assertive or passive

DATA RECORDING SHEET

The admission assessment data recording sheet is placed in the client's chart. It becomes part of the permanent health care record. The following format with additional lines for recording can be imprinted on a permanent record sheet.

Nursing History

General description of client (age, general appearance, chief concerns, etc.) _____
_____

Health-perception–health-management pattern _____
_____

Nutritional-metabolic pattern _____

Elimination pattern _____

Activity-exercise pattern _____

Sleep-rest pattern _____

Cognitive-perceptual pattern _____

Self-perception–self-concept pattern _____

Role-relationship pattern _____

Sexuality-reproductive pattern _____

Coping–stress tolerance pattern _____

Value-belief pattern _____

Examination

(See Format pp. 438–439)

FUNCTIONAL HEALTH PATTERN ASSESSMENT: INFANT AND EARLY CHILDHOOD

Use a parent report until the child can answer the items. The following includes some screening items related to parent assessment or use adult assessment (Appendix E).

I Health-perception–health-management pattern
  A Parents' report:
    1 Pregnancy/labor/delivery history (this baby, child)?
    2 Health status since birth?
    3 Adherence to routine health checks? Immunizations?
    4 Infections? Frequency? Absences from school?
    5 If applicable: Medical problem, treatment, and prognosis?
    6 If applicable: Actions taken when signs/symptoms perceived?
    7 If appropriate: Been easy to follow things doctors or nurses suggest?
    8 Preventive health practices (diaper change, utensils, clothes, etc.)?
    9 Parents smoke? Around baby?
    10 Accidents? Frequency?
    11 Crib toys (safety)? Carrying safety? Car safety?
    12 Safety practices (household products, medicines, etc.)
  B Parent (self): Parents'/family's general health status?
  C Observation
    1 General appearance of infant/child.
    2 General appearance of parent(s).
II Nutritional-metabolic pattern
  A Parents' report of
    1 Breast feeding/Bottle? Estimate of intake? Sucking strength?
    2 Appetite? Feeding discomfort?
    3 24-hour intake of nutrients?
    4 Supplements?
    5 Eating behavior?
    6 Food preferences? Conflicts over food?

7 Birth weight? Current weight?
8 Skin problems: Rashes, lesions, etc.?
B Observation
  1 Height?
  2 Weight?
  3 Skin color, hydration, rashes, lesions.
III Elimination pattern
  A Parents' report of
    1 Bowel elimination pattern (describe). Frequency? Character? Discomfort?
    2 Diaper change routine?
    3 Urinary elimination pattern (describe). Frequency of diaper change?
    4 Estimate of amount? Stream (strong, dribble)?
    5 Excess perspiration? Odor?
IV Activity-exercise pattern
  A Parents' report of
    1 Bathing routine? (When, how, where, type of soap?)
    2 Dressing routine? (Clothing, inside/outside home)
    3 Crib or other? Describe.
    4 Typical day's activity (hours spent in crib, carrying, play, type of toys).
    5 Active? Activity tolerance?
    6 Perception of baby's/child's strength ("strong/fragile")?
    7 Child: Self-care ability (bathing, feeding, toileting, dressing, grooming)?
    8 Parent (self) child care, home maintenance activity pattern.
  B Observation
    1 Reflexes (appropriate to age)
    2 Breathing pattern; rate, rhythm.
    3 Heart sounds; rate, rhythm.
    4 Blood pressure.
V Sleep-rest pattern
  A Parents' report of
    1 Sleep pattern: Estimated hours?
    2 Restlessness? Nightmares?
    3 Infant: Sleep position? Body movements?
  B Parent (self): Sleep pattern?
VI Cognitive-perceptual pattern
  A Parents' report of
    1 General responsiveness?
    2 Response to talking? Noise? Objects? Touch?
    3 Following objects with eyes? Response to crib toys?
    4 Learning (changes noted)? What teaching baby?
    5 Noises/Vocalizations?
    6 Speech pattern? Words? Sentences?
    7 Use of stimulation: Talking, games, etc.?
    8 Vision, hearing, touch, kinesthesia?
    9 Child: Name, Tell time, address, telephone number?
    10 Pain? Discomfort? (Describe)
VII Self-perception–self-concept pattern
  A Parent's report of
    1 Mood state?
    2 If child? Child's sense of worth, identity, competency?

B Child's report of
   1 Mood state?
   2 Many/few friends? Liked by others?
   3 Self-perception ("good" most of time? Hard to be "good"?).
   4 Ever lonely?
   5 Fears (transient/frequent)?
C Observation
   1 Child: Eye contact, speech pattern, posturing.
D Parent (self)
   1 General sense of worth, identity, competency?
VIII Role/relationship pattern
   A Parent's report of
      1 Family/household structure?
      2 Family problems/stressors?
      3 Family members/infant (or child) interaction?
      4 Infant/child response to separation?
      5 Child: Dependency?
      6 Child: Play pattern?
      7 Child: Temper tantrums? Discipline problems?
      8 Child: School adjustment?
   B Observation
      1 Smiling response (infant)?
      2 Social interaction (child)? Aggressive/withdrawn?
      3 Response to vocalizations? Requests?
   C Parent (self)
      1 Role engagements? Satisfaction?
      2 Work? Social? Family? Relationships?
IX Sexuality-reproductive pattern
   A Parents' report of
      1 Child's feeling of maleness/femaleness?
      2 Questions regarding sexuality? How respond?
   B Parent (self)
      1 If applicable: Reproductive history?
      2 Sexual satisfaction/problems?
X Coping–Stress tolerance pattern
   A Parents' report of
      1 Child's pattern of handling problems, frustrations, anger, etc.? Stressors? Tolerance?
   B Parent (self)
      1 Strategies for handling problems?
      2 Use of support systems?
      3 Life stressors? Family stress?
XI Value-belief pattern
   A Parent (self)
      1 Things important in life? Desires for the future?
      2 If appropriate: Perceived impact of disease on goals?

APPENDIX **G**

DIAGNOSTIC EXERCISES: LEVEL 1

A DIAGNOSTIC RECOGNITION EXERCISE

Which of the following are useful descriptions of client problems/etiological factors on which to base nursing care:

1 Needs occupational therapy/boredom
2 Impaired verbal communication/uncompensated aphasia
3 Alteration in tissue perfusion (cerebral)/arteriosclerosis
4 Alteration in nutrition: less than body protein requirements/low financial resources
5 Potential fluid volume deficit
6 Chest pain/myocardial infarction
7 Stress

B DIAGNOSTIC SELECTION EXERCISE, TYPE I

Select the best nursing diagnosis on which to base care:

Mr. G., aged 58, complains of increased, frequent urination and general malaise. He appears flushed and is having difficulty remembering events of the past 24 hrs. You note that he is exhibiting Kussmaul respirations. Blood sugar is 800 mg. percent. Mr. G.'s wife died one and one-half years ago. His son reports that "since then he's been low and drinking more heavily." There have been frequent crying episodes, eating and sleeping patterns are poor, and he has been neglecting personal hygiene. Mr. G. says he's "so lonely" without his wife.

1 Depression/loss of wife
2 Self-neglect syndrome/loss
3 Loneliness/loss of wife
4 Health management deficit/delayed grief resolution

5 Grief/loss of wife
6 Diabetes mellitus

C   DIAGNOSTIC SELECTION EXERCISE, TYPE II

Generate and evaluate diagnostic hypotheses after each set of data using list of diagnoses (Appendix A):

Mrs. A. is a 39-year-old woman. It is 9 a.m. on her second day after a hysterectomy. When you walk in the room she is wearing her own nightgown and lying supine in the bed. The bed is in disarray. Her face is flushed, she's crying, and she turns away as you approach.

Diagnostic Hypotheses to Be Investigated?

You touch her arm in a gentle way, find the skin slightly warm to the touch. She says she is having pain at the operative site.

Diagnostic Hypotheses to Be Investigated?

She begins to tell you about her husband's visit last night. She says she felt so angry but "there was no reason"; refused to kiss her husband and even "told him to go and find another woman." You recall from admission nursing history and assessment that she described her family and sexual relationships as good but that she had anticipatory anxiety, etiology undiagnosed.

Diagnostic Hypotheses to Be Investigated?

You say very gently, "When you think about it now, why do you think you were so angry?" She says, crying, "He reminds me how incomplete I am now; I'm finished as a female." You say, "Oh, no wonder you feel upset, I think we should talk about this. But first let me take your temperature and then let's sit and talk."

Diagnostic Hypotheses to Be Investigated?

T = 101°

Diagnostic Hypotheses to Be Investigated?

See Appendix O for answers.

D   DIAGNOSTIC FORMULATION EXERCISES

See Appendix H for examples.

DIAGNOSTIC EXERCISES: LEVEL 2

DIAGNOSTIC FORMULATION EXERCISES

The following three cases illustrate a basic data base collected at admission when the clients were added to a nurses' caseload. To simulate the way data were collected and hypotheses generated, stop at the end of each pattern area assessment (e.g., health perception–health management, nutritional-metabolic, etc.) to formulate any tentative nursing diagnoses that may be indicated by cues. Discard, revise, or reformulate diagnoses as you continue reading. At the end of each case, state nursing diagnoses and the data that support your admission diagnoses. A list of accepted diagnoses appears in Appendix A; diagnostic terms should be generated if the list is inadequate. Defining signs and symptoms are found in the manual accompanying this book (Gordon, 1987) or in NANDA conference proceedings: McLane, A. (1987) (Ed.). Classification of nursing diagnoses: Proceedings of the seventh conference. St. Louis, MO: Mosby. Answers (suggested diagnoses) appear in Appendix O.

CASE 1

Nursing History and Examination

First prenatal clinic visits of 24-year-old, married, former secretary with no history of chronic disease. Last menstrual period, February; expected date of confinement November 15; 5 weeks pregnant. Husband is 25-year-old machine operator who receives health care at company clinic and is in "good health."

Health-Perception–Health-Management Patter Sees self as healthy and pleased about pregnancy. Usual childhood diseases, including chicken pox, measles, mumps. No recent colds or other illnesses. Keeps healthy by "eating right" and "supporting each other." Sees this making a difference when compared to other families she knows. No use of cigarettes or drugs; one glass wine per week, socially. No pattern of breast self-exam; doesn't know how. No delay in coming to clinic when missed first period; came to clinic because parents use this hospital clinic for care.

Nutritional-Metabolic Pattern   Typical diet: *Breakfast:* orange juice, cereal with fruit, coffee, toast and butter; *Lunch:* alternate lunchmeat or cheese sandwich and salads, soft drink (no-cal) or coffee; *Dinner:* two vegetables, meat, rolls and butter, coffee, dessert or fruit; *Snacks:* 1 cookie or fruit, coffee, or soft drink. No vitamin supplements. Fluids: 1–2 glasses water, 3–4 c. coffee. Appetite good; tries to restrict calories; states has gained about 1 pound. No nausea, dental problems, skin dryness. Some tingling and fullness of breasts; lotions helpful.

Elimination Pattern   Regular bowel movements qd. No changes or discomfort. Knows that has to maintain roughage and fluid intake. Slight increase in urinary frequency; realized this is due to enlarging uterus; no problems in control. No excess perspiration or odor.

Activity-Exercise Pattern   Resigned secretarial job because of pregnancy and time pressures in job. Worked for busy executive who wanted her to stay another 4–6 months. Does housework; has restricted other exercise; drives car instead of walking; stopped playing tennis; wants to be "careful and sure nothing happens to baby." States too much activity could cause miscarriage, but doesn't know exactly how. Leisure activities: T.V., movies with husband, and visiting friends. Has felt more fatigue since stopped working; attributes this to pregnancy.

REPORTED FUNCTIONAL LEVEL

Feeding	0	Dressing	0	Home maintenance	0
Bathing	0	Grooming	0	Shopping	0
Toileting	0	General mobility	0		
		Bed mobility	0	Cooking	0

FUNCTIONAL LEVEL CODE
Level O: Full self-care
 Level I: Requires use of equipment or device
Level II: Requires assistance or supervision from another person
Level III: Requires assistance or supervision from another person *and* equipment or device
Level IV: Is dependent and does not participate

Sleep-Rest Pattern   Feels rested in a.m. Tires by afternoon and takes 2-hour nap. Sleep onset delayed since stopped work; states due to excitement of being pregnant and starts thinking about plans; can't get to sleep. No history of sleep disturbances.

Cognitive-Perceptual Pattern   No perceived hearing or vision problems, discomfort, memory changes. Learns "easily"; likes to read and then discuss questions.

Self-Perception–Self-Concept Pattern   Feels she is "easy to get along with," "bright" and "reasonably good-looking." Thinks she will be a "good, careful" mother. "Excited about changes" in her body and has been looking at maternity clothes; doesn't want to wait until dresses or slacks get tight and press on baby. No feelings of anger, depression. States "every new mother is a little fearful and anxious in case something happens to baby." Has stopped work; will devote time to "getting things ready," but friends and neighbors all work and few to talk to; day "seems long."

Role-Relationship Pattern Lives with husband; 25-year-old machine operator; married 3 years; "he is excited about baby." Both hope it is a boy. Perceives no family problems Handle problems by "attacking them"; discusses things. Social activities at tennis club; have close friends, couples same age. Moved into neighborhood 3 years ago, people friendly and help each other. No perceived financial problems. Parents and in-laws live in same town. She and husband are only children so this will be first grandchild. Client's mother had two miscarriages and client does not want this to happen to her. Parents available to help after baby born. Gets on well with parents and in-laws.

Sexuality-Reproductive Pattern Sexual relations decreased so "nothing happens to baby." Told husband this was important and he agrees. Previous sexual pattern: no perceived problems. Stopped contraceptives 6 months ago; wants three children. Menses started age 13, regular cycle 30 days; length 4 days. Last menstrual period 5 weeks. Para O, Gravida O. Plans to breast feed.

Coping–Stress Tolerance Pattern Feels "a little tense about a miscarriage," Hasn't talked to anyone about this. Usually talks over problems with husband; very supportive; but doesn't want to worry him. States they "deal with problems, not shove them under the table." Perceives this as successful but has had no big problems. No other life changes in last few years.

Value-Belief Pattern Thinks "do what you can in this life; we've no aspirations to be rich." Comes from close family and learned "family important." Methodist; practices religion and finds it supportive.

Examination

General appearance, grooming, hygiene ___Good___
Oral mucous membranes (color, moistness, lesions) ___Normal___
Teeth: dentures _0_ Cavities _0_ Missing _0_
Hears whisper? _Yes_
Reads newsprint? _Yes_ Glasses _No_
Pulse (rate) _84_ (rhythm) _Reg_
Respirations _18_ (depth) _Normal_ (rhythm) _Reg_
Breath sounds _Normal_
Blood pressure _118/70_ Hand grip _Strong_ Can pick up pencil? _Yes_
Range of motion (joints) _Full_ Muscle firmness _Firm_
Skin: bony prominence: _0_ Lesions _0_ Color changes _0_
Breasts _Firm, developed, areolas darkened, no tenderness_
Pelvis: _gynecoid (see medical exam)_
Gait _Reg_ Posture _Good_ Absent body part _0_
Intravenous, drainage, suction, etc. (specify) _0_
Actual weight _120_ Reported weight _Pregravida 119_
Height _5'6"_
Temperature _98.6°_
During history and examination:
Orientation _Yes_ Grasp ideas and questions? (Abstract, concrete) _Both_

Language spoken __Eng__ Voice and speech pattern __Normal__
Vocabulary __Good__
Eye contact __Yes__ Attention span (distraction) __Good span__
Nervous or relaxed __3__
1————————5
Assertive or passive __3__
1————————5
Interaction with family member, guardian, other (if present) ·
_____Husband not present; at work_____

Nursing Diagnoses (See Appendix O for answers.)

CASE 2

Nursing History and Examination

First admission of unconscious 5-year-old boy, with facial lacerations and linear skull fracture. To Emergency Room by ambulance after car accident; accompanied by anxious, distraught father who was not injured and provided history. Mother out of town visiting sister. (Screening assessment because of father's anxiety.)

Health-Perception–Health-Management Pattern   Previously alert, healthy child. Has had usual childhood diseases and immunizations, including tetanus; no colds this winter. States hasn't insisted son use seat belts when riding in front seat.

Nutritional-Metabolic Pattern   Appetite has been good; no vitamin supplements, no weight loss; seen by pediatrician 2 weeks ago; told developing normally.

Elimination Patterns   Bowel movements regular; no nighttime incontinence.

Activity-Exercise Pattern   Energetic 6 year old; plays actively with children in neighborhood; baseball favorite sport.

REPORTED FUNCTIONAL LEVEL

Pretrauma:

Feeding	0	Dressing	0	Home maintenance	—
Bathing	2	Grooming	2	Shopping	—
Toileting	0	General mobility	0		
		Bed mobility	—	Cooking	—

FUNCTIONAL LEVEL CODE
Level O: Full self-care
 Level I: Requires use of equipment or device
 Level II: Requires assistance or supervision from another person
Level III: Requires assistance or supervision from another person *and* equipment or device
Level IV: Is dependent and does not participate

Sleep-Rest Pattern No sleep problems; stopped naps at 4 years.

Cognitive-Perceptual Pattern Comatose since accident; no convulsions. No previous hearing, vision, or learning problems. Speech has been clear.

Self-Perception–Self-Concept Pattern Described as generally outgoing and friendly with strangers. Recently calls self "bad boy" when things go wrong. Made "big fuss" last week over skinned knee and whether "would get better."

Role-Relationship Pattern Looking forward to school in fall. Has three good friends in neighborhood. At times takes older brother's clothes to try on but relationship perceived as good. Family structure: 2 brothers 14 and 16, mother, father; paternal grandmother lives next door; other grandparents deceased. Family relationships good; no perceived problems. Father states he feels "guilty," about accident; "although not my fault"; hit from rear by another car; "Why couldn't I be the one to die"; relates unconsciousness to approaching death of child. Father pacing in room.

Sexuality-Reproductive Pattern Deferred.

Coping–Stress Tolerance Pattern Seeks parents for security when situations stressful. Father states he and wife are supportive to each other. He'll "feel better when she gets here."

Value-Belief Pattern Religion: Episcopal. Assessment deferred.

Examination

General appearance, grooming, hygiene ___ —
Oral mucous membranes (color, moistness, lesions) _Normal color; no lesions_
Teeth: dentures __0__ Cavities __0__ Missing _2 upper front_
Hears whisper? _No_
Reads newsprint? _Comatose_ Glasses __No__
Pulse (rate) __100__ (rhythm) __Reg__
Respirations __20__ (depth) __Deep__ (rhythm) __Reg__
Breath sounds __clear__ Blood pressure __98/58__ PO$_2$ _78mm_
Hand grip __Absent__ Can pick up pencil? __No__
Voluntary movement _Absent LL, LA, RL, RA_ Functional Level __4__
Range of motion (joints) _Full involuntary_ Muscle firmness _Tone decreased_
Skin: bony prominence _Intact_ Lesions _Facial lacerations_
Color changes __0__ Gait ___—___ Posture ___—___ Absent body part __0__
Intravenous, drainage, suction, etc. (specify) __I.V.__
Actual weight ___—___ Reported weight __49__
Height __36"__
Temperature __99°__
During history and examination:
Orientation _no response to stimuli_ Pupils _Equal; react to light_
Convulsions _None_ Grasp ideas and questions (abstract, concrete)? __0__
Language spoken __Eng__ Voice-speech pattern ___—___ Vocabulary ___—___
Eye contact ___—___ Attention span (distraction) ___—___
Nervous or relaxed __(Comatose)__
1————————5

Assertive or passive __(Comatose)__
1————————5
Interaction with family member, guardian, other (if present)

Nursing Diagnoses (See Appendix O for answers.)

CASE 3

Nursing History and Examination 10/27/81

Sixth admission for diabetic ketoacidosis of a 19-year-old white female with juvenile onset diabetes mellitus since age 5. Admitted with nausea and vomiting, abdominal pain, and blood glucose of 505 mgm. Medical evaluation states there is no obvious predisposing physical cause of ketoacidosis; admissions attributed to "noncompliance." Did not take insulin for 2 days prior to this admission.

Health-Perception–Health-Management Pattern States that diet, exercise, and insulin are "all important" to her health, yet doesn't follow prescribed diet, does no exercise, and only takes insulin sporadically. Feels she understands the aspects of her disease well; has been able to understand instructions given to her by doctors and nurses. Does not follow recommendations sometimes "forgets" to take insulin or because it is "too much of a pain." She states that she probably would be healthier if she were "a good little diabetic" but that she knows she isn't. Believes she is susceptible to diabetic ketoacidosis since she has had five previous admissions; says this admission was due to a "virus"; doesn't believe that not taking insulin for last 2 days could cause current problem; states she overslept (11 a.m.) and it was too late to take insulin. Takes "night dose" at 5 p.m. States once went for a week without taking insulin. Doesn't consider herself to be very healthy, would give herself a "2 on a scale of 1 to 10."

Nutritional-Metabolic Pattern Does not follow prescribed diet or count calories. *Breakfast:* Eats cereal with tea or toast, butter, and tea. *Lunch:* Eats peanut butter and butter sandwich with iced tea; usually has cereal or peanut butter again for dinner. States eats about 10 pieces of bread per day since this is what she eats whenever she gets hungry. She drinks six glasses sugar-free iced tea per day. Dislikes meat of any kind; doesn't care for poultry or fish. States that her family does not eat meals together; she gets her own meals. If her mother prepares a meat meal, she usually goes to her bedroom and feeds the meat to her cats. Usually eats alone; if does eat with parents, it's only when she makes the dessert, the only thing she knows how to cook. Has bought a vegetarian cookbook but says that she's too "lazy" to learn how to cook. Asked to see a dietician so that she can lose weight. Reports 5′ 3″, 135 lbs.

Elimination Patterns No difficulty with bowels or urination, takes no laxatives. Does not complain of polyuria despite large fluid intake (approximately 2000 cc. per day reported).

Activity-Exercise Pattern Reports no daily exercise pattern. Does not walk; feels she is weak and isn't able to do any activities. No activities outside her home. Has no physical disabilities but does not perform any activities other than watching T.V. or reading. Attended college for one semester but left and has no plans to return; unemployed.

Sleep-Rest Pattern Usually retires 1 or 2 a.m., gets up at 7 a.m. to take insulin and eat. Usually naps in the afternoon for 2 hours when has noting to do. Feels she is adequately rested. Takes no sleeping meds; no problems getting to sleep.

Cognitive-Perceptual Pattern Reports no hearing difficulties. Wears glasses all the time for nearsightedness. No difficulty with recall. Considers herself to be "rather intelligent with I.Q. of 126" yet not "smart enough to be super like 140, the gifted." States has no difficulty learning and learns well with reading materials since things that she's told sometimes "slip right through," must be interesting and challenging in order for her to give any attention to them. Points out that English and literature are her favorite subjects; reports pleasure in getting a 750 score on her SAT.

REPORTED FUNCTIONAL LEVEL

Feeding	0	Dressing	0	Home maintenance	0
Bathing	0 in bed	Grooming	0	Shopping	0
Toileting	0 in bed	General mobility	(Bed rest)		
		Bed mobility	0	Cooking	0

FUNCTIONAL LEVEL CODE
Level O: Full self-care
Level I: Requires use of equipment or device
Level II: Requires assistance or supervision from another person
Level III: Requires assistance or supervision from another person *and* equipment or device
Level IV: Is dependent and does not participate

Self-Perception–Self-Concept Pattern Considers herself to be physically weak and this prohibits her from doing things, such as joining the Army; doesn't think she could make it through basic training. She becomes annoyed at herself; considers herself to be "lazy." Believes parents are supportive enough when she needs them but states she usually doesn't tell them when things bother her and therefore remains "independent."

Role-Relationship Pattern Lives with her parents; has a brother who is in the Air Force. Related that once she told her guidance instructor that she was living as a hermit after school and then the instructor picked "up the cue and had my whole family see the school psychologist." States that psychologist helped her mother to "change a lot and stop nagging" but that it did nothing for her. Reports no family problems but states that her family is "a bunch of strangers living under the same roof." Describes family as one which doesn't outwardly show emotions but feels that they give her what she wants (such as money). Feels her family gives her enough attention but "probably I could get used to receiving more from them." States diabetes is "no big thing" to her family since she's had it since age 5; "it is considered just the way it is." Family usually doesn't visit her in the hospital unless she asks them to, says she likes it this way. Has no friends, doesn't belong to any social groups, because she "has nothing in common with people her age." Likes to talk about herself; says enjoys talking about the "concepts" she is reading (Greek mythology), whereas girls her age like to talk "about boys or what clothes are *in* this fall." She sees her life as being "boring."

Sexuality-Reproductive Pattern Reports normal menstural cycle 28 days for 5 days duration. Presently on 2d day of menstrual cycle. Had no sexual relations. Dated in high school but no dating since graduation.

Coping–Stress Tolerance Pattern States she has learned that "you can't do too much about things"; "you just wait and see what happens." Voice low during this discussion and sad facial expression. Regained composure quickly and changed subjects.

Value-Belief Pattern States that she has not yet "gotten anything out of life that I have wanted"; says she would like "to do something useful and challenging with my life" but hasn't been able to identify these things. Might consider teaching. Won't be satisfied until able to "physically do something both useful and challenging." Doesn't want to waste time doing things aimlessly.

Examination

General appearance, grooming, hygiene __Obese teenager in no acute distress; disheveled; hair__ __dull and oily (unclean), uncombed__

Oral mucous membranes (color, moistness, lesions): __Pink, moist, no lesions__

Teeth: dentures __none__ Cavities __multiple cavities__ Missing __none__

Hears whisper? __Yes__

Reads newsprint? __Yes__ Glasses __for reading and distance__

Pulse (rate) __100__ (rhythm) __Regular__

Respirations __20__ (depth) __Normal__ (rhythm) __Regular__

Breath sounds __No wheezes, rales__

Blood pressure __130/86__ Hand grip __Strong__ Can pick up pencil? __Yes__

Range of motion (joints) __Within normal limits__ Muscle firmness __Firm__

Skin: bony prominence; __Intact__ Lesions __Knotty cutaneous deposits on arms and thighs__ __from injections__

Gait __not observed__ Posture __Relaxed upright posture in bed__

Absent body part __0__

Intravenous, drainage, suction, etc. (specify) __0__

Actual weight __135__ Reported weight __135__ Height __5′3″__

Temperature __99°__

During history and examination:

Orientation: __Yes__

Grasp ideas and questions (abstract, concrete)? __Both; good abstract ability__

Language spoken __English__ Voice and speech pattern __Normal__

Vocabulary __Extensive__

Eye contact __Yes__ Attention span (distraction): __good attention span; very interested in__ __sharing information about self__

Nervous or relaxed __4__

1————————5

Assertive or passive __3__

1————————5

Interaction with family member, guardian, other (if present) __none present__

Nursing Diagnoses (See Appendix O for Answers.)

PRACTICE-BASED COMPONENTS FOR A COMPUTERIZED NURSING INFORMATION SYSTEM[1]

DATA SET ITEMS AND DEFINITIONS

The data set items that follow can be logically derived (1) from current models and standards of nursing practice and (2) from reflection on the information needed to support cognitive processes involved in patient care. Identification, demographic, medical, setting, and care provider items are required but are not unique to a nursing practice data set.

Identification Variables

1 Patient identification
Item-categories Name and assigned number.
Definition The legal name and assigned agency number of the patient.
Rationale Required for discrimination among patients during care.

Demographic Variables

2 Age
Item-categories Newborn to 120 (month/years); date of birth (month, day, year).
Definition Chronological age of the patient at admission and date of birth.
Rationale Required for application of developmental norms, health statistics, and individualization of treatment.

3 Sex
Item-categories Male or female.
Definition Predominant sexual classification based on physical characteristics.

[1]Excerpted with permission. Gordon, M. (1985). Practice-based data set for a nursing information system. *Journal of Medical Systems*, 9:45–55.

Rationale Required for application of norms, health statistics, and individualization of treatment.

4 Race/ethnicity
Item-categories DHHS or concise categories in current use.
Definition Subdivision of human population based on genetic and/or geocultural characteristics.
Rationale Required for application of norms, health statistics, and individualization of treatment.

5 Marital status
Item-categories Never married, married, separated, widowed, divorced, not determined.
Definition Current marital status on admission.
Rationale Required as contextual data relative to diagnosis, treatment and, in some cases, discharge planning.

6 Principal Residence
Item-categories Dwelling number, street address, city/town, state or foreign country, zip code.
Definition Primary, current mailing address of the patient. If no address, specify categories: city, state. If institution, specify name in addition to address.
Rationale Required for discharge planning and identification of environmental variables in diagnosis and treatment.

Setting and Care Provider Identification Variables

7 Agency subdivision
Item-categories Name of agency subdivision (determined locally).
Definition Name of recognized geographic agency subdivision (e.g., unit, clinic, or district name).
Rationale Required for further patient identification.

8 Admission and discharge date
Item-categories Month, day, year of admission and discharge.
Definition Actual month, day, year in which patient began to receive health services at the agency and month, day, year in which patient was discharged or transferred to another facility or agency.
Rationale Required variable in some instances of diagnosis and treatment. Specifies the onset and termination of nursing services.

9 Primary nurse identification
Item-categories Name or other identification of nursing care provider.
Definition Name of professional nursing care provider who is primarily responsible for care of patient from admission to discharge.
Rationale Required for designation of responsibility for diagnosis, treatment, and evaluation.

Care Provision Variables

10 Next of kin/guardian
Item-categories Name, street address, city/town, state, zip code, telephone area code, number.

Definition The name, mailing address, and telephone number of kin, close friend, or guardian.

Rationale Designation required for emergency notification. Guardian participation in treatment planning (parents) or discharge planning.

11 Functional health status

Item-categories See Table 1.

Definition Eleven categories and assessment parameters for admission-baseline data on functional health patterns.

Rationale Required as baseline and for evaluating any change that may occur during the period of hospital/clinic/community care. Documented information for legal and accreditation purposes.

12 Nursing diagnoses (See Appendix C)

Item-categories Problem, etiological or related factors, and supporting data.

Definition Actual or potential health problems for which the professional nurse is primarily accountable for the diagnosis, plan of treatment, and treatment outcomes between admission and discharge/transfer. Includes the problem, etiological or related factors, supporting data. Includes active diagnoses, conditions that develop subsequent to admission, and discharge diagnoses. Etiological categories describe the factors contributing to the problem that can be influenced by nursing intervention (e.g., probable cause). Supporting data are the assessment findings that validate the presence of the problem and etiological factors.

Rationale Required as a basis for treatment planning (etiological factors) and projecting outcomes (problems). Required for accreditation purposes, professional standards, and, in some states, legal purposes. Supporting data (subjective and objective) is required until diagnoses are standardized to assure common understanding of the diagnoses (Supporting data may always be required in teaching institutions with nursing and medical student affiliations.)

13 Projected and discharge outcomes

Item-categories Projected treatment outcomes and means of indicating presence or absence of projected outcomes at discharge.

Definition Projected outcomes are indicators of problem resolution. They are *predicted* to be attained (prognostic indicators) by discharge or other designated periods. Discharge (or periodic) outcomes are the *actual* outcomes attained by the patient. Both projected and discharge outcomes are indicators of resolution relative to the diagnoses; they are coded by diagnosis.

Rationale Desired goals or outcomes are required information for treatment planning and accreditation purposes. Projected and discharge outcome information is required for treatment evaluation and quality care review.

14 Nursing treatment orders

Item-categories Nursing treatment orders and means of designating treatments received.

Definition Definitive treatment orders coded for nursing diagnostic categories. Includes active orders, discontinued orders, and discharge orders between admission and discharge/transfer. Treatment orders are coded for the nursing diagnoses and medical diagnoses in Item 14 if the medical diagnosis or therapeutic regimen requires secondary nursing orders (e.g., observations, or individualizing of treatment or diagnostic procedures). Symbols are used to designate time (or visit) in which treatment was received by patient and for care provider identification.

Table 1

Item-Categories and Parameters: Functional Health Status Nursing History/Examination

I Health-perception–health-management pattern
  a Perception of general health status
  b Colds in past year; work/school absences
  c Health practices and effect
  d Ease of adherence to medical/nursing suggestions
  e Perceived cause of present illness
  f Actions taken when illness perceived; results
  g Personal requests regarding health management

II Nutritional-metabolic pattern
  a Typical daily food intake; supplements
  b Typical daily fluid intake
  c Weight change
  d Appetite
  e Perceived diet restrictions
  f Associated discomfort: foods, eating
  g Perceived healing ability
  h Perceived problems
  i Perceived dental problems; dentures
  j Skin color, turgor, lesions

III a Description of bowel elimination pattern: frequency, character, discomfort, control
  b Description of urinary elimination pattern: frequency, character, discomfort, control
  c Perspiration/odor

IV Activity-exercise pattern
  a Perceived energy level
  b Type and regularity of exercise pattern
  c Spare time/play activities
  d Self-care level (see code); feeding, bathing, toileting, bed mobility, dressing, grooming, general mobility, cooking, home maintenance, shopping
  e Gait, posture, ROJM, coordination

V Sleep-rest pattern
  a Perceived readiness for day's activities
  b Sleep problems: onset, early awakening, interrupted, reversal

VI Cognitive-perceptual pattern
  a Hearing; aids
  b Vision; glasses, last check
  c Memory; attention
  d Learning style; difficulties
  e Perceived discomfort or pain
  f Insight, judgment, decision making
  g Level of consciousness, orientation
  h Language spoken

VII Self-perception–self-concept pattern
  a Self-description and evaluation
  b Body/physical ability changes and self-competency evaluation
  c Frequency of anger, fear, anxiety, depression; what helps
  d Nervousness/relaxed (rating)

(continued)

Table 1

Item-Categories and Parameters: Functional Health Status Nursing History/Examination (*Continued*)

VIII Roles-relationship pattern
    a Live alone/family, family structure
    b Family problems (nuclear/extended)
    c Family problem-solving pattern
    d Family dependency needs, management
    e Family reaction to illness
    f Child-rearing/relationship patterns (problems)
    g Social group membership; frequency of loneliness
    h Perceived work/school relationship
    i Perception of neighborhood (isolated/integrated feelings)
    j Assertive/passive (rating)

IX Sexuality-reproductive pattern
    a Perceived changes/problems in sexuality, sexual relations
    b Use of contraceptives; problems
    c Menstruation onset and pattern (female)
    d Para gravida (female)

X Coping–stress tolerance pattern
    a Tension/stress management; use of drugs, alcohol, etc.
    b Significant other during stress; availability
    c Changes in life last 1–2 years
    d Problem-solving strategies; effect

XI Value-belief pattern
    a Goal achievement; goals in life
    b Perceived importance of religion
    c Desired religious practices (during hospital stay)

    Rationale Required for legal and accrediting purposes and for care and continuity of care. Required for judging responses to treatment.

15 Medical diagnosis

    Item-categories From ICDA, A.P.A., or other nomenclature system used by agency.
    Definition All physician-identified diagnoses including the primary medical diagnosis or problem, coexisting diagnoses, conditions that develop subsequent to admission, and discharge diagnoses.
    Rationale Required for predicting dysfunctional health patterns, for understanding the basis for medical treatment orders, and for discharge planning.

16 Medical treatment orders

    Item-categories Medical treatment, taxonomy in use, and means of designating treatments received (time and care provider identification).
    Definition Primary treatment orders, discontinued orders, and discharge orders formulated by a physician between admission and discharge/transfer. Symbols are used to designate time (or visit) in which treatment was received by patient and care provider designation.
    Rationale Required for legal and accrediting purposes and for care and continuity of care. Required for judging responses.

17 Diagnostic and surgical procedures

Item-categories Diagnostic procedure taxonomy, including X rays and lab tests; surgical procedure taxonomy (ICDA); dates of procedures and means of designating completion of procedures (time and care provider identification).

Definition Primary diagnostic and surgical procedure orders, discharge orders, and discontinued orders between admission and discharge. Symbols are used to designate time (or clinic visit) of order, time of completion (especially with delayed reports), and care provider identification designation.

Rationale Required for legal, accrediting, and accounting purposes and for care and continuity of care. Required for judging health status and responses.

PATIENT CLASSIFICATION: UNIVERSITY HOSPITALS OF CLEVELAND[1]

[1]Used with permission of Dr. E. J. Halloran, Senior Vice President and Director of Nursing, University Hospitals of Cleveland.

UNIVERSITY HOSPITALS OF CLEVELAND
NURSE/PATIENT SUMMARY

	RN Code Number	Other Code Number	Consultant Code Number
TODAY			
LAST NIGHT			
LAST EVENING			
Primary Nurse Code Number			

Date Today _____

DIRECTIONS: Check the items below if Actually or Potentially Present.

HEALTH PERCEPTION-MANAGEMENT
Potential for Injury . . . . _____001
Noncompliance . . . . _____002
Infection/Contagion . . . . _____003
Prolonged Disease/Disability. . . . . _____004
Instability . . . . _____005
Impaired Life Support Systems. . . . . _____006
Sanitation Deficit . . . . _____007
Socio-cultural-economic Considerations . . . . . . _____008

NUTRITIONAL-METABOLIC
Fluid
Excess Volume. . . . . _____009
Volume Deficit. . . . . _____010
Potential Volume Deficit. . . . . _____011
Bleeding . . . . _____012
Nutrition
Less Nutrition than Required. . . . . _____013
More Nutrition than Required. . . . . _____014
Potential for Excess . . . . _____015
Skin Integrity
Actual Skin Impairment . . . . _____016
Potential Skin Impairment . . . . _____017
Alterations in Oral Mucous Membrane . . . _____018
Altered Body Temperature . . . . _____019

ELIMINATION
Urinary
Incontinence. . . . . _____020
Other Altered Urinary Elim. Pattern. . . . . . _____021
Bowel
Constipation. . . . . _____022
Diarrhea . . . . _____023
Incontinence. . . . . _____024

ACTIVITY-EXERCISE
Activity Intolerance. . . . . _____025
Ineffective Airway Clearance . . . . _____026
Altered Breathing Pattern. . . . . _____027
Impaired Gas Exchange . . . . _____028
Altered Tissue Perfusion . . . . _____029
Decreased Cardiac Output. . . . . _____030
Diversional Activity Deficit . . . . _____031

SP-3530(8-85)

Altered Health Maintenance . . . . _____032
Impaired Mobility . . . . _____033
Self-Care Deficit. . . . . _____034
Impaired Home Maintenance Mgmt. . . . . _____035

COGNITION-PERCEPTION
Altered Comfort
Discomfort . . . . _____036
Pain . . . . _____037
Altered Level of Consciousness . . . . _____038
Altered Thought Process . . . . _____039
Impulsivity/Hyperactivity . . . . _____040
Altered Sensory Perception. . . . . _____041
Knowledge Deficit. . . . . _____042
Growth and Development Deficit. . . . . _____043

SLEEP-REST
Sleep Disturbance . . . . _____044

SELF-PERCEPTION/SELF-CONCEPT
Anxiety . . . . _____045
Disturbed Self-Concept . . . . _____046
Depression . . . . _____047
Fear . . . . _____048
Powerlessness . . . . _____049

ROLE RELATIONSHIPS
Grieving . . . . _____050
Altered Family Process. . . . . _____051
Altered Parenting . . . . _____052
Social Isolation. . . . . _____053
Impaired Verbal Communication . . . . _____054
Potential for Violence . . . . _____055

SEXUALITY-REPRODUCTION
Sexual Dysfunction . . . . _____056
Rape - Trauma Syndrome . . . . _____057

COPING-STRESS TOLERANCE
Ineffective Individual Coping . . . . _____058
Ineffective Family Coping . . . . _____059
Potential for Growth in Family Coping . . . . _____060

VALUE-BELIEF
Spiritual Distress . . . . _____061

MEMBERS OF THEORIST GROUP

Andrea Bircher, R.N., Ph.D.
University of Oklahoma
College of Nursing

Rosemary Ellis, R.N., Ph.D.
Case Western Reserve University
School of Nursing

Joyce Fitzpatrick, R.N., Ph.D.
Wayne State University
School of Nursing

Marjory Gordon, R.N., Ph.D.
Boston College
Graduate Medical-Surgical Nursing

Margaret Hardy, R.N., Ph.D.
Boston University
School of Nursing

Imogene King, R.N., Ph.D.
University of South Florida

Rose McKay, R.N., Ph.D.
University of Colorado
School of Nursing

Margaret A. Newman, R.N., Ph.D.
The Pennsylvania State University
College of Human Development

Dorothea Orem, R.N., Ph.D.
Consultant

Rose Marie Parse, R.N., Ph.D.
Duquesne University
School of Nursing

Martha Rogers, R.N., Sc.D.
New York University
Department of Nursing

Sr. Callista Roy, R.N., Ph.D.
Mount St. Mary's College
Department of Nursing

M. J. Smith, R.N., Ph.D.
Duquesne University
School of Nursing

Gertrude Torres, R.N., Ed.D.
Consultant

NANDA TAXONOMY I

The North American Nursing Diagnosis Association (NANDA) Taxonomy I is the first attempt at formal classification of nursing diagnoses. It represents a move from an alphabetical listing to a method of ordering diagnoses within nine human response patterns (level 1). The taxonomy builds on the work of the NANDA nurse theorist group[1] and the contributions of participants at NANDA conferences.[2] It was further developed by the NANDA Taxonomy Committee and has been endorsed by NANDA, 1986. Continued study and clinical testing by nurses will lead to refinement, revision, and expansion. The taxonomy contains the currently approved nursing diagnoses at levels 3, 4, 5, and 6, depending on their specificity. *Parentheses* indicate terms added by the taxonomy committee. *Question marks* are used to raise the possibility that gaps may exist in the taxonomy.

It may be noted that many of the concepts described as alterations (level 2) are similar to the concepts within the functional health patterns and other formats for assessment. Detailed case studies, involving synthesis of functional and dysfunctional patterns, may reveal diagnoses that describe behavior at higher levels of complexity, such as exchanging, valuing, and so forth (level I). A complete discussion of Taxonomy I is included in McLane, A. (Ed.). (1987). *Classification of nursing diagnoses: Proceedings of the Seventh Conference.* St. Louis: Mosby.

---

[1]Roy, Sr. C. (1984). Framework for classification system development. In M. J. Kim, G. K. McFarland, & A. M. McLane (Eds.). *Classification of nursing diagnoses: Proceedings of the fifth national conference.* St. Louis: Mosby.

[2]Kritek, P.B. (1986). Development of a taxonomic structure for nursing diagnoses: A review and update. In M. Hurley (Ed.). *Classification of nursing diagnoses: Proceedings of the sixth national conference.* St. Louis: Mosby; Kritek, P. B. (1984). Report of group work on taxonomies. In M. J. Kim, G. K. McFarland, & A. M. McLane (Eds.). *Classification of nursing diagnoses: Proceedings of the fifth national conference.* St. Louis: Mosby.

GUIDELINE OBSERVATIONS ABOUT NANDA NURSING DIAGNOSIS TAXONOMY I[3]

The nine major category heads in this taxonomy are viewed as nine central human response patterns. The second category level refers to "alterations," used in this context to refer to "the process or state of becoming or being made different without changing into something else." As used here, it is essentially a neutral term, and does not connote either a positive or negative change. Each subsequent lower level of the taxonomy reflects a higher degree of clinical specificity in the phenomena named. Given the incomplete nature of this taxonomy, where a given diagnosis has not yet been identified, a more generic category name may have to be used until clinically discrete phenomena are better identified.

Bracketed items in the taxonomy refer to items that have not actually been formally named, described, reviewed, or voted upon, but were viewed as necessary or desirable inclusions to create some degree of conceptual coherence. The "black boxes" or "blank boxes" are included to demonstrate the provisional nature of this first effort, and to highlight overt incompleteness. Both the boxes and the bracketed items indicate areas that still must be defined, described, and approved. They are not however in any sense exhaustive indicators of complete work.

This taxonomy includes all diagnoses formally approved by ballot after the Seventh Conference held in April, 1986. A common set of definitions for frequently used diagnosis qualifiers was also approved at the Seventh Conference.

It is recognized that several partial conceptual systems and/or constructs and mutually incompatible principles of classification are currently embedded in portions of this taxonomy. It is anticipated that these complex issues will have to be addressed and resolved in the development of subsequent taxonomies. NANDA Taxonomy II will be presented to the General Assembly in 1988, and will reflect some initial resolution of these issues.

Endorsement of this taxonomy by the NANDA General Assembly indicates an investment by NANDA in a specific taxonomy which can be tested, refined, revised, and expanded.

1 **EXCHANGING A human response pattern involving mutual giving and receiving**
   1.1 Alterations in Nutrition
      1.1.1 (Cellular)
      1.1.2 (Systemic)
         1.1.2.1 More than Body Requirements
         1.1.2.2 Less than Body Requirements
         1.1.2.3 Potential for more body requirements
         1.1.2.4 ?????
   1.2 (Alterations in Physical Regulation)
      1.2.1 (Immune)
         1.2.1.1 Potential for Infection
         1.2.1.2 ?????
      1.2.2 Alteration in Body Temperature
         1.2.2.1 Potential
         1.2.2.2 Hypothermia

[3]Guidelines excerpted from publication prepared by the NANDA Taxonomy Committee and distributed by the North American Diagnosis Association, July, 1986.

1.2.2.3 Hyperthermia
1.2.2.4 Ineffective Thermoregulation
1.2.2.5 ?????
1.3 Alterations in Elimination
　1.3.1 Bowel
　　1.3.1.1 Constipation
　　1.3.1.2 Diarrhea
　　1.3.1.3 Incontinence
　1.3.2 Urinary Patterns
　　1.3.2.1 Incontinence
　　　1.3.2.1.1 Stress
　　　1.3.2.1.2 Reflex
　　　1.3.2.1.3 Urge
　　　1.3.2.1.4 Functional
　　　1.3.2.1.5 Total
　　1.3.2.2 Retention
　1.3.3 (Skin)
　　1.3.3.1 ?????
　　1.3.3.2 ?????
1.4 (Alterations in Circulation)
　1.4.1 (Vascular)
　　1.4.1.1 Tissue Perfusion
　　　1.4.1.1.1 Renal
　　　1.4.1.1.2 Cerebral
　　　1.4.1.1.3 Cardiopulmonary
　　　1.4.1.1.4 Gastrointestinal
　　　1.4.1.1.5 Peripheral
　　1.4.1.2 Fluid Volume
　　　1.4.1.2.1 Excess
　　　1.4.1.2.2 Deficit
　　　　1.4.1.2.2.1 Actual
　　　　1.4.1.2.2.2 Potential
　1.4.2 (Cardiac)
　　1.4.2.1 Decreased Cardiac Output
　　1.4.2.2 ?????
1.5 (Alterations in Oxygenation)
　1.5.1 (Respiration)
　　1.5.1.1 Impaired Gas Exchange
　　1.5.1.2 Ineffective Airway Clearance
　　1.5.1.3 Ineffective Breathing Pattern
　1.5.2 ?????
1.6 (Alterations in Physical Integrity)
　1.6.1 Potential for Injury
　　1.6.1.1 Potential for Suffocation
　　1.6.1.2 Potential for Poisoning
　　1.6.1.3 Potential for Trauma
　1.6.2 Impairment
　　1.6.2.1 Skin Integrity
　　　1.6.2.1.1 Actual
　　　1.6.2.1.2 Potential

1.6.2.2 Tissue Integrity
    1.6.2.2.1 Oral Mucous Membrane
    1.6.2.2.2 ?????
  1.6.2.3 ?????

2 COMMUNICATING A human response pattern involving sending messages.
  2.1 Alterations in Communication
    2.1.1 Verbal
      2.1.1.1 Impaired
      2.1.1.2 ?????
    2.1.2 (Nonverbal)
  2.2 ?????
  2.3 ?????
    2.3.1 ?????
    2.3.2 ?????

3 RELATING A human response pattern involving establishing bonds
  3.1 (Alterations in Socialization)
    3.1.1 Impaired Social Interaction
    3.1.2 Social Isolation
    3.1.3 ?????
  3.2 (Alterations in Role)
    3.2.1 (Role Performance)
      3.2.1.1 Parenting
        3.2.1.1.1 Actual
        3.2.1.1.2 Potential
      3.2.1.2 Sexual
        3.2.1.1.1 Dysfunction
        3.2.1.1.2 ?????
      3.2.1.3 (Work)
    3.2.2 Family Processes
    3.2.3 ??????
  3.3 Altered Sexuality Patterns
  3.4 ?????

4 VALUING A human response pattern involving the assigning of relative worth
  4.1 (Alterations in Spiritual State)
    4.1.1 Distress
    4.1.2 ?????
  4.2 ?????
    4.2.1 ?????
    4.2.2 ?????

5 CHOOSING A human response pattern involving the selection of alternatives
  5.1 Alterations in Coping
    5.1.1 Individual
      5.1.1.1 Ineffective
        5.1.1.1.1 Impaired Adjustment
        5.1.1.1.2 ?????
      5.1.1.2 ?????
    5.1.2 Family
      5.1.2.1 Ineffective
        5.1.2.1.1 Disabled
        5.1.2.1.2 Comprised

5.1.2.2 Potential for Growth
5.1.3 (Community)
5.2 (Alterations in Participation)
5.2.1 (Individual)
5.2.1.1 Noncompliance
5.2.1.2 ?????
5.2.2 (Family)
5.2.3 (Community)
6 MOVING A human response pattern involving activity
6.1 (Alterations in Activity)
6.1.1 Physical Mobility
6.1.1.1 Impaired
6.1.1.2 Activity Intolerance
6.1.1.3 Potential Activity Intolerance
6.1.1.4 ?????
6.1.2 (Social Mobility)
6.1.2.1 ?????
6.1.2.2 ?????
6.2 (Alterations in Rest)
6.2.1 Sleep Pattern Disturbance
6.2.2 ?????
6.3 (Alterations in Recreation)
6.3.1 Diversional Activity
6.3.1.1 Deficit
6.3.1.2 ?????
6.3.2 ?????
6.4 (Alterations in Activities in Daily Living)
6.4.1 Home Maintenance Management
6.4.1.1 Impaired
6.4.1.2 ?????
6.4.2 Health Maintenance
6.4.3 ?????
6.5 Alterations in Self-Care
6.5.1 Feeding
6.5.1.1 Impaired Swallowing
6.5.1.2 ?????
6.5.2 Bathing/Hygiene
6.5.3 Dressing/Grooming
6.5.4 Toileting
6.6 Altered Growth and Development
6.6.1 ?????
6.6.2 ?????
7 PERCEIVING A human response pattern involving the reception of information
7.1 Alterations in Self-Concept
7.1.1 Disturbance in Body Image
7.1.2 Disturbance in Self-Esteem
7.1.3 Disturbance in Personal Identity
7.1.4 ?????

7.2. Sensory Perceptual Alteration
    7.2.1 Visual
        7.2.1.1 Unilateral Neglect
        7.2.1.2 ?????
    7.2.2 Auditory
    7.2.3 Kinesthetic
    7.2.4 Gustatory
    7.2.5 Tactile
    7.2.6 Olfactory
7.3 (Alterations in Meaningfulness)
    7.3.1 Hopelessness
    7.3.2 Powerlessness
    7.3.3 ?????
8 KNOWING A human response pattern involving the meaning associated with information
8.1 Alterations in Knowledge
    8.1.1 Deficit
    8.1.2 ?????
    8.1.3 ?????
8.2 (Alterations in Learning)
    8.2.1 ?????
    8.2.2 ?????
8.3 Alterations in Thought Processes
    8.3.1 (Confusion)
    8.3.2 ?????
    8.3.3 ????
9 FEELING A human response pattern involving the subjective awareness of information
9.1 Alterations in Comfort
    9.1.1 Pain
        9.1.1.1 Chronic
        9.1.1.2 (Acute)
        9.1.1.3 ?????
    9.1.2 (Discomfort)
9.2 (Alterations in Emotional Integrity)
    9.2.1 Anxiety
    9.2.2 Grieving
        9.2.2.1 Dysfunctional
        9.2.2.2 Anticipatory
        9.2.2.3 ?????
    9.2.3 Potential for Violence
    9.2.4 Fear
    9.2.5 Post-Trauma Response
        9.2.5.1 Rape Trauma Syndrome
            9.2.5.1.1 Rape Trauma
            9.2.5.1.2 Compound Reaction
            9.2.5.1.3 Silent Reaction
        9.2.5.2 ?????

DIAGNOSIS QUALIFIERS[1]

The following are definitions of terms used to qualify diagnoses:

Actual Existing at the present moment; existing in reality

Potential Can, but has not yet, come into being; possible

Ineffective Not producing the desired effect; not capable of performing satisfactorily

Decreased Smaller; lessened; diminished; lesser in size, amount, or degree

Increased Greater in size, amount or degree; larger, enlarged

Impaired Made worse, weakened; damaged, reduced; deteriorated

Depleted Emptied wholly or partially; exhausted of

Deficient Inadequate in amount, quality, or degree; defective; not sufficient; incomplete

Excessive Characterized by an amount or quantity that is greater than is necessary, desirable, or useful

Dysfunctional Abnormal; impaired or incompletely functioning

Disturbed Agitated; interrupted, interfered with

Acute Severe but of short duration

Chronic Lasting a long time; recurring; habitual; constant

Intermittent Stopping and starting again at intervals; periodic; cyclic

[1]NANDA Taxonomy Committee, 1986.

NANDA GUIDELINES AND REVIEW CYCLE FOR PROPOSED NEW NURSING DIAGNOSES[1]

DEVELOPMENT/SUBMISSION GUIDELINES FOR PROPOSED NEW NURSING DIAGNOSES

Introduction

The North American Nursing Diagnosis Association (NANDA) solicits proposed new nursing diagnoses for review by the Association. Such proposed diagnoses undergo a systematic review process which concludes with a mail ballot vote by the entire membership. Acceptance of the proposed diagnosis by mail ballot establishes the diagnoses for inclusion in NANDA's official list of diagnoses. Such acceptance indicates NANDA's view that the diagnosis shows readiness for use and continuing development by the discipline.

To assist interested parties in submitting proposed diagnoses, the NANDA Diagnosis Review Committee, which is charged with overseeing this process, has prepared a set of guidelines for submission. These guidelines are designed to assure consistency, clarity, and completeness of submissions. Diagnoses submitted which do not meet the guidelines will be returned to the person submitting them for appropriate revision to assure that the review process can be initiated. Proposed diagnoses are reviewed by the Diagnoses Review Committee and their clinical technical review task forces and by the NANDA Board prior to general assembly review and comment and membership vote.

---

[1]The following guidelines and review cycle were prepared by the NANDA Diagnosis Review Committee and distributed by the North American Nursing Diagnosis Association, 1985. To obtain copies and updates on guidelines and review cycle write to: North American Nursing Diagnosis Association, St. Louis University, School of Nursing, 3525 Caroline Ave., St. Louis, MO 63104.

Nursing Diagnosis Defined

Several definitions of nursing diagnoses exist in the nursing literature. The following are provided as four possible ways of conceptualizing a nursing diagnosis.

1 "A nursing diagnosis is a clinical judgment about an individual, family or community which is derived through a deliberate, systematic process of data collection and analysis. It provides the basis for prescriptions for definitive therapy for which the nurse is accountable. It is expressed concisely and it includes the etiology of the condition when known." (Shoemaker, 1984, p. 94)

2 "Nursing diagnosis is a concise phrase or term summarizing a cluster of empirical indicators representing patterns of unitary man." (Roy, 1982, p. 219)

3 "Nursing diagnoses made by professional nurses describe actual or potential health problems that nurses, by virtue of their education and experience, are capable and licensed to treat." (Gordon, 1976, p. 1299)

4 "A nursing diagnosis is a concise phrase or term summarizing a cluster or set of empirical indicators, representing normal variations and altered patterns (actual or potential) of human functioning which nurses by virtue of education and experience are capable and licensed to treat." (McLane, 1979, p. 33)

Proposed New Nursing Diagnosis:
Required Components for Submission

1 *Name* This part provides a name for the diagnosis, a concise phrase, term, or label.

2 *Definition* This part provides a clear, precise definition of the named diagnosis. The definition expresses the essential nature of the diagnosis named and delineates its meaning. The definition should enable one to differentiate this diagnosis from all others.

3 *Defining characteristics* This part provides a list of observable cues that the client presents which substantiate for the nurse that the nursing judgment (i.e., the selected diagnosis) appropriately labels and describes the client state, the phenomena of concern. Cues must be both listed and defined. Cues are separated into two positions or sets: major and minor.

    a *Major defining characteristics:* those which appear to be present in all clients experiencing the phenomena of concern.

    b *Minor defining characteristics:* those which appear to be present in many clients experiencing the phenomena of concern.

4 *Substantiating/supportive materials* This part provides documentation which substantiates the existence, nature and characteristics of the phenomena of concern. Minimal validation documentation is a listing of references demonstrating a reasonable review of relevant literature. Narrative materials accompanying such a reference list may not exceed 1500 words.

Proposed New Nursing Diagnosis:
Optional Components for Submission

1 *Supplemental Information* The following types of supplemental information may be submitted to further clarify the nursing phenomena identified by the proposed nursing diagnosis.

a Related Factors In some cases, there may be specific factors which appear to show some type of patterned relationship with the phenomena of concern, named as a nursing diagnosis. Where this situation exists, it may be helpful to name and describe these. Such factors may be described variously as antecedent to, associated with, related to, contributing to, or abetting.

b Sources of Variance In some cases, unique sources of variance in the experience of the phenomena may be possible. Where this situation exists, it may be helpful to identify these. Such sources of variance may include developmental stage variance, ethnic or cultural variance, levels of risk variance, acuity variance, and multi-diagnosis variance.

2 *Supplemental Validation* If it is available, supplemental validation of the nursing diagnosis may be submitted. This may include research abstracts, brief reports of validation projects, or reports of intervention or treatment studies. These must be brief in character, not exceeding 1500 words.

References

Gordon, M. (1976). Nursing diagnosis and the diagnostic process. *American Journal of Nursing,* 76: 1298–1300.

McLane, A. (1979). A taxonomy of nursing diagnoses: Toward a science of nursing. *Milwaukee Professional Nurse,* 20: 33.

Roy, C. (1982). Theoretical Framework for Classification of Nursing Diagnosis. In M. J. Kim & D. A. Moritz. (Eds.), *Classification of nursing diagnoses: Proceedings of the third and fourth national conferences. New York: McGraw Hill, pp. 215–221.*

Shoemaker, J. (1984). Essential features of nursing diagnosis. In M. J. Kim, G. K. McFarland, & A. M. McLane. (Eds.), *Classification of nursing diagnoses: Proceedings of the fifth national conference. St. Louis: Mosby, pp. 104–115.*

REVIEW CYCLE

The North American Nursing Diagnosis Association (NANDA), in an effort to meet its purpose "to develop, refine, and promote a taxonomy of nursing diagnostic terminology of general use to professional nurses" has developed a formal cycle of diagnosis review to enable the process of incorporation of new diagnoses submitted by interested parties. This process is cyclic in character, assuring continuous development and refinement of the taxonomy.

Step 1   Receipt of Diagnoses

Diagnoses may be entered into the review cycle on the initiative of either NANDA or other individuals or groups.

A NANDA initiates this process by soliciting diagnoses, advertising its interest in diagnoses, publishing their guidelines for submission, and responding to inquiries concerning such guidelines.

B Individual nurses or nurse groups initiate this process by submitting a diagnosis for review. When a submission is received by NANDA, it is initially reviewed for compliance with submission guidelines. Those submissions which involve only a suggested name or are only partially developed are returned to the person submitting the recommendation with a request for completion as described in the guidelines. Those submissions which meet criteria for the guidelines then enter the review process. The person submitting the suggested diagnosis receives a copy of the diagnosis review cycle at this time, to facilitate an understanding of NANDA's policies and procedures.

Step 2 Diagnoses Enter the Public Domain

NANDA formally recognizes all diagnoses under review as part of the public domain. As such, any diagnosis submitted for review is briefly reported in the *NANDA Nursing Diagnosis Newsletter* when it enters the review cycle. Persons submitting diagnoses are advised of this fact and are asked to indicate in writing their acceptance of this policy on a form provided by NANDA.

It is recognized, however, that individuals have often invested considerable time and energy in an effort to delineate one or more diagnoses. Therefore, the publication of a diagnoses entering the review cycle will include the name of the person(s) submitting this diagnosis, assuring them of recognition of their efforts. This will also improve networking and communication among members actively engaged in exploring common or comparable diagnoses.

Step 3 Diagnoses Are Reviewed by Clinical/Technical Task Forces

The NANDA Diagnosis Review Committee (DRC) is charged with the task of reviewing proposed diagnoses and recommending their acceptance, modification, or rejection to the NANDA board. This committee's work is guided by the advice and critique of clinical/ technical task forces who review diagnoses.

A Each diagnosis accepted for review is assigned by the chairperson of DRC to a member of that committee. This person serves as a primary or lead reviewer of the diagnosis and the chairperson of the clinical/technical review task force, which will review the diagnosis.

B The clinical/technical review task force is a panel created to review a specific diagnosis based on individual clinical and technical expertise. Task force members are drawn not only from the NANDA membership, but also from expert groups in organizations such as the Canadian Nurses' Association and the American Nurses' Association. NANDA board members who do not serve on the DRC are ineligible to serve on these task forces. Task forces are created as needed and appropriate by the DRC.

C Members of the various task forces receive diagnoses for critique and review with an evaluation form provided. This evaluation form enables reviewers to assess the degree to which the diagnosis submitted meets the criteria of the submission guidelines. Task force members are given 2 weeks to respond to a request for a review. These reviews are forwarded to the primary reviewer.

D Based on task force members' advice and comments, the primary reviewer prepares a diagnosis proposal for each diagnosis. These are presented at a meeting of the DRC.

Step 4 Diagnoses Are Reviewed by the NANDA Diagnosis Review Committee

The DRC convenes to review, discuss, and take action on the proposals for new diagnoses prepared by the primary reviewers of the clinical/technical task forces. Three possible outcomes emerge from this process.

A The DRC accepts the proposed diagnosis or makes minor changes,
or

B The DRC substantively alters the diagnosis as submitted by the original proposer, based on reviewer advice. The DRC then accepts the proposed diagnosis,
or

C The DRC rejects the diagnosis and identifies specific reasons for the rejection. In this case, the original proposer of the diagnosis is provided with specific recommendations for improvement.

The DRC notifies the original proposer of the diagnosis of their action at this time. They concurrently forward their recommendations to the NANDA board.

Step 5 Diagnoses Are Reviewed by the NANDA Board

The NANDA board receives the recommendations of the DRC, and convenes to review, discuss, and take action on the DRC recommendations. Once more, three possible outcomes emerge from this process.

A The board accepts the DRC recommendation,
or

B The board returns the diagnosis to the DRC with comments for revision and recommendations for change,
or

C The board rejects the DRC recommendation and identifies specific reasons for the rejection.

The DRC then notifies the original proposer of the board's action, and prepares accepted diagnoses for general assembly review and comment.

Step 6 Diagnoses Are Reviewed by the General Assembly

The general assembly has the authority to review and comment on proposed diagnoses for the DRC's actions prior to the submission to the membership for acceptance. The DRC prepares proposed diagnoses for this review and comment. The DRC therefore engages in the following activities.

A The DRC groups the diagnoses as possible or appropriate for general assembly review.

B The DRC structures time for review and comment by the general assembly during the national conference, advising the original proposer of the diagnosis of this action.

C The DRC develops policies, procedures and protocols for general assembly review and comment and conducts these sessions accordingly.

D The DRC collects general assembly comments and incorporates these into proposed diagnoses as appropriate and feasible.

E The DRC reports these changes to the board.

Step 6 Diagnoses Are Voted Upon by the NANDA Membership

The DRC prepares diagnoses for a NANDA membership vote. This includes several activities.

A The DRC creates a mail ballot of proposed diagnoses to be distributed to all current NANDA members.

B The DRC oversees the distribution and tallying of ballots. They record any suggestions for needed subsequent revision of any given diagnosis.

C The DRC communicates information on the outcome of balloting to the original proposer of the diagnosis. Unapproved diagnoses can be revised and reenter the cycle. Approved diagnoses become a part of the approved NANDA taxonomy.

D The DRC forwards the approved diagnoses to the national conference proceedings editor for inclusion in the proceedings and to the taxonomy committee for inclusion in the NANDA taxonomy.

E The DRC prepares a cycle report for the board.

Step 8 The Cycle Is Reactivated

The entire diagnosis review cycle is then reactivated. The *NANDA Nursing Diagnosis Newsletter* is the official vehicle for communication with the membership about the process, guidelines, timeliness, changes, and necessary publicity. Changes in accepted diagnoses undergo this same process and utilize the same review procedures.

ANSWERS TO DIAGNOSTIC EXERCISES

A DIAGNOSTIC RECOGNITION EXERCISE (APPENDIX G)

Item 1 *Needs occupational therapy/boredom* is not a nursing diagnosis. Need for care is described before describing the problem. If signs of boredom are present, further investigation is required.

Item 2 *Impaired verbal communication/uncompensated aphasia* represents a useful description on which to base care; it is a nursing diagnosis. The client would be helped to compensate for aphasia.

Item 3 *Alteration in tissue perfusion (cerebral)/arteriosclerosis* is a serious condition but usually not within the diagnostic competencies of a nurse. If this diagnostic judgment is made, the client should be referred for medical evaluation. Probably the client has nursing diagnoses but they are not described by this label. Alteration in tissue perfusion is accepted for clinical testing (see Appendix A), but it is difficult to justify that nursing care can resolve this problem.

Item 4 *Alteration in nutrition: less than body protein requirements/low financial resources* is a nursing diagnosis which employs accepted diagnostic labels. A more concise description would be, protein deficit/low financial resources.

Item 5 *Potential fluid volume deficit* is a well-formulated potential problem that provides a basis for care when risk factors are delineated.

Item 6 *Chest pain/myocardial infarction* is a concise expression of the accepted diagnostic category, alteration in comfort: pain. A modifier (chest) is employed to specify anatomical location. The stated etiology does not provide a basis for nursing intervention because nurses do not treat a myocardial infarction. If chest pain is a new symptom or current orders for pain medication or other drugs are inadequate to control pain, these observations should be referred to the physician. The pain may also signify decreased activity tolerance or a pain self-management deficit that requires health education. Further data are needed to determine if this is chronic pain (angina) or a sign of a complication. Chest pain/myocardial infarction represents inadequate formulation of a nursing diagnosis and inadequate assessment.

Item 7 *Stress* is not a useful description of a problem. The term represents an inference that requires further exploration to identify the problem and etiology before a plan of care can be designed.

B DIAGNOSTIC SELECTION EXERCISE, TYPE I

Item 1 *Depression/loss of wife* represents inadequate problem formulation. Data suggest depression is a sign of another problem.

Item 2 *Self-neglect syndrome/loss* represents superficial problem formulation. Data suggest this is a sign of another problem.

Item 3 *Loneliness/loss of wife* represents superficial problem formulation. Does not provide a basis for clustering all the related data.

Item 4 *Health management deficit/delayed grief resolution* is the best nursing diagnosis within the set on which to base care. Permits clustering all data in one concise expression and focusing nursing care on grief resolution.

Item 5 *Grief/loss of wife* does not adequately represent the data available; grief is an expected reaction to loss of a wife, therefore no problem is communicated on which to base care.

Item 6 Diabetes Mellitus is a medical diagnosis, not a nursing diagnosis. Disease-related nursing care can be organized on the basis of this description.

C DIAGNOSTIC SELECTION EXERCISE, TYPE II

Diagnostic hypotheses generated from the *first set* of data include: (1) *wound infection* (Is flush due to fever and a possible wound infection?), (2) *atelectasis* (Is flush due to fever and possible pulmonary complications? This complication is of low probability in lower abdominal surgery.), (3) *urinary retention* (Are the cues—bed in disarray, lower abdominal surgery, crying, and face flushed—signs of discomfort due to retention? This is a low probability on the second day unless there has been a postoperative history of retention.), (4) *incisional pain* (Are the signs of discomfort caused by pain? A likely pain site is the operative wound.), or (5) *fluid volume deficit* (Is flush and signs of discomfort on the second post-operative day caused by a history of low fluid intake?). The cues bed in disarray, face flushed, and crying at 9 a.m. suggest the possibility of sleep disturbance related to any of the above hypotheses. Adding the cues—turns away as you approach and hysterectomy—suggests unexpressed anger and situational depression over loss. A hypothesis to direct cue search could be formulated broadly as *ineffective coping related to loss* or more specifically as *perceived sexuality impairment.*

The test for skin warmth evident in the *second set* of data further supports the hypotheses—wound infection, pulmonary complications and fluid volume deficit. Pain at the operative site is a cue that also points to wound infection or to incisional pain without the presence of infection.

The *third set of cues* supports the hypothesis of *perceived sexuality impairment.* Information in the *fourth data set* suggests the nurse is testing the hypothesis of perceived sexuality (or reproductive) impairment. A likely etiological hypothesis is *loss (hysterectomy).* Note the priority for hypothesis investigation; the plan is to investigate previously generated hypotheses related to conditions manifesting fever—wound infection, atelectasis, and fluid volume deficit.

In the *fifth data set* information is obtained to support the hypotheses—wound infection, fluid volume deficit, and the low probability hypothesis of *pulmonary complications.* Amount and sufficiency of last voiding would decrease the risk of missing the problem of urinary retention. The nurse would quickly collect further data on these possibilities and call a physician.

Pain perception may be heightened by the psychological problem. A judgment has to be made whether to: (1) collect further data related to pain management, (2) offer the client the postoperative narcotic ordered, or (3) offer the opportunity to discuss perceptions and feelings about sexuality or reproductive loss, or (4) a combination of these actions.

Data support tentative nursing diagnoses formulated either as *perceived sexuality or reproductive impairment/loss (hysterectomy)* or as *ineffective coping/perceived loss of sexuality.* Further data would help formulate the diagnosis more specifically or data may support the possibility of a normal process of grieving. Pain management and any surgical-related care would be determined after medical evaluation of the client.

D DIAGNOSTIC FORMULATION EXERCISES (APPENDIX H)

Case 1: Nursing Diagnoses

1 Problem: *Anticipatory anxiety (miscarriage)*
Etiological Factors: *Identification with Mother's Miscarriage; Knowledge Deficit (Activity Tolerance and Health Management During Pregnancy)*

States too much activity could cause miscarriage; activity (tennis, walking, sexual) self-restricted "so nothing happens to baby."
Client's mother had two miscarriages and client doesn't want this to happen.
Wants to be "careful and sure nothing happens to baby."
Resigned secretarial job because of pregnancy, time pressures in job; expected date of confinement—35 weeks.
Sleep onset delayed "since stopped work."
Increase of fatigue attributed to pregnancy.
Thinks she will be "good, careful mother."
Using maternity clothes before clothes get tight and press on baby.
"Every new mother is a little fearful and anxious in case something happens to baby."

Medical exam: no health problems; pregnancy progressing normally.
Will devote time to "getting things ready;" friends and neighbors work; few to talk to; days "seem long," afternoon naps, 2 hrs.

2 *Health Management Deficit/Lack of Knowledge* (Breast Self-Exam)

No pattern of breast self-exam.
States doesn't know how to examine.

Case 2: Nursing Diagnoses

1 Problem: *Potential Airway Obstruction*

Comatose
Drooling at intervals
Unresponsive to stimuli
PO$_2$ 78 mm

2 Problem: *Total Self-Care Deficit (Level 4)*
Etiological Factors: *Comatose State*

Unresponsive to stimuli
No voluntary movement of extremities

3 Problem: *Parental Guilt*
Etiological Factors: *Perceived Responsibility (Accident); Fear of Child's Death*

Hasn't insisted son use seat belts.
States feels "guilty about accident, although not my fault."
"Why couldn't I be the one to die"; relates coma to approaching death.
Father pacing in room states will "feel better" when mother returns from out of town trip to visit sister.

Case 3: Nursing Diagnoses

These data describe a complex client-situation. Although a great deal of information was collected, more is needed for diagnosis. The case demonstrates that in complex situations, all the data needed cannot be collected in a busy hospital unit at admission. Secondly, time is needed to think about alternative interpretations and what diagnostic hypotheses would direct further cue-search.

Further data on family dynamics, support systems, and the client's insight and inclination to deal with problems are needed. Historically, focusing on noncompliance/knowledge deficit has not been effective (sixth admission for ketoacidosis). Underlying problems exist.

Ethically it is important to remember that this 19-year-old client's rights should not be violated in data collection. Calling the family to verify data or to gather further information without this client's knowledge could be viewed as a violation of rights. It may also jeopardize the nurse-client relationship. When encountering a client who volunteers the type and amount of information previously presented, the question *why* should be raised. Does the behavior signify a plea for help, a testing of the nurse's reaction, or both? Mutual understanding needs to exist regarding the client's choice to deal with her life situation. If help is being requested then the problems interfering with her disease management, as well as general health management, can be further explored and identified. At some point the client and nurse may decide that one or both parents should be included.

Noncompliance (disease management) is a presenting problem but probably only a sign of more serious problems. Nurses perceiving themselves to have inadequate diagnostic or treatment skills in the possible developmental problems that this client and family exhibit may seek consultation. A mental health–clinical nursing specialist may be consulted.

Two possible hypotheses can serve as a basis for (1) clustering current data and (2) guiding further cue search.

Chronic Situational Depression

19 year old

Disheveled; hair dull and oily (unclean)

Sixth admission for diabetic ketoacidosis (blood glucose 505 mgm.)

Doesn't consider self healthy; would give herself "2 on a scale of 1 to 10"

Usually eats alone

States she has learned that "you can't do too much about things", "You just wait and see what happens"

Voice low during this discussion and sad facial expression

Feels she is physically weak and not able to do any activities

Not yet "gotten anything out of life that I have wanted"

Would like to do something "useful and challenging with my life" but hasn't been able to identify these things

No friends; doesn't belong to any social groups because "has nothing in common with people her age"

Perceives her life as "boring"

No insulin taken 2 days prior to admission; doesn't believe this could cause her current problem

Overslept (11 a.m.) and too late to take insulin; night dose at 5 p.m.

States once went week without taking insulin

States diet, exercise, insulin important to health

States doesn't follow diet; forgets to take insulin; too much of a "pain"

No exercise; takes insulin sporadically

States understands her disease

Believes susceptible to ketoacidosis (five previous admissions)

Knotting, cutaneous deposits on arms and thighs from injecting

No daily exercise

Asked to see dietician so that she can lose weight

Weight (reported 135 lbs.); Height 5′ 3″

Attended college for one semester; no plans to return

Unemployed 19 year old

Considers self "rather intelligent; IQ of 126; not smart enough to be super like 140, the gifted"

Pleased with 750 score on SAT

States things must be interesting and challenging in order to hold attention

English and literature are favorite subjects

Might consider teaching
Not satisfied until able to "physically do something both useful and challenging
Doesn't want to waste time doing things aimlessly
Likes to talk about self and "concepts" she is reading about (e.g. Greek mythology); girls her age talk "about boys, clothes"
Dated in high school; not dating since graduation

Dysfunctional Family Dynamics

Perceives family as "a bunch of strangers living under the same roof",; don't show emotions but give her what she wants (such as money)
States family gives enough attention but "probably I could get used to receiving more from them"
Usually eats alone
No activities outside home
Psychologist helped mother to "change a lot and stop nagging"
Lives with parents; brother in Air Force
Believes parents are supportive when needs them
Usually doesn't tell parents when things bother her and therefore remains "independent"
States family does not eat meals together; gets own meals
Bought vegetarian cookbook (doesn't eat meat); says too "lazy" to learn to cook
Diabetes "no big thing" to family as she has had it since age 5
Family doesn't visit hospital unless asked; likes it that way

ANNOTATED BIBLIOGRAPHY

The following references to nursing diagnosis and related areas are supplementary to the chapter bibliographies. Citations are organized with three broad areas: diagnosis, process, and application. Each area has further subdivisions.

DIAGNOSIS

I Concept of Nursing Diagnosis

Baer, C. L. (1984). Nursing diagnosis: A futuristic process for nursing practice. *Topics in Clinical Nursing,* 5:89–98. Discussion of nursing diagnosis and the criteria for a profession. Views nursing diagnosis as having the potential to influence nursing autonomy. A summary of advantages and disadvantages of using nursing diagnosis is given.

Bircher, A. (1975). On the development and classification of diagnoses. *Nursing Forum,* 14:10–29. Proposes a mastery-competency classification system based on the organizing principle of Maslow's hierarchy of human needs. Defines nursing diagnosis, discusses the potential problems and dangers inherent in making a diagnosis, and outlines the values of nursing diagnosis.

Bonney, V., & Rothberg, J. (1963). *Nursing diagnosis and therapy: An instrument for evaluation and assessment.* New York: National League for Nursing. Contains early definition of nursing diagnosis and tool for assessment of functional problems. Assessment form was developed to facilitate planning for nurse staffing for chronically ill and disabled clients.

Carnevali, D. L. (1984). Nursing diagnosis: an evolutionary view. *Topics in Clinical Nursing,* 5:10–29. Discussion of the evolution of nursing diagnosis, the nursing domain for diagnosis, evolution of the diagnostic reasoning process, the relation of nursing values to nursing diagnosis, and the evolution of nursing diagnosis. Offers predictions regarding the future of nursing diagnosis.

Carpinito, L. J. (1985). Altered thoughts or altered perceptions? *American Journal of Nursing,* 85:1283. Examination of two nursing diagnoses and suggestions for their use in clinical settings.

Chambers, W. (1962). Nursing diagnosis. *American Journal of Nursing,* 62:102–104. Early article on diagnosis that emphasizes the elements of observation, interpretation, and identifying nursing problems.

Clark, J. (1978). Should nurses diagnose and prescribe? *Journal of Advanced Nursing,* 4:485–488. Discusses value of nursing diagnoses and concludes that nurses should diagnose and prescribe if competent.

Craig, J. L. (1983). Ten reasons why we need nursing diagnosis. *RNABC News,* (Canada) (September), pp. 9–11. Good summary of the reasons nursing diagnosis is needed for professional activities.

Evans, S. L. (1979). Descriptive criteria for the concept of depleted health potential. *Advances in Nursing Science,* 1:67–74. Presents the concept of depleted health potential, its criteria and suggestions for use as a diagnosis.

Gebbie, K. M. (1984). Nursing diagnosis: What is it and why does it exist? *Topics in Clinical Nursing,* 5:1–9. Discussion of the concept of nursing diagnosis, the reasons for its emergence, the contribution it has made to nursing care, and the consequences both positive and negative of its use.

Gebbie, K. A., & Lavin, M. A. (1974). Classifying nursing diagnoses. *American Journal of Nursing,* 44:250–253. Report of the first national conference on nursing diagnosis and the diagnoses identified.

Gleit, C. J., and Tatro, S. (1981). Nursing diagnoses for healthy individuals. *Nursing and Health Care,* 2:456–457. Suggests more liberal use of nursing diagnosis with well patients. Views this as promoting high-level wellness and a more cost-effective health care system.

Gordon, M. (1982). Conceptual issues in nursing diagnosis. In N. Chaska (Ed.), *The nursing profession: A time to speak.* New York: McGraw-Hill. Identifies issues in identification, standardization, and classification of nursing diagnoses. States first step in implementing nursing diagnosis is for nurses to recognize their autonomy and accountability in practice.

Gordon, M. (1979). The concept of nursing diagnosis. In Symposium on the Implementation of Nursing Diagnosis. *Nursing Clinics of North America,* 14:487–496. Discussion of the concept of nursing diagnosis and related issues. Progress up to 1979 in identification and classification is summarized; resources for implementation are cited.

Gordon, M. (1978). Classification of nursing diagnosis. *Journal of New York State Nurses' Association,* 9:5–9. Identifies four major areas of nursing practice which require clinical diagnosis and eight issues in practice which could be clarified by use of standardized nomenclature.

Gordon, M. (1976). Nursing diagnosis and the diagnostic process. *American Journal of Nursing,* 76:1276–1300. Defines nursing diagnosis in terms of concept and structure (PES) and discusses the diagnostic process.

Gordon, M., Sweeney, M. A., & McKeehan, K. (1980). Development of nursing diagnoses. *American Journal of Nursing,* 80:699. Discusses historical development of nursing diagnosis from 1960 to 1980. Traces changes in form and focus.

Gould, M. T. (1983). Nursing diagnoses concurrent with multiple sclerosis. *Journal of Neurosurgical Nursing,* 15:339–345. A descriptive study identifying nursing diagnoses which are concurrent with the medical diagnosis of multiple sclerosis.

Hardy, E. (1983). The diagnostic wheel: Identifying care that is unique to nursing. *Canadian Nurse,* 79:38–40. Describes implementation of an experimental nursing assessment form and diagnostic wheel composed of fifteen alterations in living patterns divided into four major areas of concern. Examples of its use are given.

Jacoby, M. (1983). (Diagnostics). The dilemma of physiological problems: Eliminating the double standard. *American Journal of Nursing,* 85:281–285. Explores the conceptual focus of nursing diagnosis, particularly the issue of physiological problems. Stresses the need for clinical research to validate the situations and populations in which nurses diagnose and independently treat physiological malfunctions and potential malfunctions.

Jones, P. E. (1979). A terminology for nursing diagnosis. *Advances in Nursing Science,* 2:1–16. Reviews methods of describing nursing practice and taxonomy development. Describes a study to identify and validate diagnostic categories.

Jones, P. E., & Jakob, D. F. (1983). *Definition of nursing diagnosis, phase 3 and final report.* Toronto, Canada: Faculty of Nursing, University of Toronto. Defines nursing diagnosis and presents detailed report of a study of clinicians' diagnoses. Presents listing of nursing diagnoses, many of which are currently classified by the NANDA.

Kim, M. J. (1985). (Diagnostics) The dilemma of physiological problems: Without collaboration, what's left? *American Journal of Nursing,* 85:281–284. Discusses the need for identification and classification of physiological problems nurses use in practice. Stresses the need to represent the diversity in nursing practice by including the collaborative, or interdependent, domain of practice.

King, L. S. (1967). What is a disgnosis? *Journal of the American Medical Association,* 202:714–717. Examines the concept of diagnosis and presents the view that diagnosis is not confined just to medicine.

Lash, A. A. (1978). Re-examination of nursing diagnosis. *Nursing Forum,* 17:332–343. Reviews differences between medical diagnosis and nursing diagnosis in the literature from 1953 to 1976. Views nursing diagnosis as offering autonomy and independent decision making which is necessary to the profession and professional nursing practice.

Levine, M. (1965). Trophicognosis: An alternative to nursing diagnosis. In American Nurses' Association, *Exploring progress in medical-surgical nursing. ANA regional clinical conference,* vol. 2, Kansas City, MO: American Nurses Association, pp. 55–70. Early paper on nursing diagnosis advocating use of a different term.

Mundinger, M., & Jauron, G. (1975). Developing a nursing diagnosis. *Nursing Outlook,* 23:94–98. Proposes two part structure for nursing diagnosis and the use of "related to" instead of "due to." Discusses problems encountered in defining and instituting nursing diagnosis and gives examples of mistakes made by beginning diagnosticians.

Myers, N. (1973). Nursing diagnosis. *Nursing Times,* 69:1299–1230. Emphasizes the importance of diagnosis. Defines nursing diagnosis.

Price, M. R. (1980). Nursing diagnosis: Making a concept come alive. *American Journal of Nursing,* 80:668–674. Discussion of structural components of nursing diagnoses, common errors in diagnosis, steps in the diagnostic process, and how to use a diagnosis.

Proder, B. (1975). What you should know about nursing diagnosis. *Medical Record News,* (August) p. 87–90. Supports the need for a classification system and presents an approach for manual collection of data on patients with nursing diagnosis.

Rothberg, J. S. (1967). Why nursing diagnosis? *American Journal of Nursing,* 67:1040–1042. Argues that diagnosis is essential to professional practice and that nursing diagnosis ensures focus on the individual. Presents an early definition of the concept.

Soares, C. A. (1978). Nursing and medical diagnoses: A comparison of essential and variant features. In N. Chaska. (Ed.), *The nursing profession: Views through the mist.* New York: McGraw-Hill. Outlines the diagnostic process in nursing and compares to the diagnostic process in medicine. States that a nursing diagnosis must include the statement of the problem (a conflict in needs) and the indirect or direct causes associated with the problem.

See Chapter 1 and 2 Bibliographies.

II Legal and Professional Accountability in Nursing Diagnosis

Bruce, J. A., & Snyder, M. (1979). The legal side: The right and responsibility to diagnose. *American Journal of Nursing,* 82:645–646. Discusses the legal applicability of nursing diagnosis and the professional right to use nursing diagnosis.

Connecticut Nurses' Association. (1975). Do nurses diagnose? *Connecticut Nursing News,* 48:7. Discusses the confusion that has resulted in various court cases due to the absence of a uniform definition of "diagnosis."

Cushing, M. (1983). Expanding the meaning of accountability. *American Journal of Nursing,* 83:1202–1203. Description of three court cases showing the increase in court decisions in favor of holding nurses accountable for exercising their judgment as health care professionals.

Cushing, M. (1982). Matter of judgment. *American Journal of Nursing,* 82:990. Discussion and examples of the legal aspects of clinical judgment.

Hershey, N. (1976). The influence of charting upon liability determinations. *Journal of Nursing Administration,* 6:35–38. Discusses the importance of charting when a legal issue arises.

Hull, R. T. (1981). Responsibility and accountability analyzed. *Nursing Outlook,* 29:707–712. An examination of the structure and function of responsibility that leads to a schema to help clarify some current questions and issues.

Newton, L. H. (1979). To whom is the nurse accountable? A philosophical perspective. *Connecticut Medical Supplement,* 43:7–9. Discusses the dilemmas of accountability with which nurses are faced because of six types of accountability applicable in four different concepts of health care.

Shoemaker, J. (1979). How nursing diagnosis helps focus your care. *RN,* 42:56–61. Describes nursing diagnosis as a simple, practical way of improving care. Steps in the diagnostic process and required diagnostic skills are discussed.

Warren, J. J. (1983). Accountability and nursing diagnosis. *Journal of Nursing Administration,* 83:34–37. Addresses the fact that a taxonomy of nursing diagnoses improves communication within the domain of nursing practice and when implemented could improve nursing care and document nursing accountability.

See Chapter 9. Bibliography.

III Nursing Diagnosis: Research Methods

Alexander, C. S., & Becker, H. J. (1978). The use of vignettes in survey research. *Public Opinion Quarterly,* 42:93–104. Methodology applicable to the study of nursing diagnosis is discussed.

Brown, M. (1974). The epidemiological approach to the study of clinical nursing diagnosis. *Nursing Forum,* 13:346–359. Discusses the epidemiological method for establishing the prevalence, distribution, and causality of a nursing diagnosis. Outlines five criteria for the development of a taxonomy of nursing diagnoses.

Fehring, R. J. (1986). Validating diagnostic labels: Standardized methodology. In M. Hurley. (Ed.), *Classification of nursing diagnoses: Proceedings of the sixth conference.* St. Louis: Mosby. Discusses methods to establish reliability and validity estimates for diagnostic categories. Presents methods of handling data which result in reliability and validity scores for diagnostic categories.

Gordon, M. (1985). Nursing diagnosis. In H. H. Werley & J. J. Fitzpatrick. (Eds.), *Annual Review of Nursing Research,* vol. 3. New York: Springer-Verlag. Reviews major studies in nursing diagnosis (large sample studies). Concludes that diversity in aspects of methodology, analysis, and reporting does not facilitate combining results on the clinical validity and epidemiology of nursing diagnoses.

Gordon, M. (1980). Predictive strategies in diagnostic tasks. *Nursing Research,* 29:39–45. Report of a study of diagnostic strategies used to identify postsurgical complications. Methods are applicable to the study of nursing diagnostic reasoning.

Gordon, M., Sweeney, M., & McKeehan, K. (1980). Methodological problems and issues in identifying and standardizing nursing diagnosis. *Advances in Nursing Science,* 2:1–15. Identifies conceptual issues in research on nursing diagnosis and presents three models for identifying and validating diagnostic categories. Interrater reliability of diagnosticians is discussed.

Gould, M. T. (1983). Nursing diagnoses concurrent with multiple sclerosis. *Journal of Neurosurgical Nursing,* 15:339–345. A descriptive study identifying nursing diagnoses which are concurrent with the medical diagnosis of multiple sclerosis.

Halloran, E. J. (1980). Analysis of variation in nursing workload by patient medical and nursing condition. (Doctoral Dissertation, University of Illinois, College of Nursing.) *Dissertation Abstracts International,* 41:3385B. Presents data that contribute to information about epidemiology of nursing diagnoses; major purpose was to study nurse workload.

Hoskins, L. M., McFarlane, E. A., Rubenfeld, M. G., Walsh, M. B., & Schreier, A. M. (1986). Nursing diagnosis in the chronically ill: Methodology for clinical validation. *Advances in Nursing Science,* 8:80–89. Describes a study which identified 50 nursing diagnoses in a chronically ill population, validated the diagnoses, and identified the defining characteristics of these diagnoses. Focuses on the methods used to derive and validate the nursing diagnoses.

Jones, P. E., & Jakob, D. F. (1983): *Definition of nursing diagnosis, phase 3 and final report.* Toronto, Canada: Faculty of Nursing, University of Toronto. Presents detailed report of a study of clinicians' diagnoses.

Nursing Clinics of North America, (1985). vol. 20, December. Entire issue on studies of diagnostic categories.

Tanner, C. A., & Geddis-Hughes, A. M. (1984). Nursing diagnosis: Issues in clinical practice research. *Topics in Clinical Nursing,* 5:30–38. Stresses that if nursing diagnosis is to positively influence practice, the existing nomenclature must be critically

evaluated and systematically tested. Stresses that the measurements used to identify diagnoses must be relevant to everyday practice, reliable, valid, and sensitive.
See Chapter 11 Bibliography.

IV Diagnostic Classification System Development

Process of Development

Adelotte, M. K. (1987). Nursing taxonomies: State of the art. In A. McLane. (Ed.). *Classification of nursing diagnoses: Proceedings of the seventh conference.* St. Louis: Mosby. Comprehensive review of taxonomy development and the difficulties in developing the discipline of nursing. Places taxonomy development in the context of development of nursing knowledge, its domains, its classifications, and its language.

Feinstein, A. R. (1979). Clinical biostatistics: What are the criteria for criteria? *Clinical Biostatistics,* 25:108–113. Presents an outline of the criteria for developing diagnostic criteria used in clinical decision-making, many of which are adaptable to nursing diagnosis.

Gebbie, K. A. (1976). Development of a taxonomy of nursing diagnoses. In J. Walter, G. Pardee, & D. Molmo. (Eds.), *Dynamics of problem-oriented approaches: Patient care and documentation.* Philadelphia: Lippincott. Advocates development of nomenclature by utilizing inductive and deductive reasoning and a classification system for taxonomy preparation.

Gebbie, K., & Lavin, M. A. (1973). Classifying nursing diagnosis. *Missouri Nurse,* 42:10–14. The first contemporary article suggesting classification of nursing diagnoses. Defines nursing diagnosis, reviews status, and makes recommendations for future development.

Kritek, P. B. (1986). Struggle to classify our diagnoses. *American Journal of Nursing,* 86: 722–723. Discussion of nursing diagnosis taxonomic development and problems encountered.

Kritek, P. B. (1978). The generation and classification of nursing diagnoses: Toward a theory of nursing. *Image,* 10:33–40. Describes the current effort to classify diagnoses as first-level theory building.

McKay, R. P. (1977). Research Q & A: What is the relationship between the development and utilization of a taxonomy and nursing theory? *Nursing Research,* 26:222–224. Defines taxonomy and classification system. Discusses major tasks in development of a taxonomy of nursing diagnoses and its relevance to theory development.

Neumann, P. G. (1974). An attribute frequency model for the abstraction of prototypes. *Memory and Cognition,* 2:241–248. Discussion and results of research to abstract prototype categories.

Roy, Sr. C. (1975). A diagnostic classification system for nursing. *Nursing Outlook,* 23:90–94. Explores the rationale for a classification system in nursing. Lists principles of ordering a taxonomy and the deductive approach to its development. Discusses the implications of a diagnostic classification system in nursing practice, education, and research.

Silva, M.C. (1986). Research testing nursing theory. *Advances in Nursing Science,* 9:1–11. Examines 62 studies testing aspects of 5 conceptual models. Discusses factors impeding this research and suggests implications for future work.
See Chapter 11 Bibliography.

Considerations in Development

Dracup, K. (1983). Editorial: Nursing diagnosis: A rose by any other name. *Heart and Lung,* 12:211. Comments on the use of terminology in a profession. Includes questions raised at a critical care conference regarding "physiological diagnoses."

Douglas, D., & Murphy, E. K. (1985). Nursing process, nursing diagnosis, and emerging taxonomies. Identifies issues in taxonomy development. In J. McCloskey & H. Grace. *Current issues in nursing practice* (2d ed.). Boston: Blackwell Scientific. Views current taxonomy development as expanding, clarifying, and defining the concepts underlying nursing process and nursing diagnosis.

Edel, M. K. (1985). Noncompliance: An appropriate nursing diagnosis? *Nursing Outlook,* 33:183–185. Discusses compliance and its interpretations, to evaluate noncompliance as a nursing diagnosis. Concluded that elimination of noncompliance as a nursing diagnosis would encourage greater therapeutic alliances with patients, giving patients greater choices in alternative treatments.

Fawcett, J. (1984). The metaparadigm of nursing: Present status and future refinements. *Image,* 16:84–89. The central concepts and themes of the discipline of nursing are identified and formalized as nursing's metaparadigm. Examples are given, and refinements are proposed.

Feild, L., & Winslow, E. H. (1985). Moving to a nursing model. *American Journal of Nursing,* 85:1100–1101. Presents excerpts and a summary of a position paper on medical-surgical nursing which describes the current transition from a medical to nursing model of practice. Views the nursing model as the focus for nursing diagnosis. Notes that the medical model is useful in working with physicians in the diagnosis and treatment of disease but it is the nursing model that will help nurses achieve autonomy and control of their practice.

Gleit, C. J., & Tatro, S. (1981). Nursing diagnoses for healthy individuals. *Nursing and Health Care,* 2:456–457. Suggests classification of wellness diagnoses. Emphasis on wellness can lead to a more cost-effective health care system.

Good, M. (1985). (Letters) Noncompliance may be an appropriate diagnosis. *Nursing Outlook,* 33:267. Response to a paper by Edel (listed above). Suggests that nurses let go of their negative view of the word compliance, and view it from the perspective of self care. Also see letter by R. (Toth) Haddon.

Gordon, M. (1985). Diagnostic category development. In J. McCloskey & H. Grace. *Current Issues in Nursing Practice,* (2d. ed.). Boston: Blackwell Scientific. Discusses category development in the context of clinical reasoning and factors that require attention in development and refinement.

Hagey, R. S., & McDonough, P. (1984). The problem of professional labeling. *Nursing Outlook,* 32:151–157. Discusses the problems that can occur in diagnostic labeling when used to save time or meet institutional obligations. Provides many points for thought and discussion.

Jacoby, M. (1983). (Diagnostics) The dilemma of physiological problems: Eliminating the double standard. *American Journal of Nursing,* 85:281–285. Explores the conceptual focus of nursing diagnosis, particularly the issue of physiological problems. Stresses the need for clinical research to validate the situations and populations in which nurses diagnose and independently treat physiological malfunctions and potential malfunctions.

Jones, P. E., & Jakob, D. F. (1983). *Definition of nursing diagnosis, phase 3 and final report.* Toronto, Canada: Faculty of Nursing, University of Toronto. Defines nursing diagnosis and presents detailed report of a study of clinicians' diagnoses. Presents listing of nursing diagnoses, many of which are currently classified by the NANDA.

Jones, P., & Jakob, D. (1981). Nursing diagnosis: Differentiating fear and anxiety. *Nursing Papers (McGill University)*, 14:20–29. Results of a study that suggests nurses commit diagnostic errors in the identification of fear and anxiety. Suggestions presented for improving diagnostic accuracy.

Kim, M. J. (1985). (Diagnostics) The dilemma of physiological problems: Without collaboration, what's left? *American Journal of Nursing*, 85:281–284. Discusses the need for identification and classification of physiological problems nurses use in practice. Stresses the need to represent the diversity in nursing practice by including the collaborative, or interdependent, domain of practice.

Kritek, P. K. (1985). Nursing diagnosis in perspective: Response to a critique. *Image*, 17:3–8. Analyzes and discusses issues raised in a paper published by Shamansky and Yanni (see below).

Loomis, M. E., & Wood, D. J. (1983). Cure: The potential outcome of nursing care. *Image*, 15:4–7. Presents a method of classification and proposes that in the diagnosis and treatment of human responses, nurses are capable of curing the actual or potential health problem.

Lunney, M. (1982). Nursing diagnosis—refining the system. *American Journal of Nursing*, 82:456–460. Suggests a naming system for nursing diagnoses which includes (1) the broad pattern or process which is altered or dysfunctional and (2) the specific factors contributing to the unhealthful response that are the focus of intervention.

Martens, K. (1986). Let's diagnose strengths, not just problems. *American Journal of Nursing*, 86:192–193. Stresses the importance of identifying positive resources in the client-situation and suggests that nursing diagnosis be expanded to include these strengths; gives examples of diagnostic statements of this type.

McKay, R., & Segall, M. (1983). Methods and models for the aggregate. *Nursing Outlook*, 31:328–334. Presents a model for community nursing that incorporates nursing diagnosis as an element to be identified in community research and education.

Newman, M. A. (1984). Nursing diagnosis: Looking at the whole. *American Journal of Nursing*, 84:1496–1499. Discusses a model incorporating patterns developed for a taxonomy of nursing diagnoses.

Pridham, K. E., & Schutz, M. E. (1985). Rationale for a language for naming problems. *Image*, 17:122–126. Suggests that many of the experiences patients have, which nursing addresses, defy classification. Views current diagnoses as relevant to other disciplines as well as nursing, thus not helpful in defining nursing as a distinct discipline. Presents criteria for a nomenclature system.

Roy, Sr. C. (1975). A diagnostic classification system for nursing. *Nursing Outlook*, 23:90–94. Explores the rationale for a classification system in nursing. Lists principles of ordering a taxonomy and the deductive approach to its development. Discusses the implications of a diagnostic classification system in nursing practice, education and research.

Shamansky, S. L., & Yanni, C. R. (1983). In opposition to nursing diagnosis: A minority opinion. *Image*, 15:47–50. Examines the premises underlying nurses' diagnoses and their impact on clinicians and the health care delivery system.

Shoemaker, J. K. (1984). Essential features of a nursing diagnosis: In M. J. Kim, G. McFarland, & A. McLean (Eds.), *Classification of nursing diagnoses: Proceedings of the fifth national conference.* St. Louis: Mosby, pp. 104–115. Report of a consensus study on characteristics of nursing diagnosis. Presents definition that relates nursing diagnosis to nursing process components.

Simmons, D. A. (1980). *Classification scheme for client problems in community health nursing.* Rockville, MD: U.S. Government Printing Office. Nomenclature and classification system developed and tested by the Visiting Nurse Service of Omaha to describe nursing problems in community health and to be used in computerized clinical information systems. Many diagnostic categories are similar to the NANDA listing of diagnoses.

Soares, C. A. (1978). Nursing and medical diagnoses: A comparison of essential and variant features. In N. Chaska. (Ed.), *The nursing profession: Views through the mist.* New York: McGraw-Hill. Presents a framework for classification of nursing diagnoses.

Stanitis, M. A., & Ryan, J. (1982). Noncompliance: an unacceptable diagnosis? *American Journal of Nursing,* 82:941–942. Discusses the diagnosis of noncompliance and concludes that it is a negative, counterproductive label that may lead to inappropriate nursing behaviors.

Suppe, F., & Jacox, A. K. (1985). Philosophy of science and the development of nursing theory. In H. H. Werley & J. J. Fitzpatrick (Eds.), *Annual review of nursing research,* vol. 3. New York: Springer-Verlag. Views taxonomy as a type of conceptual framework and reviews literature on diagnostic taxonomy in context of philosophy of science and nursing theory development. Includes review of evaluation of theories and conceptual frameworks.

Vincent, P. (1985). (Letters) Noncompliance may be an appropriate diagnosis. *Nursing Outlook,* 33:266. Response to a paper by Edel (see above). Suggests the issue to be debated is not *if* compliance is an appropriate nursing diagnosis but *when* it is appropriate. Also see author's response, p. 266.

See Chapter 11 Bibliography.

Reports on Classification System Development (NANDA)

Gebbie, K. A., (Ed.). (1976). *Summary of the second national conference: Classification of nursing diagnoses.* St. Louis: National Group for Classification of Nursing Diagnoses. Contains accepted nursing diagnoses, 1975.

Gebbie, K. A., & Lavin, M. A. (Eds.). (1975). *Classification of nursing diagnoses: Proceedings of the First National Conference.* St. Louis, MO: Mosby. Reports the first organized effort to classify diagnoses at the First National Conference on Classification of Nursing Diagnoses (1973) and the diagnoses that resulted. Includes papers on various classification systems in medicine, the nature of classification, and implications for practice, education, and research. Contains diagnoses identified, 1973.

Hurley, M. (Ed.). (1986) *Classification of nursing diagnoses: Proceedings of the sixth conference.* St. Louis: Mosby. Contains accepted nursing diagnoses, 1984. Includes papers on classification, taxonomic structure, quality assurance, DRGs, implementation, and computerization. Research papers are included on specific nursing diagnoses, use in practice, diagnostic process, and research methodology.

Kim, M. J., McFarland, G., & McLane, A. (Eds.). (1984). *Classification of nursing diagnoses: Proceedings of the fifth national conference.* St. Louis: Mosby. Contains new nursing diagnoses accepted in 1982 and papers on classification development and issues, research, implementation, and use in related areas of practice. First bylaws of the newly designated North American Nursing Diagnosis Association.

Kim, M. J., & Moritz, D. A. (Eds.). (1982). *Classification of nursing diagnoses: Proceedings of the third and fourth national conferences.* New York: McGraw-Hill. Contains accepted nursing diagnoses, 1980. Papers included on various subjects related to nursing diagnosis, issues in implementation, and research.

McLane. A. J. (Ed.). (1987). *Classification of nursing diagnoses: Proceedings of the seventh conference*. St. Louis: Mosby. Includes major papers presented, developments in diagnosis and taxonomy, research papers and abstracts, and current listing of nursing diagnoses, 1986.

See Chapter 11 Bibliography.

PROCESS

Aspinall, M. J. (1975). Development of a patient-completed questionnaire and its comparison with the nursing interview. *Nursing Research,* 24:377–381. Study to compare effectiveness of assessment by questionnaire and by interview. More errors were made by unstructured interview and this method consumed more time. Important limitations of the study are cited.

Aspinall, M. J., & Tanner C. A. (1981). Decision making for patient care: applying the nursing process. New York: Appleton-Century-Crofts. Chapter on clinical decision making provides overview of the subject. Remaining chapters are on specific clinical topics, some of which are nursing diagnoses.

Benner, P. (1984). *From novice to expert*. Menlo Park, CA: Addison-Wesley. Major work on the description of clinical judgment and expertise of nurses. Defines seven domains of competencies in nursing practice.

Bieri, J., Atkins, A., Briar, S., Leaman, R., Miller, H., & Tripoldi, T. (1966). *Clinical and social judgment*. New York: Wiley. Report of some of the early formulations of information processing theory as applied in clinical judgment. Reports of methods applicable to nursing studies of judgment.

Billings, R. S., & Marcus, S. A. (1983). Measures of compensatory and noncompensatory models of decision behavior: Process tracing versus policy capturing. *Organizational Behavior and Human Performance,* 31:331–352. Presents models for studying decisions that are applicable to the study of clinical judgment in nursing.

Buckhout, R. (1974). Eyewitness testimony. *Scientific American,* 231:23–31. Discussion of biases in observation which are applicable to data collection in nursing.

College of Nursing, Texas Women's University. (1979). *Nursing diagnoses*. (Monograph, Fall 1979.) Denton, TX: College of Nursing. Overview of status of nursing diagnosis. Reports of three research studies (concept attainment, relation between logical reasoning and diagnosis, and a study of restlessness).

Detmer, D. E., Fryback, D. G., & Gassner, K. (1978). Heuristics and biases in medical decision-making. *Journal of Medical Education,* 53:682–683. Discusses the biases in clinical reasoning. Applicable to nursing diagnosis.

deChesnay, M. (1983). Problem solving in nursing. *Image,* 15:8–11. Levels of problems and the nursing process linked to a change theory to explain the dynamics of labeling clients as difficult patients.

Doona, M. E. (1976). The judgment process in nursing. *Image,* 8:27–28. Discusses the importance of clinical judgment in nursing and analyzes phases and types of judgment.

Eckman, P., & Friesen, W. V. (1975). *Unmasking the face: Guide to recognizing emotions from facial expressions*. Englewood Cliffs, NJ: Prentice-Hall. Assessment guidelines for identifying facial expressions and underlying feelings. Also presents information about emotional states and skill training exercises.

Einhorn, H. J., & Hogarth, R. M. (1985). Ambiguity and uncertainty in probabilistic inference. *Psychological Review,* 94:433–461. A study of how people make decisions under ambiguous and uncertain conditions, such as clinical practice situations.

Elstein, A. S., Holmes, M. M., Ravitch, M. M., Rovner, D. R., Holzman, G. B., & Rothert, M. L. (1983). Medical decisions in perspective: Applied research in cognitive psychology. *Perspectives in Biology and Medicine,* 26:486–501. Description of a cognitive model for describing clinical diagnosis in the professions.

Gordon, M. (1980). Predictive strategies in diagnostic tasks. *Nursing Research,* 29:39–45. Report of a study of nurses' hypothesis testing strategies. Implications for nursing history and diagnosis are discussed.

Grier, M. R. (1984). Information processing in nursing practice. In H. H. Werley & J. J. Fitzpatrick (Eds.), *Annual Review of Nursing Research,* vol. 2. New York: Springer-Verlag. Major review of studies using the information processing model of judgment and decision making.

Hammond, K. R. (1966). Clinical inference in nursing: A psychologist's viewpoint. *Nursing Research,* 15:27–38. One of a series of articles often quoted as the first studies of clinical judgment in nursing. Presents an analysis of cognitive tasks encountered by nurses. Views these tasks as complex because nurse must think "as" the doctor thinks when making judgments.

Keren, G. (1984). On the importance of identifying the correct problem space. *Cognition,* 16:121–128. Discusses the concept of the problem space in cognitive processing of information.

Knill-Jones, R. P. (1977). Clinical decision making. II. Diagnostic and prognostic inference. *Health Bulletin,* 35:213–222. Application of probability and decision theory to clinical inference.

Koran, L. M. (1975). The reliability of clinical methods, data, and judgments. *New England Journal of Medicine,* 293:695–701. Points out the difficulties in the reliability of clinical judgments.

Lazare, A. (1976). The psychiatric examination in the walk-in clinic: Hypothesis generation and hypothesis testing. *Archives of General Psychiatry,* 33:96–102. Useful in regard to the discussion of hypothesis generation and testing.

Levine, R. F. and Crosley, J. M. (Spring 1986). Focused data collection for the generation of nursing diagnoses. *Journal of Nursing Staff Development,* 56–64.

McCarthy, M. M. (1981). The nursing process: Application of current thinking in clinical problem solving. *Journal of Advanced Nursing,* 6:173–177. Explores the components of nursing process from a problem solving perspective. Relates current research in medical problem solving to nursing. No discussion of nursing diagnoses.

McGuire, C. H. (1985). Medical problem solving: A critique of the literature. *Journal of Medical Education,* 60:587–594. Review of research findings. Suggests that current research in medical problem solving consists of small samples and microscopic analyses which have not contributed to understanding of problem solving.

Moritz, D. A. (1979). Nursing histories: A guide, yes; a form, no. *Oncology Nursing Forum,* 6:18–19. Use of a checklist for nursing histories is viewed as a questionable practice. Argues that the way each area in an assessment is pursued and described varies with the concerns and patterns encountered in clients.

Nu, N. V. (1979). Medical problem-solving assessment: A review of methods and instruments. *Evaluation and the Health Professions,* 2:281–307. Review of instruments and methods employed to measure problem solving.

Pendelton, S.H. Diagnostics: Clarification or obfuscation? *American Journal of Nursing,* 86:944. Discussion of common errors in diagnosis, such as assuming not diagnosing, insufficient data, non-nursing problems, nonspecific problems, circular statements.

Phillips, L. R., & Rempusheski, V. F. (1985). Decision-making model for diagnosing and intervening in elder abuse and neglect. *Nursing Research,* 34:134–139. Presents a model for decision making in suspected elder abuse that includes variables influencing decision making. Model is adaptable to nursing diagnosis of other conditions.

Putzier, D. J., & Padrick, K. P. (1984). Nursing diagnosis: A component of nursing process and decision making. *Topics in Clinical Nursing,* 5:21–29. Describes use of nursing diagnosis in each step of nursing process. Views nursing diagnosis as the pivotal factor in decision making. Contrasts this to symptom management and gives some case studies in application.

Rogers, J. C. (1983). Clinical reasoning: Ethics, science, art. *American Journal Occupational Therapy,* 37,601–616. Excellent paper on aspects of clinical reasoning. Discussed in the context of clinical reasoning in occupational therapy.

Rosenhan, D. L. (1973). On being sane in insane places. *Science,* 179:250–258. Report of a study involving pseudopatients in a psychiatric hospital and the influence of setting on diagnosis. Demonstrates how preconceptions can influence judgment and labeling of clients.

Simon, H. A. (1974). How big is a chunk? *Science,* 183:482–488. Discusses the concept of chunking information. Applicable to information processing in diagnostic judgment.

Spector, R. (1986). *Cultural diversity in health and illness.* New York: Appleton-Century-Crofts. Useful ideas about culture and symptoms and influences of culture in judgments about others.

See Chapter 6, 7, and 8 Bibliographies.

III APPLICATION

I Specialties and Settings

Bryant, S. O., & Kopeski, L. M. (1986). Psychiatric nursing assessment of the eating disorder client. *Topics in Clinical Nursing,* 8:57–66. Identifies nursing diagnoses within functional health patterns. Provides psychiatric nursing criteria for the clinical assessment of the anorexic and bulemic client.

Clark, S. R. (1984). Nursing diagnosis: Its application in an ambulatory-care setting. *Topics in Clinical Nursing,* 5:57–66. Shows, through example, the use of nursing process and nursing diagnosis in the ambulatory care setting.

Dalton, J. (1985). Descriptive study: Defining characteristics of the nursing diagnosis cardiac output, alterations in, decreased. *Image,* 17:113–117. Study of nurses use of this diagnosis. Discusses need for further refinement, legal issues related to misdiagnosis, and relates data to NANDA taxonomy.

Davidson, S. B. (1984). Nursing diagnosis: Its application in the acute-care setting. *Topics in Clinical Nursing,* 5:50–56. Attempts to clarify the differences between what nurses diagnose and what physicians diagnose. Use of a conceptual framework and diagnostic process.

Dwyer, J. M. (1986). *Manual of gynecologic nursing.* Boston: Little, Brown. Incorporation of nursing diagnosis in gynecological nursing.

Fredette, S., & Gloriant, F. S. (1981). Nursing diagnosis in cancer chemotherapy. *American Journal of Nursing,* 81:2013–2022. Discusses the concept of nursing diagnosis and identifies diagnoses occurring in patients undergoing cancer chemotherapy.

Gleit, C. J., & Tatro, S. (1981). Nursing diagnoses for healthy individuals. *Nursing and Health Care,* 2:456–457. Suggests more liberal use of diagnosis as a basis for activities related to promotion of high level wellness. Suggests use of wellness diagnoses can lead to a more cost-effective health care system.

Guzzetta, C. E., & Dossey, B. M. (1983). Nursing diagnosis: framework, process and problems, *Heart and Lung,* 12:281–291. Discusses nursing diagnosis, diagnostic process, and issues related to classification.

Hauck, M. R., & Roth, D. (1984). Application of nursing diagnoses in a pediatric clinic. *Pediatric Nursing,* 10:49–52. Suggests that nursing diagnoses can help nurses analyze their observations and identify interventions. View nursing diagnosis as enhancing accountability, responsibility, and pride in nursing care.

Heart and Lung (1985), vol. 4. Four articles related to critical care in a symposium on nursing diagnosis.

Johnson, M. (1984). Theoretical basis for nursing diagnosis in mental health nursing. *Issues in Mental-Health Nursing,* 6:53–71. Discusses nursing diagnosis and diagnostic process in the context of the adaptation model and functional patterns.

Kim, M. J. (1983). Nursing diagnosis in critical care. *Dimensions of Critical Care Nursing,* 2:5–6. Discussion of nursing diagnosis and the issues surrounding diagnosis in critical care.

Lister, D. W. (1983). The nursing diagnosis movement and the occupational health nurse. *Occupational Health Nursing,* 31:11–14. Discusses what nursing diagnosis is and how its implementation is beneficial to nursing care.

Maas, M. L., & Specht, J. P. (1985). Implementation of nursing diagnosis: Maturation of a professional model of practice. In J. McCloskey & H. Grace, *Current Issues in Nursing Practice.* (2d ed.). Boston: Blackwell Scientific. Discusses development of a professional model of practice and the implementation of nursing diagnosis.

McKay, R., & Segall, M. (1983). Methods and models for the aggregate. *Nursing Outlook,* 31:328–334. Discusses how and why graduate programs in public health nursing should clarify the relationship between community and aggregate.

Occupational Health Nursing (1985), vol. 33, no. 8. Entire issue on diagnosis.

Parisi, B. (1983). Nursing diagnosis: Application for renal nurses. *Dialysis and Transplantation,* 12:362,366,370–371. The structure of nursing diagnosis and its application to the overall nursing process is defined, and a case report is presented as a learning exercise.

Rantz, M., Miller, T., & Jacobs, C. (1985). Nursing diagnosis in long term care. *American Journal of Nursing,* 85:916–917, 926. Report of implementation of nursing diagnosis and interdisciplinary care planning in a nursing home. Identifies five common diagnoses in long term care.

Simmons, D. A. (1980). *Classification scheme for client problems in community health nursing.* Rockville, MD: U.S. Government Printing Office. Nomenclature and classification system developed and tested by the Visiting Nurse Service of Omaha to describe nursing problems in community health and to be used in computerized clinical information systems. Many diagnostic categories are similar to the NANDA listing of diagnoses.

Steele, J. E. (1984). The social policy statement: Assuring a positive future for nurse practitioners. *Nurse Practitioner,* 9:15–16, 68. Discusses the ANA Social Policy Statement in relation to nurse practitioners' practice in ambulatory care.

Taylor, J. W. (1985). Nursing management of stroke: Part I. Acute care. *Cardiovascular Nursing,* 21:1–5. Identifies nursing diagnoses commonly occurring in patients in the acute phase after a stroke.

Tilton, C., & Maloff, M. (1982). Diagnosing the problems in stroke. *American Journal of Nursing,* 82:597–601. Identifies nursing diagnoses commonly occurring with cerebrovascular accidents.

Young, M. S., & Lucas, C. M. (1984). Nursing diagnosis: Common problems in implementation. *Topics in Clinical Nursing,* 5:68–77. Discusses implementing nursing diagnosis in the health care setting, including particular problems of implementation and possible solutions to these problems.

II Care Delivery

Gordon, M. (1985). Practice-based data set for a nursing information system. *Journal of Medical Systems,* 9:43–55. The purpose of this paper was to examine the assumption that nursing practice components are not sufficiently clarified to develop specifications for a nursing data set within a nursing information system.

Halloran, E. J. (1983). RN staffing: More care—less cost. *Nursing Management,* 14:18–22. A study on type of staffing and related cost showing that a more highly qualified staff (more RNs) can lead to greater attention to total patient needs and decreased cost of nursing care.

Halloran, E., & Halloran, D. C. (1985). Exploring the DRG/Nursing equation. *American Journal of Nursing,* 85:1093–1095. Report of a study demonstrating that predicting total hospital costs may be more accurate using a combination of nursing diagnosis and DRGs, as opposed to using either one alone.

Long Island Jewish–Hillside Medical Center. (1985). *Computerized nursing care planning: utilizing nursing diagnosis.* Washington, DC: Oryn Publications. Computer system incorporating nursing diagnoses. Includes screens for diagnostic categories and information on signs and symptoms, related factors, patient outcomes, nursing care plan, specificities, and evaluations, each validated by consensus of nurse experts.

McCourt, A. E. (1981). The measurement of functional deficit in quality assurance. *Quality Assurance Update,* 5:1–3. Presents a scale for measuring self-care deficits and relates precision in measurement to quality assurance.

Werley, H. H., & Grier, M. R. (1981). *Nursing information systems.* New York: Springer. Report of a research conference on nursing information systems, June, 1977. Sections on nursing diagnoses, clinical decision making, standardization of nomenclature, use of diagnosis in client classification nurse staffing, and other topics related to clinical information processing.

Westfall, U. E. (1984). Nursing diagnosis: its use in quality assurance. *Topics in Clinical Nursing,* 5:78–88. Clarifies the terms nursing diagnosis and quality assurance by exploring definitions, interrelationships of the two, and operational problems encountered when linking the two.

Young, D. E., & Ventura, M. R. (1980). Application of nursing diagnosis in quality assessment research. *Quality Assurance Update,* 4:1–4. Discusses the application of nursing diagnosis in development of diagnostic outcome and process criteria for three accepted nursing diagnoses. Argues that combining medical and nursing diagnoses more clearly defines the population to be assessed than using medical diagnosis alone.
See Chapter 9 and 10 Bibliographies.

III Education

Fredette, S., & O'Connor, K. (1979). Nursing diagnosis in teaching and curriculum planning. *Nursing Clinics of North America,* 14:541–552. Discussion of nursing diagnosis as the focus of theoretical and clinical study in educational programs. Examples given of increasing competency in diagnosis as learner proceeds in the educational program.
Gaines, B. C., & McFarland, M. B. (1984). Nursing diagnosis: its relationship to and use in nursing education. *Topics in Clinical Nursing,* 5:39–49. Reviews the concepts and presents a study of the use of nursing diagnosis in schools of nursing.
Howe, K. R., Holmes, M., & Elstein, A. S. (1984). Teaching clinical decision making. *Journal of Medicine and Philosophy,* 9:215–228. Outlines the process and presents teaching methodologies that are also applicable to nursing.
Jacoby, M. K., & Adams, D. J. (1981). Teaching assessment of client functioning. *Nursing Outlook,* 29:248–250. Discusses systematic ordering of data in nursing diagnosis and offers guidelines for students.
Kemp, V. H. (1985). Concept analysis as a strategy for promoting critical thinking. *Journal of Nursing Education,* 24:382–384. Describes the process of concept analysis and identifies the usefulness of this strategy for the development of critical thinking which is an essential component of scientific inquiry.
Lee, H. A., & Strong, K. A. (1985). Using nursing diagnosis to describe the clinical competence of baccalaureate and associate degree graduating students: a comparative study. *Image,* 17:82–85. Report of a study comparing conceptions of clinical competence of professional and technical nursing students with the expectations of their nursing faculty using a nursing diagnosis framework.
Morris, J. L. (1982). Nursing diagnosis: A focus for continuing education. *Journal of Continuing Education,* 13:33–36. Report of a continuing education program that uses nursing diagnosis as a focus. Describes implementation of the focus in programming.
Watts, F. N. (1980). Clinical judgment and clinical training. *British Journal of Medical Psychology,* 53:95–108. Detailed exploration of the process of clinical judgment and review of research and theory on the teaching of clinical judgment.

NAME AND TITLE INDEX

SUBJECT INDEX